Automated Scoring
of Complex Tasks
in Computer-Based Testing

Automated Scoring
of Complex Tasks
in Computer-Based Testing

Edited by

David M. Williamson
Isaac I. Bejar
Educational Testing Service

Robert J. Mislevy
University of Maryland

LEA
2006
LAWRENCE ERLBAUM ASSOCIATES, PUBLISHERS
Mahwah, New Jersey   London

Camera ready copy for this book was provided by the editors.

Lawrence Erlbaum Associates, Inc., Publishers
10 Industrial Avenue
Mahwah, New Jersey 07430
www.erlbaum.com

Cover design by Kathryn Houghtaling Lacey

CIP information for this volume may be obtained by contacting the
Library of Congress

ISBN 0-8058-4634-4 (cloth : alk. paper)
ISBN 0-8058-5977-2 (pbk. : alk. paper)

Books published by Lawrence Erlbaum Associates are printed on acid-
free paper, and their bindings are chosen for strength and durability.

Printed in the United States of America
10 9 8 7 6 5 4 3 2 1

Contents

v

Preface

The increasing availability and capability of computers and associated technologies (e.g., the internet) is fueling a trend toward more innovative constructed-response tasks in computer-based testing (CBT), both for learning and for making important decisions about people. If such assessment tasks are to be used successfully with more than a handful of examinees, automated scoring is required. But few professionals have experience and expertise in developing and implementing valid automated scoring systems for innovative CBT tasks. This lack of general expertise in the area of automated scoring is due in part to a lack of examples of "best practice" in the design, implementation, and evaluation of automated scoring systems for innovative CBT tasks.

This volume provides examples of such best practices as they are currently understood and is intended to provide researchers and practitioners with an understanding of current automated scoring methods and domains of application. Further, it provides a unifying conceptual framework for understanding the role of automated scoring in constructing valid assessments. While there is often a technology component to the design of such assessments, the emphasis of this volume is on the goals of measurement and how the statistical methods and the technology interact to achieve those goals rather than on the sophistication of the technology itself. The volume is intended for audiences with an applied interest in automated scoring, and who have a fundamental grasp of statistical methods and measurement principles such as reliability, validity, and test use. The authors contributing to this volume are leaders in innovative approaches to automated scoring for their domains of interest and communicate their understanding in an accessible way for the intended audiences.

Psychometricians and educational researchers may be the primary readers of the volume since their research agendas and/or professional responsibilities may encompass similar goals and challenges to those represented in the volume. Specifically, they may have responsibility for designing a valid test of a performance-oriented construct and may be considering emerging technologies and/or statistical methods. This is reflected in the fact that many of the contributors to the volume are themselves doctoral degree holders in educational measurement or related fields.

Though not designed as a textbook, the emphasis on applied measurement of performance-oriented domains may lend to its use as a supplemental text in graduate level courses in educational measurement, educational statistics, or psychometric degree programs. Similarly, certain chapters may be useful in graduate level courses that directly relate to the methodologies (e.g., multiple regression) under study.

Cognitive scientists, information technologists, and education specialists who are interested in the development of cognitively-oriented tutoring systems are likely to find the volume useful for examples of potential models for decision-making logic constructed as part of the design of learning systems.

The volume may also be appreciated by those who hold doctoral degrees and conduct research in performance-oriented domains requiring the integration of complex information, particularly if measurement of ability in the domain is a goal. Examples of such domains may include medical practice, operation of sophisticated mechanical and electrical equipment, and engineering. Similarly, those with advanced degrees in statistical methods may find the volume useful as a set of examples in establishing measurement goals in the context of a domain and applying a variety of statistical methods to reach those goals.

In providing a survey of methods and domains of application, this volume emphasizes variety in the methods used for automated scoring and in the types of assessment domains to which the methods are applied. In so doing, it provides a broad survey of successful applications and lessons learned for considering one's own potential research agenda into automated scoring. There are, of course, other research efforts and implementations not reported here that may target automated scoring methodologies for a single measurement domain (e.g., scoring of essays) or, conversely, a single methodology applied to a variety of situations that may be related to the goals of automated scoring (e.g., books devoted to a methodologies such as regression, neural networks, and Bayesian inference).

The volume opens with an introduction that reminds the reader of the motivations and challenges of automated scoring for CBT and touches on the history of technological innovations applied to the automated scoring of multiple-choice tests. The following chapter elaborates the tenets of Evidence Centered Design (ECD), a framework of models for assessment design that guide development and ensure the construct validity of an assessment and, as part of that framework, the design of the automated scoring mechanisms. The models and relationships of ECD are intended to serve as a unifying framework for considering how scoring methods meet assessment needs and comparing the similarities and distinctions among methods and applications across chapters. As part of the ECD chapter, a distinction is made between task-level scoring, called evidence identification, and test-level scoring, called evidence accumulation. Although common usage of the term "automated scoring" can be applied to both or either of these components of scoring, the distinction is useful in understanding the role of an automated scoring procedure in the context of the larger assessment.

Each subsequent chapter addresses a different methodology used in automated scoring, progressing in sequence from the more common and well-known methods toward newer and less widely implemented approaches. The methodological chapters begin with a review of human scoring and some of the principles that make such human scoring, somewhat paradoxically, both the gold standard against which to compare all automated scoring methods and the baseline against which automated scoring methods are intended to provide substantial improvements. The review of some basic characteristics of human scoring serves as a backdrop for evaluating the goals and characteristics of subsequent chapters.

The initial methodological chapters deal with techniques for automated scoring that rely on well-known methods with a relatively extensive history, either in inference processes for other applications, including artificial intelligence systems, or for scoring more traditional tests. Chapter 4 presents a natural extension of human logic into rule-based systems. This is illustrated through the application of a rule-based logic system for scoring architectural designs for the Architect Registration Examination; a national professional registration assessment used in the licensure of architects. This rule-based system was designed to mimic the logic of expert human graders, including key components of modeling the uncertainty in evaluation expressed by such expert committees. Chapter 5 describes a regression-based method used to score the diagnostic behaviors of aspiring physicians interacting with simulated patients administered by the National Board of Medical Examiners as part of the battery of assessments used for medical licensure. Chapter 6 applies another well-known methodology, item response theory (IRT), in a form that addresses the persistent problem of conditional dependence in simulation-based task design and scoring. The model, referred to as Testlet Response Theory, is presented and discussed by the originators of the method.

The remaining methodological chapters address techniques that are less well known to the field of educational measurement or which involve complexities that require additional consideration in their implementation. Chapter 7 presents an application of Bayesian networks to assessment for learning targeted at computer network troubleshooting proficiency in simulated environments for Cisco Learning Institute. Bayesian networks are a method borrowed from the field of artificial intelligence and are only recently being applied to problems in educational measurement. The newness of this methodology and its application in this chapter serves as a contrast to applications of more well-known methods in previous chapters. Chapter 8 presents another relatively new and innovative methodology, neural networks. Neural networks are a pattern recognition method modeled after the learning behavior and "firing" of neurons in cognition. In assessment, the statistical methods that mimic this neural activity cluster the patterns of test performance they observe based on what is learned and represented in the neural network. These clusters serve as the basis for scoring. In Chapter 9 the author takes up the ambitious goal of summarizing current automated scoring methods for the domain of essay grading, a domain which currently boasts a number of commercially available methods as well as numerous methods emerging from ongoing research. The methods vary considerably, and in fundamentally meaningful ways, in their approach to scoring textual responses. This chapter summarizes characteristics of the different methods and provides references for further study on specific methods to the interested reader.

The new and innovative nature of automated scoring of constructed response tasks in CBT provides the opportunity for two concluding chapters. The first, Chapter 10, provides a methodological overview and commentary on the volume that offers a final perspective on the contrasting features of each approach to automated scoring. In addition, this discussion of contrasting features of methodologies also offers a comparison of some characteristics of the ECD framework for assessment design to another assessment framework: the Berkeley Assessment and Evaluation Research (BEAR) Assessment System. The volume closes with Chapter 11; a vision for the future development of automated scoring methods that provides some perspective and direction for the next steps in targeting further development of automated scoring systems for constructed response tasks in computer based testing.

Obviously, this volume would not exist without the expertise and dedication of the contributors and their colleagues who facilitated their work, both directly and through financial support. The goals and direction of the volume were sharpened substantially by the sound advice of Gregory Chung, Mark Reckase, and Mark Shermis during their reviews; for which we are very grateful. We also gratefully acknowledge Janice F. Lukas for her editorial expertise in ensuring that our ideas are expressed far more effectively than we could have achieved on our own. Additionally, we thank Debra Riegert at LEA for her guidance and patience. Finally, and most significantly, we thank our families for their support and encouragement during the production of the volume.

—David M. Williamson
—Robert J. Mislevy
—Isaac I. Bejar

1

Automated Scoring of Complex Tasks in Computer-Based Testing: An Introduction

David M. Williamson
Isaac I. Bejar
Educational Testing Service

Robert J. Mislevy
University of Maryland

> *Part of the inhumanity of the computer is that, once it is competently programmed and working smoothly, it is completely honest.*—Isaac Asimov; retrieved November 9, 2005, from www.quotationspage.com.

Our society is undergoing a seemingly continuous technological revolution, with digital innovations and expansions of computer capabilities now a constant aspect of modern life. Computational advances offer an unprecedented array of analytical methodologies to educational assessment. Given this plethora of delivery options, interactive task technologies, and analytical tools, how can measurement professionals make best use of emerging technologies to meet previously unattainable assessment goals? The key is not novel technology or sophisticated analysis per se, but an understanding of how these innovations can contribute to a coherent assessment argument. This volume presents a number of cutting-edge computerized assessments at the intersection of advances in analytical methods (both well-known and novel) for automated scoring and assessment design and delivery. Each chapter presents a different assessment, each with its own particular score reporting goals, constructs of interest, assessment tasks, and automated scoring methodologies. Although the specifics of the technologies and analytical methods vary from one example to the next, they share a reliance on principles of assessment design and an emphasis on how the innovative aspects of their designs contribute to the analytical argument of assessment. Together, they provide the reader with both an understanding of automated scoring technologies for complex computerized assessment tasks in computer-based testing and an approach to assessment design that clarifies the role these technologies play in an assessment argument.

The technological advances of the past decade are a catalyst for change in educational measurement. They allow increased flexibility, complexity, interactivity and realism of computer-administered assessment tasks, including multimedia components. Coupled with capabilities for internet delivery and its implications for large-scale on-demand administration, the potential wealth of data that can be tracked and recorded from such administrations appears capable of revolutionizing assessment. Such a revolution relies, in part, on the promise of a standardized automated analytical approach to measuring previously elusive constructs and complex problem-solving behavior. Of course, this promise depends on the ability of the measurement profession to address new challenges in the practice of educational measurement posed by such an approach to assessment. That is, just how do we make sense of rich data from complex tasks?

One key to leveraging the expanded capability to collect and record data from complex assessment tasks is implementing *automated scoring algorithms* to interpret data of the quantity and complexity that can now be collected. By *automated scoring* we mean any computerized mechanism that evaluates qualities of performances or work products. Automated scoring may be used to alleviate or supplement scoring typically conducted by human raters (e.g., by replacing one of two human graders in a scoring program or by producing computer-generated annotations of a response for consideration by a human grader), or to evaluate qualities too tedious or too difficult for humans to carry out in practice. Pioneering efforts, with Page (1966) representing some of the earliest work, have developed the field to the point that automated scoring of complex constructed response computer-based testing (CBT) tasks is operational in high-stakes assessments, as well as in classroom and other learning environments. This volume offers a survey of current methods for automated scoring and the domains in which they have been applied or are being developed. It provides examples of the range of methods that can be brought to bear in making sense of complex assessment data, the range of domains and the nature of tasks that can be used, and a survey of challenges that have been encountered.

In order to meaningfully discuss the automated scoring of complex assessment data, one must first determine what types of data may be appropriately characterized as complex. We offer the following characteristics as a guideline for distinguishing relatively complex assessment task data. For each conditionally independent[1] task, the task and resultant data may be considered "complex" if each of the following conditions are met:

1.   Completing the task requires the examinee to undergo multiple, non–trivial, domain–relevant steps and/or cognitive processes[2].

2.   Multiple elements, or features, of each task performance are captured and considered in the determination of summaries of ability and/or diagnostic feedback.

3.   There is a high degree of potential variability in the data vectors for each task, reflecting relatively unconstrained work product production.

4.   The evaluation of the adequacy of task solutions requires the task features to be considered as an interdependent set, for which assumptions of conditional independence typically do not hold.

Of course, there is no implication that complex tasks must be computerized. To the contrary, it has been traditionally necessary for assessments requiring the use of complex tasks (e.g., for writing ability, architectural design, foreign language proficiency, etc.) to administer and score those tasks by non–computerized means. It is only with the technological advances of the past decade that the development of computerized simulations that adequately present stimulus material and capture relevant response patterns has been recognized as a potential means of assessment for these domains. It is in the context of those technological advances that automated scoring becomes feasible, if nothing else because the availability work products in digital form are a prerequisite to economical implementation of automated scoring.

Educational measurement has a long-standing relationship with the multiple-choice item, and with good reason! Multiple-choice items are well known for their capabilities as expedient, efficient, relatively easy to develop, administer and score, and generally effective means for assessing ability in many domains. Despite these advantages, multiple-choice items are the subject of criticism. Because the multiple-choice format looks very different from—and more mechanical than—the real-world tasks for which they are applied as predictors or as diagnostic tools, these tests are often characterized as irrelevant and trivial (e.g., Fiske, 1990) by both the lay public and by other professionals in

---

[1] We specify conditionally independent to recognize that many tasks treated as independent may be based on some parent situation, passage, diagram, scenario, etcetera., that induce a conditional dependency among tasks as a result of being based on a common stimulus. Chapters 6 and 7 address modeling the dependencies among evaluations of multiple aspects of the same task performance.

[2] This may correlate with extended time required to complete a task.

the field. That is, they lack face-validity. For example, in a field such as engineering, addressing a real-world problem can take hours, days, or even years and require the integration of knowledge and skills that cannot be represented in simple multiple-choice formats. In cases such as these, an ideal assessment might be an unbiased observation of individuals as they worked over time to obtain an accurate understanding of the individual's strengths and weaknesses (Martin & VanLehn, 1995).

An approximation to the goal of naturalistic generation, in which the examinee must formulate, rather than recognize, an answer, is found in the development of the complex constructed-response task (Bennett & Ward, 1993). Constructed response tasks are believed to be more capable of capturing evidence about cognitive processes than multiple-choice items (Ackerman & Smith, 1988; Ward, Frederiksen, & Carlson, 1980) and are therefore more likely to measure important abilities and knowledge that are untapped by multiple-choice items. The use of complex constructed-response items may also provide an important educational benefit: These item formats permit the opportunity to examine the strategies that examinees use to arrive at their solution, which lends itself to collecting and providing diagnostic information to the candidate that is not easily provided by traditional multiple-choice formats (Birenbaum & Tatsuoka, 1987). Furthermore, it has been argued that the use of the constructed-response format would provide better evidence of the intended outcomes of educational interventions more clearly than multiple-choice assessments (Breland, Camp, Jones, Morris, & Rock, 1987; Frederiksen & Collins, 1989). Constructed response formats offer better evidence for measuring change on both a quantitative (e.g., Strategy A was employed on four occasions, with two effective results) and a qualitative (e.g., Strategy A was used before instruction and Strategy B afterward) level (Mislevy, 1993). By linking characteristics of cognitive processing to expected observable behaviors, it becomes possible to describe proficiency in terms of the cognitive components and skills (e.g., McNamara, 1996; Sheehan & Mislevy, 1990).

The successful implementation of complex constructed-response tasks relies on cognitive modeling at some level, so that the assessment system reflects students' strengths and weaknesses. That a thoughtful psychological model undergirds the construction and scoring of tasks does not imply that fine-grained measurement models must be used to report data. They might, if the assessment needs to provide diagnostic inferences for individual students. But they might not, if only high-level summative decisions are required. The point is that there must be a consideration of the targets of inference that are important for test (and therefore task) design. The measurement model that is appropriate to the purpose of assessment could be as simple as a single unidimensional estimate of domain ability or as complex as an extensive cognitive diagnosis model and intervention matrix underlying an intelligent tutoring system.

When finer-grained inferences are required, the psychological, and subsequently the measurement, models are constructed to allow an evaluation of the critical aspects of knowledge and skill. In these cases, the orientation of the models and their associated tasks differs from traditional emphasis on a purely correct or incorrect response and instead are also designed to address Thompson's (1982) question, "What can this person be thinking so that his actions make sense from his perspective?" (p. 161). Once such a model is constructed, its utility extends beyond the application in cognitive assessment in that tests of the model with regard to patterns of predicted and observed responses from individuals possessing different understanding of the domain ought to serve as a validation process for the cognitive theory of performance on which the model was constructed (Gitomer & Yamamoto, 1991).

Although complex constructed-response items are used routinely in some large-scale testing programs (e.g., the College Board's Advanced Placement Program), their use engenders complications. The most fundamental of these complications is this: Although complex tasks provide evidence of constructs or cognitive processes that are difficult or impossible to address with multiple-choice items, the speed with which examinees can respond to multiple-choice items allows more tasks to be administered in a given time. Therefore, the use of multiple-choice items allows for greater breadth of domain coverage and potentially greater reliability (from a standard test theory perspective; Bennett, 1993b).

Even when complex constructed-response items are clearly preferable to multiple-choice, robust implementation of scoring using human judges requires detailed and defensible scoring rubrics. Ensuring timely scoring for high volume assessments requires a large number of judges and the associated costs of housing, meals, travel and honoraria. The consistency and potential biases of judges must be monitored to maintain the scale stability and interjudge agreement (Bennett, 1993b; Braun, 1988). A human scoring program for constructed response requires a substantial scoring apparatus (see discussion in chap. 3, this volume) to insure fair and valid scoring. With such efforts, human scoring can be an expensive undertaking. But without these efforts, the value of the assessment itself can be jeopardized by threats to the operational quality of scores, as illustrated by experience described in Koretz, Stetcher and Diebert (1992). Furthermore, most current large-scale implementations of human scoring miss an opportunity to glean educational value from constructed response tasks; that is, a qualitative analysis that would be the basis of diagnostic score reports based on features of the performance (Bennett, 1993a).

These demands of complex constructed response suggest the potential value of computerized delivery and automated scoring to reduce the time and expense of scoring, to maintain tractability and consistency of scoring, and to permit the introduction of qualitative analyses. Indeed, these types of computerized scoring of complex open-ended items are currently being implemented, with the goal of providing many of the advantages described earlier (e.g., Bejar, 1991; Braun, Bejar, & Williamson, chap. 2, this volume; Kenney, 1997; Margolis & Clauser, chap. 5, this volume; Martinez & Katz, 1996; Stevens & Casillas, chap. 8, this volume; Williamson, Almond, Mislevy, & Levy, chap. 7, this volume; Williamson, Bejar, & Hone, 1999 and 2004).

Despite this enthusiasm over the potential of automated scoring, it would be naïve to think computerized delivery and scoring are a panacea, or even a new idea (see, e.g., Hubbard, Levit, & Barnett, 1970). Nevertheless, the prevailing trend of technological innovation enables assessment researchers to consider possibilities that were previously beyond their capabilities. The proliferation of personal computers, remote assessment capacity through the internet, multimedia applications and even video imaging have dramatically expanded the realm of possibilities for innovations in assessment format and administration. Even the conception of what constitutes relevant assessment data has expanded, with new capabilities for tracking such aspects as individual mouse clicks, voice data, digital imaging, and even iris focal points during assessment. This technology has completely solved the problem of data collection; it is now possible to collect vast quantities of performance data, in excruciating detail, with complete accuracy during performance assessment via computerized simulations. The challenge now rests more squarely on the need to make sense of this mountain of data, or rather, to use prior conceptualizations to selectively collect only that data that is meaningful with respect to some pre-established assessment hypotheses. Towards this end, the primary interest of harnessing technology for educational assessment is perhaps best stated by Thornburg (1999):

> The key idea to keep in mind is that the true power of educational technology comes not from replicating things that can be done in other ways, but when it is used to do things that couldn't be done without it. (p. 7)

Although the focus on complex constructed response tasks, particularly with computerized simulations, in computer-based testing may be the current vanguard of automated scoring in educational measurement, it would appear that an interest in automated scoring has shadowed every item type used in educational measurement. A passage from Greene (1941) illustrates the fact that researchers have always sought ways of using emerging technological tools to automate and improve on human scoring processes:

> The International Business machine (I.B.M.) Scorer (1938) uses a carefully printed sheet … upon which the person marks all his answers with a special pencil. The sheet is printed with small parallel lines showing where the pencil marks should be placed to indicate true items, false items, or multiple-choices. To score this sheet, it is inserted in the machine, a lever is moved, and the total score is read from a dial. The scoring is accomplished by electrical contacts with the pencil marks. … Corrections for guessing can be obtained by setting a dial on the machine. By this method, 300 true–false items can be scored simultaneously. The sheets can be run through the machine as quickly as the operator can insert them and write down the scores. The operator needs little special training beyond that for clerical work. (p. 134)

Today we may read this passage with a wry smile, given our perspectives on the evolution from these beginnings to large-scale administration with our "special pencils" now standardized as the No. 2, and onward to computerized administration and adaptive testing. However, the fundamental characteristics that we still find to be compelling motivators and issues of interest for modern automated scoring development are also expressed in this early discussion, including the speed and efficiency of operation, the alleviation of the need for highly qualified scorers, and immediate score reporting based on selection of a statistical model (in this case, including a correction for guessing). In addition, the questions and concerns are likewise similar as with modern approaches to automated scoring, including the need for programming the machine to identify correct responses and accommodation of response variations (such as differential use of the special pencils or changing answers), as well as the need for special hardware (the pencil, the carefully printed sheets, the scoring machine, etc.). Although the envelope has now been stretched to the point that these advantages and issues in automated scoring are now directed at the scoring of far more complex tasks than true-false and multiple-choice, this has been accomplished through a long series of incremental improvements, a path down which we continue to travel for the automated scoring of ever more complex and innovative assessment tasks.

While technological advances have inspired research into their application in assessment, new technology is an enabler of assessment innovation, not a solution in itself. Despite early visions of computerized simulations in assessment (e.g., Hubbard, Levit, & Barnett, 1970), it has taken many years for operational assessment to materialize. The technological challenges of programming, task development and administration via computer proved much more readily addressed than fundamental measurement challenges, as noted by Melnick (1996):

> Complex test stimuli result in complex responses which require complex models to capture and appropriately combine information from the test to create a valid score. It is amazing to me how many complex "testing" simulation systems have been developed in the last decade, each *without* a scoring system. (p. 117)

The lesson learned from this experience, and a thrust of this volume, is that it is not new technology or analytical methods alone that determine the success of assessment innovations, but the integration of these advances with all other aspects of a sound and formalized assessment design. In this respect, the technological capacity to develop realistic simulations that incorporate an increasing variety of media and response formats has, to date, exceeded the pace of development of assessment methodologies for interpreting such assessment data. This discrepancy between technological capability for task design and delivery and the infrastructure of measurement has highlighted the need for new approaches to measurement. The challenge faced by such a new approach is to create a conceptual and analytical assessment design that incorporates simulation tasks to produce a coherent, valid assessment rather than a colorful, but psychometrically sparse, set of exercises. This may require revisiting the fundamental assumptions about educational measurement that have grown from a rich history of multiple-choice testing, causing us to question whether strict adherence to traditional metrics for evaluating test performance is akin to an effort to build a mechanical horse rather than the automobile.

Such efforts to revisit and reevaluate approaches to measurement in technology rich environments, both from the conceptual perspective and from the perspective of innovative statistical methods in measurement, have been underway for a number of years. Some notable milestones in the evolution of this perspective include the Hydrive project's use of interactive simulations for troubleshooting aircraft hydraulics (Mislevy & Gitomer, 1996; Steinberg & Gitomer, 1996), The National Council of Architectural Registration Boards (NCARB) implementation of tasks requiring examinees to build architectural designs using a computer-aided design (CAD) interface for the Architect Registration Examination (ARE) (Kenny, 1997), the National Board of Medical Examiners (NBME) incorporation of simulated patients in the assessment of physician ability for medical licensure (Clauser, Margolis, Clyman, & Ross, 1997), and Cisco Learning Institute's use of simulated network environments in the NetPass assessment of computer networking ability (Bauer, Williamson, Steinberg, Mislevy, & Bejar, 2001), among others.

The key to leveraging new technologies to improve assessment is formally incorporating automated scoring into the validity argument for assessment tasks, and the assessment itself, for its intended purpose. That is, automated scoring is not simply an application of technological advances, but is a (significant) part of an overall validity argument for use of an assessment (Bennett & Bejar, 1998). Bennett and Bejar (1998) argued that a substantial part of the value of automated scoring is the inherent demands such scoring make on the explicit nature of the validity argument and the interactions of this argument with other elements of the assessment design. The automated scoring component of an assessment must be integrated within an overall chain of evidential reasoning connecting observations from assessment tasks with inferences about people. With respect to constructing a strong validity argument for use of automated scoring, what is needed most is a framework for understanding the role of automated scoring in the argument. Part of this need for a new framework within which to evaluate the adequacy of an assessment design includes the need to address some fundamental questions for which there are currently no absolute answers:

1. What constructs demand the use of complex simulations and extended problem-solving tasks rather than their relatively direct and efficient multiple-choice counterparts?

2. How are we to make sense of the rich and interrelated data obtained from complex assessment simulations?

3. What statistical methods are available and effective in drawing conclusions from this complex data? Indeed, what is "scoring" when the rich assessment data recorded is parsed, combined, evaluated with multiple iterations of if–then rule application and recombination into new variables before being used to report a result?

4. What constitutes an assessment "task" when a single "prompt" might initiate a 2-hour long exercise in complex problem solving resulting in megabytes of assessment data, with dozens of extracted variables?

5. What is the best way to deal with the potential for construct-irrelevant variance that can result from many elements of observable data stemming from a common task?

These are just some of the critical questions illustrating the thorny, and often unexplored, issues researchers have encountered when developing and implementing automated scoring systems.

The preceding discussion emphasizes the point that technology itself is not a solution leading to better assessment. Instead, it is the *strategic use* of technology in a coherent assessment design that leads to successful innovations in assessment. Such a coherent design requires an understanding and incorporation of many more measurement issues than simple applications of technology. No one component, be it the technology of interactive tasks, computerized adaptive testing, voice-recognition technology, text parsing, or other automated scoring technologies, will ensure a successful assessment. All of these elements must be woven together into an assessment design that makes best use of their particular contributions to achieve a particular measurement goal that requires these capabilities.

Reflecting this importance of a framework that specifies the role each design element plays in achieving the goals of measurement, this volume begins with a presentation of the fundamental framework of evidence-centered design (ECD) as the organizational theme for better understanding how automated scoring systems contribute to and function within the assessment design and how, as a reflection of these design decisions, they differ from each other in goals and function. A key emphasis of this chapter is that it's not so much the empirical method of automated scoring that is critical, but rather how this selected method fits into the assessment argument. This theme is revisited in subsequent chapters to provide a unifying theme to the volume and to facilitate comparisons of methods across chapters.

With the primary concepts of ECD outlined, the next chapter uses this emphasis on understanding and modeling the analytical argument represented in scoring methods to revisit issues in human scoring of complex tasks. The human scoring chapter (chap. 3) recalls commonly held assumptions and procedures surrounding human scoring. It questions the degree to which such approaches satisfy the demands of a transparent argument represented by the scoring processes of an assessment design. Specifically, this chapter calls into question assumptions commonly made about the sufficiency of human scoring, and argues for a greater understanding and modeling the cognitive processes of human graders engaged in scoring.

The remaining chapters present assessment designs that exemplify the convergence of psychometric methods, measurement principles, and technology in applied practice. These chapters survey the current automated scoring methodologies being applied for complex assessment tasks in fielded assessment systems and those under current development. Each chapter of this volume represents a different approach to addressing the kinds of goals for automated scoring exemplified by the earlier quote from Greene. For each of the approaches presented, the purpose and context of the assessment is presented to ground an understanding of how the automated scoring serves the needs of the assessment design, as seen through the lens of Evidence-Centered Design (see chap. 2). This series of chapters begins with a presentation of rule-based and so called "mental model" scoring, as a set of essentially if–then logic rules for automated scoring. Chapter 3 presents the regression-based scoring for the patient management problems of the National Board of Medical Examiners (NBME) Primum® Computer-Based Case Simulations, perhaps the most well-researched operational automated scoring program. Chapter 6 explores the potential for Testlet Response Theory, an extension of Item Response Theory to account for violations of the assumption of conditional independence of responses. Chapter 7 presents an overview of issues and the array of methodologies for automatic scoring of essays. Following this is a presentation of the use of neural networks for understanding complex problem solving in educational settings. The final methodological chapter presents the development of an assessment of computer networking ability scored using Bayesian networks. Chapter 10 is an informed commentary on chapters 2 through 9 from a methodological and applied measurement perspective. The volume closes with a chapter on the importance of, and some proposed goals for, future development and continued progress of automated scoring methodologies for educational measurement.

Each of these methods and content areas has been selected for inclusion in this volume as part of an effort to provide examples of the wide range of methodologies being applied and investigated as general approaches to automated scoring. Further, it represents the array of content domains for which automated scoring is a sufficiently promising possibility to inspire dedicated research and applied measurement programs. The chapters have been organized to represent a progression, beginning with foundations of design and modeling, moving to examples of innovative application of fundamental and relatively well-known analytical methodologies, and subsequent chapters presenting more innovative and less common analytical methods. A number of promising and operationally fielded automated scoring systems are not represented in this volume, but are nonetheless very well-researched and exciting innovations in measurement that the interested reader is advised to seek out for additional understanding of issues and advances in the field. These include an edited volume on automated scoring for essays (Shermis & Burstein, 2003) and applications of Bayesian networks to the field of Physics learning systems (VanLehn & Niu, 2001), to name just two. With this goal of providing a survey of current methods and applications of automated scoring, we hope that this volume provides both a sound grounding in the current state-of-the-art of automated scoring as well as providing inspiration and direction for further research with the hope that the future will allow a better understanding of what it means for an automated scoring system to be considered competently programmed and working smoothly.

REFERENCES

Ackerman, T. A., & Smith, P. L. (1988). A comparison of the information provided by essay, multiple-choice, and free response writing tests. *Applied Psychological Measurement, 12*(2), 117–128.

Bauer, M., Williamson, D. M., Steinberg, L. S., Mislevy, R. J., & Behrens, J. T. (2001, April). *How to create complex measurement models: A case study of principled assessment design.* Paper presented at the annual meeting of the American Educational Research Association, New Orleans, LA.

Bejar, I. I. (1991). A methodology for scoring open-ended architectural design problems. *Journal of Applied Psychology, 76,* 522–532.

Bennett, R. E. (1993a). On the meanings of constructed responses. In R. E. Bennett & W. C. Ward (Eds.), *Construction versus choice in cognitive measurement: Issues in constructed response, performance testing, and portfolio assessment* (pp. 1–27). Hillsdale, NJ: Lawrence Erlbaum Associates.

Bennett, R. E. (1993b). Toward intelligent assessment: An integration of constructed-response testing, artificial intelligence, and model-based measurement. In N. Frederiksen, R. J. Mislevy, & I. Bejar (Eds.), *Test theory for a new generation of tests* (pp. 99–123). Hillsdale, NJ: Lawrence Erlbaum Associates.

Bennett, R. E., & Bejar, I. I. (1998). Validity and automated scoring: It's not only the scoring. *Educational Measurement: Issues and Practice, Winter 1998,* 9–17.

Bennett, R. E., & Ward, W. C. (Eds.) (1993). *Construction versus choice in cognitive measurement: Issues in constructed responses, performance testing, and portfolio assessment.* Hillsdale, NJ: Lawrence Erlbaum Associates.

Birenbaum, M., & Tatsuoka, K. K. (1987). Open-ended versus multiple-choice Response formats— It does make a difference for diagnostic purposes. *Applied Psychological Measurement, 11,* 385–395.

Braun, H. I. (1988). Understanding scoring reliability: Experiments in calibrating essay readers. *Journal of Educational Statistics, 13,* 1–18.

Breland, H. M., Camp, R., Jones, R. J., Morris, M. M., & Rock, D. A. (1987). *Assessing writing skill.* (Research Monograph NO. 11). New York: College Entrance Examination Board.

Clauser, B. E., Margolis, M. J., Clyman, S. G., & Ross, L. P. (1997). Development of automated scoring algorithms for complex performance assessments. *Journal of Educational Measurement, 34,* 141–161.

Fiske, E. (1990, March 5). How to learn in college: Little groups, many tests. *The New York Times,* pp. A1, A2.

Frederiksen, J. R., & Collins, A. (1989). A systems approach to educational testing. *Educational Researcher, 18(9),* 27–32.

Gitomer, D. H., & Yamamoto, K. (1991). Performance modeling that integrates latent trait and class theory. *Journal of Educational Measurement, 28(2),* 173–189.

Greene, E. B. (1941). *Measurements of human behavior.* New York: The Odyssey Press.

Hubbard, J. P., Levit, E. J., & Barnett G, O. (1970). Computer-based evaluation of clinical competence. *Bulletin of the American College of Physicians, 11*, 502–505.

Kenney, J. F. (1997). New testing methodologies for the Architect Registration Examination. CLEAR Exam Review, 8(2), 23–28.

Koretz, D., Stecher, B., & Diebert, E. (1992). *The Vermont portfolio assessment program: Interim report on implementation and impact, 1991–92 school year.* (CSE Technical Report No. 350). Los Angeles, CA: National Center for Research on Evaluation, Standards, and Student Testing.

Martin, J., & VanLehn, K. (1995). Student assessment using Bayesian nets. *International Journal of Human–Computer Studies, 42,* 575–591.

Martinez, M. E., & Katz, I. R. (1996). Cognitive processing requirements of constructed figural response and multiple-choice items in architecture assessment. *Educational Assessment, 3*(1), 83–98.

McNamara, T. F. (1996). *Measuring second language performance.* New York: Longman.

Melnick, D. (1996). The experience of the National Board of Medical Examiners. In E. L. Mancall, P. G. Vashook, & J. L. Dockery (Eds.), *Computer-based examinations for board certification* (pp. 111–120). Evanston, IL: American Board of Medical Specialties.

Mislevy, R. J. (1993). Foundations of a new theory. In N. Frederiksen, R. J. Mislevy, & I. Bejar (Eds.), *Test theory for a new generation of tests* (pp. 19–39). Hillsdale, NJ: Lawrence Erlbaum Associates

Mislevy, R. J., & Gitomer, D. H. (1996). The role of probability-based inference in an intelligent tutoring system. *User-Modeling and User-Adapted Interaction, 5,* 253–282.

Moncur, Michael (2005). Isaac Asimov–US science fiction novelist & scholar. Retrieved November 9, 2005, from www.quotationspage.com.

Page, E. B. (1966). Grading essays by computer: Progress report. *Notes from the 1966 Invitational Conference on Testing Problems*, 87–100.

Shermis, M. D., & Burstein, J. (2003). *Automated essay scoring: A cross-disciplinary perspective.* Hillsdale, NJ: Lawrence Erlbaum Associates.

Steinberg, L. S., & Gitomer, D. G. (1996). Intelligent tutoring and assessment built on an understanding of a technical problem-solving task. *Instructional Science, 24,* 223–258.

Thompson, P. W. (1982). Were lions to speak, we wouldn't understand. *Journal of Mathematical Behavior, 3,* 147–165.

Thornburg, D. D. (1999). *Technology in K–12 Education: Envisioning a new future.* Retrieved April 8, 2004, from http://www.air.org/forum/Thornburg.pdf.

VanLehn, K. & Niu, Z. (2001). Bayesian student modeling, user interfaces and feedback: A sensitivity analysis. *International Journal of Artificial Intelligence in Education, 12*(2), 154–184.

Ward, W., Frederiksen, N. & Carlson, S. (1990). Construct validity of free response and machine scoreable forms of a test. *Journal of Educational Measurement, 17,* 11–29.

Williamson, D. M., Bejar, I. I., & Hone, A. S. (1999). 'Mental model' comparison of automated and human scoring. *Journal of Educational Measurement, 36,* 158–184.

Williamson, D. M., Bejar, I. I., & Hone, A. S. (2004). Automated Tools for Subject Matter Expert Evaluation of Automated Scoring. *Applied Measurement in Education, 17*(4), 323–357.

2

Concepts, Terminology, and Basic Models of Evidence-Centered Design

Robert J. Mislevy
University of Maryland

Linda S. Steinberg

Russell G. Almond
Janice F. Lukas
Educational Testing Service

> *What is wanted is simple enough in purpose—namely, some method which will enable us to lift into consciousness and state in words the reasons why a total mass of evidence does or should persuade us to a given conclusion, and why our conclusion would or should have been different or identical if some part of that total mass of evidence had been different.*—J. H. Wigmore (1937, p. 8)

Evidence-centered design[1] (ECD) is an approach to constructing and implementing educational assessments in terms of evidentiary arguments. The application of ECD in assessment design has several desirable properties for the relationship between assessment tasks and constructs of interest, innovative task types, item generation, and validity argumentation. The investigative process of ECD helps define the construct of interest and provide explicit evidential linkages between characteristics of assessment tasks as evidential components of proficiencies that define the targeted assessment construct. The ECD process provides an evidential focus that both provides direction for and increases the probability of success of efforts to produce innovative task types. The key is targeting the critical task characteristics and reducing the tendency to pursue false avenues in task design. The emphasis on task construction and models for their construction also facilitates item generation efforts, whether manual or automated. The development and evaluation of automated scoring algorithms for complex tasks is facilitated by ECD's attention to identifying the elements of a

---

[1] A glossary of ECD terms is included at the end of this chapter.

complex work product that constitute evidence, and characterizing the strength of this evidence about the proficiencies that have been targeted for the assessment's purpose. In combination, these characteristics also provide a substantial basis for validity arguments from a construct-representation perspective.

This chapter introduces the basic concepts of ECD, including some of the terminology and models that have been developed to implement the approach. Our goal is to provide a framework for assessment design that helps to disambiguate the role of automated scoring methods from other critical stages of assessment design and the interaction of these design components, as well as delineating the stages of automated scoring processes. This disambiguation is particularly useful for complex simulation scoring in which the simulation task design and the scoring methodology are often intimately intertwined. It is in the area of complex responses and atypical assessment designs that the ECD process has its greatest benefits. Given the complexity of automated scoring development and implementation, the emerging field of automated scoring can only benefit, we would argue, by the availability of shared terminology. Shared terminology helps the assessment designer sort out assessment purpose, targeted proficiencies to be measured, elements of task design, and evidential value of responses. A shared conceptual framework based on the role of the procedures and shared protocols provides a better understanding of how scoring processes communicate with or substitute for one another. We offer the framework of ECD as a step in this direction, and as a common means of communication in this volume to describe and compare automated scoring methods and their current applications in educational measurement.

In accordance with this emphasis on automated scoring, this chapter is focused on models that comprise the *Conceptual Assessment Framework*, or CAF, and the *four-process delivery architecture* for assessment delivery systems. The reader interested in a more complete treatment of ECD is referred to Mislevy, Steinberg, and Almond (2002), for connections to the philosophy of argument and discussions of the earlier stages of design, and to Almond, Steinberg, and Mislevy (2002) for amplification on delivery system architecture.

The chapter begins with a rationale for assessment as a special case of an exercise in evidentiary reasoning, with validity as the grounds for the inferences drawn from assessment data (Cronbach, 1989; Embretson, 1983; Kane, 1992; and Messick 1989, 1994). ECD provides a structural framework for parsing and developing assessments based on evidentiary reasoning, and this section outlines some of the benefits that result from this perspective on assessment design. The next section provides a brief overview of the models that make up the design blueprint (the Conceptual Assessment Framework or CAF). This is followed by a presentation of the four-process delivery architecture describing how ECD components function in operational assessment. In the final section, the elements of previous sections are revisited with additional discussion in the context of two hypothetical assessment systems. This discussion (and examples) illustrates how automated scoring can play roles in either task-level or test-level scoring processes, or both. As a simple running illustration, we use examples based on the paper and pencil (P&P) and the computer adaptive (CAT) versions of the Graduate Record Examination (GRE). As this is written, the GRE is comprised of three domains of items, concerning verbal, quantitative, and analytic reasoning skills. In each case, a student responds to a number of items in the domain, and an estimate of a single proficiency with regard to that domain is reported. As an existing assessment, this example is meant to provide a concrete illustration from a relatively familiar context for the ECD terminology, rather than to illustrate assessment design in action. The succeeding chapters in this volume take up the challenge of describing in terms of ECD assessments that use a variety of statistical scoring methods.

ASSESSMENT AS EVIDENTIARY ARGUMENT

Advances in *cognitive psychology* deepen our understanding of how students gain and use knowledge. Advances in *technology* make it possible to capture more complex performances in assessment settings by including, for example, simulation, interactivity, collaboration, and constructed response. Automated methods have become available for parsing complex Work products and identifying educationally meaningful features of them. The challenge of assessment design is in knowing just how to put all this new knowledge to work to best serve the purposes of an assessment; that is, in support of valid measurement.

Familiar schemas for designing and analyzing tests produce assessments that are useful because they are coherent for many of the purposes for which they were developed (e.g., efficient nationwide testing with little technological support), but they are limited by the constraints and purposes under which they evolved: Unidimensional characterizations of participants (i.e., examinees), for example; conditionally independent responses, multiple-choice responses, and the absence of evolving interactions between participants and task situations. Progressing beyond traditional constraints requires not only the means for doing so (through advances such as those mentioned above) but schemas for producing assessments that are coherent for new and more ambitious assessment goals supported by emerging technologies; that is, for assessments that may indeed gather complex data to ground inferences about complex student models, to gauge complex learning or evaluate complex programs—but which build on a sound chain of reasoning from observed actions and results to what we subsequently infer about the ability of the participant, much like the chain of reasoning required to make sound evidentially based decisions in the field of jurisprudence (Schum, 1989), from which some of these concepts of evidentiary reasoning have evolved.

Recent work on validity in assessment lays the conceptual groundwork for such a scheme. The contemporary view focuses on the support—conceptual, substantive, and statistical—that assessment data provide for inferences or actions (Messick, 1989). From this perspective an assessment is a special case of evidentiary reasoning, the essential form of which was laid out by Messick (1994):

> A construct-centered approach [to assessment design] would begin by asking what complex of knowledge, skills, or other attribute should be assessed, presumably because they are tied to explicit or implicit objectives of instruction or are otherwise valued by society. Next, what behaviors or performances should reveal those constructs, and what tasks or situations should elicit those behaviors? Thus, the nature of the construct guides the selection or construction of relevant tasks as well as the rational development of construct-based scoring criteria and rubrics. (p. 17)

This perspective is valuable because it is a universal approach that helps organize thinking for assessments for all kinds of purposes, using all kinds of data, task types, scoring methods, and statistical models. We can ask of a simulation task, for example, just what knowledge and skills it is meant to reveal? Do the scoring methods actually recognize the clues that are present in performances? Does the format introduce requirements for extraneous knowledge? Every decision in the assessment design process influences the chain of reasoning from examinees' behaviors in the task setting to conclusions about what they know or can do. Obviously, these decisions and chains of inferential reasoning have an impact on choices about scoring methodology and, for automated scoring, provide a framework for evaluation of the method to determine appropriateness and applicability. From an evidentiary reasoning perspective, this framework provides a basis and procedure for examination of the impact of scoring method on the inferences that must ultimately be drawn.

As powerful as it is in organizing thinking, simply having an evidentiary reasoning point of view isn't as helpful as it could be in carrying out the actual work of designing and implementing assessments. A more structured framework is needed to provide common terminology and design objects that make the design of an assessment explicit and link the elements of the design to the processes that must be carried out in an operational assessment. Such a framework not only makes the underlying evidentiary structure of an assessment more explicit, but also makes the operational elements of an assessment, including task elements and models for acquiring domain expertise, easier to reuse in other applications (e.g., educational products and tutoring systems) and easier to share across domains and with other professionals. The evidence-centered design (ECD) models developed in Mislevy, Steinberg, and Almond (2003) and Almond, Steinberg, and Mislevy (2002) are intended to fill this gap. A glossary at the end of this chapter provides definitions of key ECD terminology.

In simplified form, the ECD process consists of an interdependent series of assessment design steps, with subsequent steps continuing to influence the outcomes of previous work and vice versa. As in any complex problem of design under constraints, the process is iterative and cyclical, with results and insights from any part of the work able to prompt us to rethink or to revise other parts. Although we can present the issues in a linear order, we certainly don't expect to address them in such strict linear sequence. The key questions for exploring and explicating assessment designs are these:

a.   Why are we assessing? (*Purpose Definition*)

b.   What will be said, done, or predicted on the basis of the assessment results? (*Claims* and *Score Reporting*)

c.   What portions of a field of study or practice does the assessment serve? (*Domain Analysis*)

d.   Which knowledge and proficiencies are relevant to the field of study or practice? (*Domain Model*)

e.   Which knowledge or proficiencies will be assessed? (*Student Model*)

f.   What behaviors would indicate levels of proficiency? (*Evidence Models*)

g.   How can assessment tasks be contrived to elicit behavior that discriminates among levels of knowledge and proficiency? (*Task Models*)

h.   How will the assessment be conducted and at what point will sufficient evidence be obtained? (*Assembly Models*)

i.   What will the assessment look like? (*Presentation Models*)

j.   How will the assessment be implemented? (*Delivery System Model*)

An evolving assessment design iteratively cycles through these questions to provide a set of answers in terms of design elements, consistent with one another, coherent as an expression of an assessment argument, and able to address an assessment's purpose within its constraints. Designing assessments in concert with this conceptual approach and implementing them in a common infrastructure provides several practical benefits. It makes explicit the choices and the accompanying rationale of good test developers. It lays out the validity argument that underlies a test. It promotes the reuse of assessment elements and processes. Finally, it provides a roadmap for addressing unfamiliar constructs, data, purposes, task types, and content areas. All of these elements are important for automated scoring of complex constructed response data, for without these design structures and rationales it can become difficult, if not impossible to work through the assessment and scoring algorithm logic. Nor do complex simulation assessments typically have the degree of transparency of traditional test designs that facilitates reverse engineering a final configuration to infer key design decisions. The following section highlights some of the basic ECD structures that provide the context for discussion of automated scoring methods and how they function in practice.

BASIC ECD STRUCTURES

Overview

Although the full ECD framework starts with the initial analysis of a substantive domain and assessment purposes, in this discussion we focus on the two components that are closest to the implemented assessment, and therefore provide the best basis for discussion of automated scoring methods. They are the Conceptual Assessment Framework (CAF) and the Four-Process Delivery Architecture for assessment delivery systems. Again, the interested reader is referred to Mislevy, Steinberg, and Almond (2003) for a discussion of the design process from start to finish. Suffice it to say here that in any particular assessment, the objects in the CAF models described in general terms in the following section will need to be designed to address the purposes of that particular assessment. For this discussion, in line with the Messick citation quoted earlier, we presume that all of the characteristics of tasks have been selected to provide the opportunity to get evidence about the targeted knowledge and skill; all of the scoring procedures are designed to capture, in terms of observable variables, the features of student work that are evidentially relevant to that end; and the characteristics of students reflected as student model variables summarize evidence about the relevant knowledge and skills from a perspective and at a grain size that suits the purpose of the assessment.

Figures 2.1 and 2.2 depict the main ECD models for design and delivery respectively, that is, the CAF and the four-process delivery architecture. We look at their contents and their connections more closely in the following sections. In a nutshell, the CAF models lay out the blueprint for the design structures of an assessment, and their interrelationships convey the substantive, statistical, and operational aspects of the design. The CAF models provide the technical detail required for implementation: specifications, operational requirements, statistical models, details of scoring rubrics, and so on. The four processes of the delivery system carry out, examinee by examinee, the functions of selecting and administering tasks, interacting as required with the examinee to present materials and capture Work products, evaluating responses from each task, and accumulating evidence across tasks.

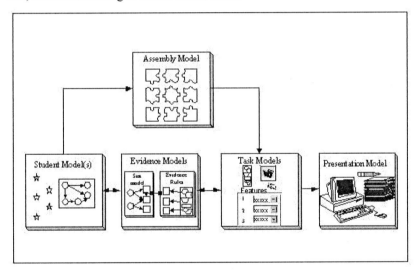

FIG. 2.1. The principle design objects of the conceptual assessment framework (CAF). These models are a bridge between the assessment argument and the operational activities of an assessment system. Looking to the assessment argument, they provide a formal framework for specifying the knowledge and skills to be measured, the conditions under which observations will be made, and the nature of the evidence that will be gathered to support the intended inference. Looking to the operational assessment, they describe the requirements for the processes in the assessment delivery system.

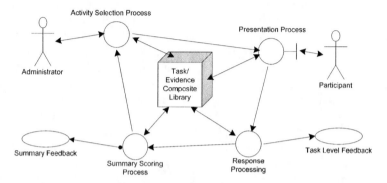

FIG. 2.2. The four principle processes in the assessment cycle. The Activity Selection Process selects a task (tasks include items, sets of items, or other activities) and directs the Presentation Process to display it. When the participant has finished interacting with the item, the Presentation Process sends the results (a work product) to the Response Scoring Process. This process identifies essential observations about the results and passes them to the Summary Scoring Process. All four processes can add information to a database of results as required in a given assessment system. The Activity Selection Process then makes a decision about what to do next, based on the current beliefs about the participant or other criteria.

The Conceptual Assessment Framework

The blueprint for an assessment is called the Conceptual Assessment Framework (CAF). To make it easier to focus on key design decisions and processes (and deal with each of them individually when appropriate) and to rearrange the pieces of the framework as needed, the framework is broken up into a number of pieces called *models*. Each model provides specifications that answer such critical questions as "What are we measuring?" or "How do we measure it?"

What Are We Measuring? The Student Model. A student model defines one or more variables related to the knowledge, skills, and abilities we wish to measure. A simple student model characterizes a student in terms of the proportion of a domain of tasks the student is likely to answer correctly. A more complicated model might characterize a student in terms of degree or nature of knowledge of several kinds, each of which may be required in different combinations in different tasks.

In each of the three GRE domains, the student model consists of a single unobservable variable, a proficiency in that domain. Quantitative reasoning will be used as an example, but the same structure is used for the verbal or analytical measures. Any student's value on this variable is not known, and indeed can never be known with certainty. At any point in time, our state of knowledge about its value is expressed by a probability distribution across the range of values it might take. Figure 2.3 depicts the student model for this example: A single proficiency variable, denoted θ, and an associated probability distribution that contains the assessors knowledge about an examinee's θ, at any given point in time. The mean of this distribution is a point estimate of the examinee's ability, and its standard deviation is a measure of its accuracy—that is, how much evidence the estimate is based on.

At the beginning of the assessment, the probability distribution representing what is known about ability of a particular examinee is uninformative. We update this distribution in accordance with behaviors we see the examinee make in various situations we have structured; that is, when we see her responses to some GRE Quantitative test items. In succeeding chapters, we see student models with multiple latent variables, each representing some aspect of knowledge, skill, or ability posited to influence performance. In each case, however, the idea is the same as with this simple univariate student model. These variables are how we characterize students' knowledge or ability. We don't get to observe them directly; we express what we do know about them in terms of a probability distribution; and evidence in the form of behavior in assessment situations allow us to update our knowledge, by updating the probability distributions accordingly.

Where Do We Measure It? The Task Model. Task models describe how to structure the kinds of situations we need to obtain the kinds of evidence we need to support our claims about student model variables. They describe the Presentation Material that is presented to the participant and the Work products that are generated in response. They also contain task model variables that describe features of tasks as well as how those features are related to the Presentation Material and Work products, and may additionally provide information about the focus or amount of evidence a task can provide about student model variables. Those features can be used by task authors to help

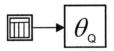

FIG. 2.3. The student model for the GRE Quantitative Measure.

structure their work, by psychometricians to help reduce the number of pretest participants needed (Mislevy, Sheehan, & Wingersky, 1993), and by test assemblers to help ensure that a particular form of the assessment is balanced across key kinds of tasks.

A task model does not represent a single task, but rather a family of potential tasks waiting to be constructed. Tasks are made from task models by selecting and completing variables in the specification made by the task model (i.e., finding or authoring presentation material and setting the values of the task model variables). A typical assessment will have many task models representing different families of related tasks.

A task model in the GRE describes a class of test items. There is some correspondence between task models and GRE item types, such as sentence completion, passage comprehension, and quantitative comparison. Different item types will generally require different task models, because different sets of variables needed to describe their distinct kinds of stimulus materials and presentation formats, and different features may be important in modeling item parameters or controlling item selection. The same task models will be required for paper and pencil (P&P) and CAT for using what are the same items from the perspective of content, even though specifications for presenting and managing the item are wholly different in the two modes; these functions are handled in the presentation model (discussed in a later section). In the P&P GRE, a student is administered a pre-assembled test containing more than 100 test items. In the computer adaptive test (CAT) GRE, items are selected one at a time to administer from a large pool of items based on updated values of the student model variables (via the assembly model, also discussed in a later section).

How Do We Measure It? The Evidence Model. Evidence models provide detailed instructions on how we should update our belief about the student model variables given a performance in the form of examinees' Work products from tasks. An evidence model contains two parts, which play distinct roles in the assessment argument:

- Evidence Rules describe how the observable variables that summarize an examinee's performance on a particular task will be evaluated from the Work product that was produced. These observables are the primary outcomes from task performances, and they provide information both for updating our belief about student model variables and for providing task-level feedback. In an operational assessment, Evidence Rules guide the Response Scoring Process. It is important to note that Evidence Rules concern the *identification* and *summary of evidence within tasks*, in terms of observable variables. Many of the automated scoring procedures that are discussed in this volume concern this stage of an assessment; that is, identifying, extracting, summarizing, or evaluating the key features of performance in a student's work.

For GRE items, Work product is the student response (A, B, C, D, or E) and the Evidence Rule is the rule determining the observable variable associated with each item (correct or incorrect). The Evidence Rule in this example takes the form IF (student response) equals (key) THEN observable variable equals "correct" ELSE observable variable equals "incorrect".[2]

- The measurement model part of the evidence model provides information about the connection between student model variables and observable variables. Psychometric models are often used for this purpose, including the familiar classical test theory and item response theory, and less familiar latent models and cognitive diagnosis models. In an operational assessment, measurement models guide the Summary Scoring process. It is important to note that measurement models concern the accumulation and synthesis of evidence across tasks, in terms of student model variables. Some of the automated scoring procedures in this volume concern this stage of an assessment, namely, synthesizing nuggets of information in the form of values of observable variables over tasks.

The difference between what is described in Evidence Rules and the measurement model is especially important for understanding automated scoring because the term "automated scoring" is colloquially applied to procedures that may play either of these two distinct roles, or collapse them into a single undifferentiated algorithm. By clearly differentiating these roles, we will find it easier to understand the role a given automated scoring procedure is playing in a particular assessment. This helps us understand and compare alternative procedures.

It is useful to think of the logic of evaluation rules as working from a particular piece of student work, so a summary of its key aspects. There may be multiple stages of evaluation rules, such as in automated essay scoring (Chap. 9) that start by extracting lexical and syntactic features of text, then producing a score from them using regression models or neural networks. Measurement models, in contrast, concern the distribution of possible values of key features of performances; think of data that are the input into a psychometric-style model for scores-on-tasks as a function of characteristics of students. Whatever level of summary of performance from individual tasks that is then aggregated across tasks is the boundary between the evaluation rules and the measurement

---

[2] This evidence rule is simplified and ignores the additional observable variable outcome possibilities of "omitted" and "not reached" for items skipped by examinees or not reached in the allotted time for assessment, respectively.

model—the demarcation between *evidence identification* for individual tasks and *evidence accumulation* over tasks.

Whether a given process on the path from performance to inference, automated or otherwise, is evidence identification or evidence accumulation is determined by its role in the assessment argument. To illustrate that the same data can be input to either identification or accumulation, consider an assessment comprised of sets of questions about stimuli, such as paragraphs or designs that contains several flaws that need to be identified and corrected. Typically the questions in a set are treated as if they met the local independence assumption of item response theory and the outcome of each question is passed to the IRT measurement model that updates the corresponding student model.

However, it has been observed that there can be dependencies among items relating to common stimuli (see Chap. 6 on Testlet Response Theory). One way to remove the dependencies is to summarize performance on the set as the number of questions answered correctly. A second phase of item-level scoring—simply summarizing performance within the set—produces the set score. The set score is then passed to a graded-response IRT measurement model to update the student model.

These two approaches to dealing with sets of questions illustrate the contextually determined nature of the boundary between evidence identification and evidence accumulation. In the first case, evidence identification is implemented as a scoring procedure for each question and evidence accumulation is the aggregation of the outcome from the set, which is passed to measurement model consisting of a dichotomous IRT model. In the second case evidence identification is the scoring of individual items for a set *and* a subsequence count summarizing the set, which is passed to a graded-response IRT model for evidence accumulation.

Continuing with our GRE example, in the P&P GRE, a student is administered a preassembled test containing more than 100 test items. She answers all items to produce a Work product, a string of A's, B's, C's, D's, and E's. The evidence rule is applied to each item in turn with the appropriate evidence rule data (the correct answer for that item) to determine which items were answered correctly. The results for each item are used to estimate her θ through the statistical relationships in the measurement model (in this case IRT parameterizations represented in Fig. 2.4). Similarly, for the computerized adaptive test (CAT) form of GRE, items are selected one at a time to administer and after each item administration the Evidence Rules and measurement model are applied and her θ estimate updated, with the resultant value used to help select the next item to administer in order to be more informative the value of

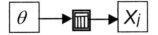

FIG. 2.4. The Measurement Model used in GRE-CAT.

her θ. Figure 2.4 shows the measurement model used in the GRE CAT. It gives the probability for a correct or incorrect response to a particular Item j, as a function of a student's θ. When it comes time to update belief about a student's θ based on a response to this item, this fragment is joined with the student model discussed above and the updating procedures discussed in Chapter 6 enter into play.

How Much Do We Need to Measure?   The Assembly Model.
Assembly models describe how the student models, evidence models, and task models must work together to form the psychometric backbone of the assessment. Targets describe how accurately each student model variable must be measured, and constraints describe how tasks must be balanced to properly reflect the breadth and diversity of the domain being assessed.

In both the P&P and CAT versions of the GRE, assembly rules govern the mix of item types, the content of reading passages, numbers of items that use geometric figures, abstract versus concrete concepts, sentence complexity, and many other task features. Statistical features of items such as their difficulty are also taken into account, but in different ways as befit the way they are presented. P&P test forms are all constructed to match the same targeted distributions of item difficulties and overall accuracy. GRE CAT test forms are custom-matched to each individual student to increase information about that student in light of their unfolding sequence of responses. Students doing well tend to be administered harder items, whereas students doing poorly tend to be administered easier ones.

How Does It Look? The Presentation Model.   Today's assessments
often get delivered through many different means. Examples include paper and pencil, stand-alone computer or the Web, hand-held devices, assessments being read aloud over the phone, or portfolios assembled by the students. A presentation model describes how the tasks appear in various settings, providing a style sheet for organizing the material to be presented and captured. The same GRE items can be administered under either P&P or CAT formats, but they ways they are composited or rendered on a computer screen require wholly

different sets of instructions—in one case directions to the printer, in the other case code to the computer that will display them.

How Do We Put It All Together? The Delivery System Model.

The delivery system model describes the collection of student, evidence, task, assembly, and presentation models necessary for the assessment and how they will work together. It also describes issues that cut across all of the other models, things like platform, security, and timing (i.e., tuning the ways in which the common models are used for different assessment purposes).

Breaking the assessment specification up into many smaller pieces allows it to be reassembled in different configurations for different purposes. For example, a diagnostic assessment requires a finer grain size student model than a selection/placement assessment. If we want to use the same tasks in both the diagnostic and selection assessment, we must use the same task models (written generally enough to address both purposes). However, we want different evidence models, each one appropriate to the level of detail consistent with the purpose of the assessment. And given Evidence Rules that specify Work products coming in, evaluations that must be made, and observable variables that come out, one can compare alternative methods for evaluating the observables—human scorers versus automated essay scoring, for example.

Comparing with the standard high-stakes GRE, for example, a practice test for the GRE would require different processes and different interactions among them in a delivery system that focused on diagnostic reports and instructional, even item-level, feedback. Such changes might include more detailed student model variables for reporting to an examinee, a different measurement model that related performance to these more detailed facets of knowledge, and additional kinds of presentation material that referring examinees to sources of additional study or on-the-spot instruction.

Four-Process Architecture for Assessment Delivery

Assessments are delivered in a variety of platforms. P&P tests are still the most widely used; oral exams have a long history, and the use of computer-based tests is growing rapidly. New ways to deliver tests are making an appearance as well—over the Web, over the phone, and with hand-held devices.

To assist in planning for all these diverse ways of delivering a test, ECD provides a generic framework for test delivery: the Four-Process Delivery Architecture. The Four-Process Delivery Architecture shown in Figure 2.2 is an idealized system representing activities that take place in an assessment cycle; any realized assessment system must contain these four processes in some form or other. They are essential to making the observations and drawing the inferences that comprise an assessment argument. This is true whether some of the processes are collapsed or degenerate in a given system, and regardless of whether they are carried out by humans, computers, or human-computer interactions.

How Is the Interaction with the Examinee Handled? The Presentation Process.

The Presentation Process is responsible for presenting the task and all supporting presentation material to the student and for gathering up the Work products. Examples include a display engine for computer-based testing, a simulator that can capture an activity trace, and a system for distributing test booklets and capturing and scanning the answer sheets. In the P&P GRE, the presentation process concerns administering preassembled test booklets to examinees and collecting their bubbled-in answer sheets. In the CAT, presentation concerns presenting a customized sequence of items to an examinee one at a time, in each instance capturing a response to be evaluated on the spot that will guide the selection of the next item.

How Is Evidence Extracted Evidence from a Task Performance? The Response Scoring Process.

The Response Scoring Process is responsible for identifying the key features of the Work product which are the observable outcomes for one particular task. The observable outcomes can go back to the participant for task level feedback and/or on to the Summary Scoring process. Examples include matching a selected response to an answer key, running an essay through an automated scoring engine such as Educational Testing Service's e-Rater, and having a human rater score a student portfolio according to a rubric. The Evidence Rules from the CAF specify how this is to be accomplished. The Response Scoring Process can consist of multiple stages, such as when lexical and syntactic features are identified in an essay and a regression model is used to summarize them into a single score for the task response. A variety of approaches can embody this process: linear regression of work-product features, artificial neural nets, rule-based decision algorithms, and holistic judgments by human raters are all methods by which response processing can be accomplished. Many procedures that are commonly called automatic scoring constitute response scoring in the assessment, or a subset of multiple stages required in a multi-stage Response Scoring Process. Examples from this volume include Braun, Bejar, and Williamson (Chap. 4 this volume,

Margolis and Clauser (Chap. 5 this volume), and Williamson, Almond, Mislevy, and Levy (Chap. 7 this volume).

The logical content of the Response Scoring Process is the same in GRE CAT and P&P forms: The student's answer is compared with the key. The implementation is rather different for the two modes of administration, however. In the P&P version, sophisticated algorithms and sensitive machine are employed to determine, via relative intensities of light reflection, which answer bubble the student marked. In the CAT version, the character that corresponds to the location where the student clicked a mouse button to indicate an answer choice is compared with the character stored in memory as the key. Note that an automated scoring process is employed either way!

How Is Evidence Accumulated Across Tasks? Summary Scoring.

This process is responsible for accumulating the observable outcomes across multiple tasks to produce section and assessment level scores. Examples include the IRT engine used in GRE-CAT testing, process counting up the number of "right" answers, and the Bayesian network summary scoring approach described in Williamson et al (Chap. 7 this volume). The measurement model in the CAF associated with a particular task specifies how this is to be accomplished. Some procedures referred to as automated scoring constitute a summary scoring process, whereas others combine summary scoring with some or all of response scoring. Examples from this volume include Wainer et al (Chap. 6) and Stevens and Casillas (Chap. 8).

What Happens Next? Activity Selection.

The activity selection process is responsible for deciding what the next task should be and when to stop the assessment. When making these decisions, adaptive assessments consult the current state of what is known about a student, in terms of the values of the student-model variables as they have been updated by the Summary Scoring process. An instructional system will also make decisions about switching between assessment and instruction modes. Examples of activity selection processes include simple linear sequencing (the P&P GRE, although the student may chose the order in which to answer items within each section as it is administered), computerized adaptive item selection (the GRE CAT), and student choice as to when to move on in a self-paced practice system.

Where Do Processes Get the Information They Need? Task/Evidence Composite Library.

All four process require certain kinds of data in order to do their jobs: The Presentation Process requires the text, pictures, and other material to be displayed; the Response Scoring Process requires the "key" or other evidence rule data against which to evaluate the Work products; the Summary Scoring process requires the parameters that provide the "weights of evidence" for each task; and the Activity Selection process requires classification and information codes used to balance the assessment form. The Task/Evidence Composite Library is a unified database that stores this information. In the P&P GRE, some of this information is used once to assemble forms, and others are used later to score responses and accumulate evidence when completed forms are returned. In the GRE CAT, the information must be available during testing because item selection, task scoring, and test scoring are all being carried out as testing proceeds from one item to the next.

We have suggested, without providing all the details, the clear mapping between the design models built in the Conceptual Assessment Framework and the Four-Process Delivery Architecture for assessment delivery systems. All of the design decisions made in the blueprint are reflected either directly in the implementation or in one of the processes leading up to the implementation. Again, further discussion and examples are available in Almond, Steinberg, and Mislevy (2003).

Pretesting and Calibration

In order to score an assessment, the Response Scoring Process or the Summary Scoring Process (or both) may need to build in empirical information from previous administrations of the tasks. In the case of Response Scoring, this information is incorporated into Evidence Rules. In the case of Summary Scoring, it appears in scoring weights or item parameters in psychometric, regression, or neural network models. We refer to a start-up set of data from which to estimate these values as pretest data, and the operation of determining the values as calibration.

An example for Response Scoring occurs in automatic scoring of essays. Lexical and syntactic features of essays can be extracted directly from essays, but how should they be combined to produce a score for a given essay? A common way to solve this problem is to obtain a pretest sample of essays written to the same prompt (or to the family of prompts for which a scoring rule is desired), and have them rated by human experts. The calibration procedure can then be fit using a regression model for human scores as a function of lexical and syntactic features. Several models may be fit and compared, and the regression function found most satisfactory for the pretest sample can then be applied to automatically score new essays for which only the features are known. As mentioned above, and further elaborated in Chapters 4 through 9, this combination could be carried out by other means such as artificial neural networks, logical rules, and human judgment.

An example for Summary Scoring occurs routinely in computerized adaptive testing based on item response theory (IRT), such as the GRE CAT. A collection of items may be administered to a pretest sample of students. Calibration consists of fitting the IRT model to the data, which provides estimates of item parameters that characterize the relationship of the response (the observable variable) to each item and the IRT proficiency variable, which is the single variable in the student model in such an assessment. The resulting item parameters can then be used to test future students, not only for summary scoring but for activity selection as well. This is because the item parameters indicate how much information an item is likely to provide for a student about something is already known from previously acquired data.

Validation

Validity is paramount among the principles of psychometrics, for validity speaks directly to the extent to which a claim about a student, based on assessment data from that student, is justified (Messick, 1989). Establishing validity entails making the warrant explicit, examining the network of beliefs and theories on which it relies, and testing its strength and credibility through various sources of backing. It requires determining conditions that weaken the warrant, exploring alternative explanations for good or poor performance, and feeding them back into the system to reduce inferential errors.

Embretson (1983) distinguished between validity arguments that concern why data gathered in a certain way ought to provide evidence about the targeted skill knowledge, and those that investigate relationships of resulting scores with other variables to support the case. These are, respectively, arguments about "construct representation" and arguments from "nomothetic span." ECD provides a framework for expressing a construct representation argument for validity—for building validity into an assessment from the start. Although this is a great strength of principled assessment design, it is not sufficient to establish validity. More traditional validation studies based on nomothetic arguments, using scores from individual items or assessments, remain essential: Do item and test scores correlate with what they should? Do they improve instruction decisions as intended? Do task scores agree with external evidence about the quality of performances? This requirement is not diminished by automated scoring methods, and indeed may become all the more important when high-stakes evaluations take place outside the immediate watch of humans. Validity studies of inferences involving automated scoring are only beginning to appear. Some are noted in the various chapters in this volume. Bennett's discussion (Chap. 11 this volume) makes a case for vigorous research in this direction.

EXAMPLES OF ASSESSMENT FOR TWO DIFFERENT PURPOSES

We have now described the basic objects of the ECD design models and delivery architecture, and along the way looked at how these ideas play out in the familiar context of the GRE assessment. We now go back for a closer look at the delivery processes and cycles related to somewhat less typical assessments for two different purposes. We consider a high-stakes selection test and a drill-and-practice tutoring system for Chinese character reading and writing. These examples, although relatively easy to describe even to people with no experience with East Asian languages, are singularly useful in helping us address a number of interesting design issues, including the impact of different purposes on assessment design and delivery, as well as dealing with automated scoring and non-traditional types of data, including audio and pictures.

A High-Stakes Assessment

For the sake of familiarity, we look first at an assessment system design for high-stakes selection testing (Fig. 2.5). All elements of an assessment's design flow from the purpose of the assessment—in particular, the nature of the claims relevant to make as a result of a participant's engagement with the assessment, as well as the timing, nature, and granularity of feedback. For our high-stakes selection example, a single score (together with information that facilitates interpretation in terms of comparison with a typical test-taking population) delivered at the end of the assessment will suffice. Because no task-specific diagnostic feedback is called for, responses can be evaluated as either correct or incorrect. Our high-stakes selection example also comes with some typical operational constraints: it must be delivered to a large population of test-takers, only a limited amount of time is available to cover a potentially large domain, and it must be scored inexpensively and quickly.

Working through the design process (which we do not describe here), we identify the salient claims about students' knowledge and skill, evidence, and tasks for our purpose, and blend these requirements with the constraints just described. The result is a set of models that represents the specifications for this assessment.

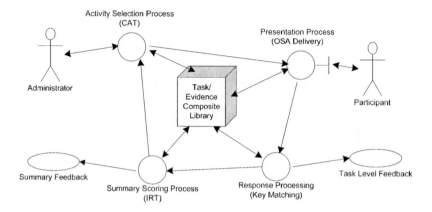

FIG. 2.5. Assessment cycle objects specialized to a high-stakes selection assessment.

- What we want to measure is represented by the student model for Overall Mastery. In this student model we have a single student model variable, which indicates the participant's overall level of mastery. This can be supported by familiar unidimensional IRT-based statistical processes. Task model variables can be used to help predict the parameters of each item. The IRT summary-scoring process is used to accumulate information across tasks only as to an overall proficiency in the domain of tasks, and is not capable of providing detailed across-task feedback.

- Tasks that can elicit appropriate evidence can be generated from a Phonetic Transcription[3] task model. The participant is presented a picture of one or more characters and is requested to type a phonetic transcription. The resulting Work product from this task is a string of characters that can be matched to a key.

- Evidence to support inferences related to mastery is evaluated by the evidence model for Correct/Incorrect Key Matching. In this evidence model, we have a simple algorithm that matches a selected response containing the desired evidence against a key to produce a Boolean value (representing "Correct" or "Incorrect") for a single observable for each task, which is used to update the single student model variable.

We cycle through the Delivery Processes as follows:

1. We start with the Activity Selection Process. After taking care of the administrative requirements, its job is to select the next task (or item) from

---

[3] Phonetic transcription is mapping from the sounds a language uses to construct words to a unique strings of symbols. Pronunciation guides in dictionaries provide familiar examples; for example, one phonetic transcription of "river" is 'ri-v&r.

the Task/Evidence Composite Library. In doing this, it may examine the values of certain task model variables, for example, to ensure breadth of content or prevent task overlap. In an adaptive assessment, it also consults the current estimate of the student's overall proficiency to select a task that is particularly informative in light of what we know about the participant's preceding responses.

2.   When the Activity Selection Process has selected a task, it sends an instruction to the Presentation Process. The Presentation Process uses the task model to determine what Presentation Material is expected for this task and what Work products will be produced (in this case, a string giving the short response). It might also consult with task model Variables to set options for the presentation of the task (e.g., use of different screen resolutions).

3.   The participant interacts with the Presentation Process to produce some kind of response, which in this case is just the character string. This is stored in a Work product, which is sent to the Response Scoring Process to start the scoring process.

4.   The Response Scoring Process looks at the Evidence Rule Data to ascertain the "key," or correct answer, for this item. It then checks the Work product against this data using the Evidence Rules to set the observables to appropriate values. Since the correct response is a targeted string of Roman characters that represents a phonetic stream, the assessment designer has a choice to make at this point in response scoring: Either an exact match can be demanded, or a match to one of the close acceptable alternatives in a library, or a match based on an algorithm of closeness to the target. Judgments such as this must be evaluated in light of the intent of measurement and whether exact matching is important for the student to achieve? However resolved, only the final evaluation of the observable "IsCorrect" is relevant for operation with the Overall Proficiency student model.

5.   The Summary Scoring Process takes the observable and uses it to update the Scoring Record. For the Overall Proficiency schema, the student model contains only a single variable, the IRT student proficiency parameter θ. The Weights of Evidence in this case are the IRT item parameters; for example, difficulty, discrimination, and guessing under the three-parameter logistic model. Evidence Accumulation is accomplished through successive products of the likelihood functions induced by each item response; from a

Bayesian perspective, successive updating of the probability distribution that reflects current belief about the participant's θ.

6. The Activity Selection Process can now select the next task, or decide to stop. In making this decision, it can use the updated distribution for θ, either to select an item likely to be particularly informative about the participant in light of what is known thus far, or to terminate testing because a predetermined level of accuracy has been achieved.

For this testing purpose, we can use mostly off-the-shelf components. The Activity Selection Process can be an adaptive item selection algorithm or a linear one. The Summary Scoring Process is just the standard IRT scoring process. The Presentation Process could be a standard computer-based client interface with a few customizations (e.g., support for Chinese fonts). One big difference from most current delivery architectures is that we have separated the first scoring step (Response Processing) from presentation of the task (Steps 3 and 4). This may not seem consequential because this example Step 4 is so simple: Just compare a string to a target. However, doing this gives us quite a bit of flexibility to use the tasks for other purposes where a more sophisticated Response Scoring Process, with multiple observables being evaluated, would be required.

Separating the stages has some important implications for modularity. None of these processes needs to be computer-based; some or all could be manual processes. We are free to implement the four processes in a way that best meets the needs of a particular assessment. We could obtain a spoken rather than written Work product, for example, from similarly constructed tasks and use them to evaluate spoken Chinese and character recognition jointly. In that case, we could use a pronunciation scoring process based on human raters or one based on computer speech recognition, without affecting the other processes within the system. Alternatively, we could swap out an English language-based presentation process and replace it with one in which directions were localized for a different region. Distinguishing the separate pieces conceptually maximizes the potential for reuse even if we ultimately decide to implement them in the same (human or computer) process.

A Drill-and-Practice Tutoring System

To illustrate how components can be reused, we will look at a delivery system specialized for a drill-and-practice tutoring system (Fig. 2.6). The design for a drill-and practice example poses different requirements than for the preceding high-stakes example. Now we need to be able to deliver across-task feedback on multiple aspects of proficiency, as well as task-specific diagnostic feedback. Because task-specific feedback is called for in addition to scoring, responses

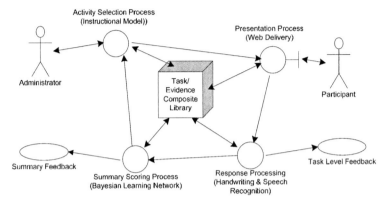

FIG. 2.6. The Assessment Cycle specialized for a tutoring system. The new processes enable diagnostic task-based feedback and accumulation of evidence about multiple skills to support more targeted and informative summary feedback.

will be evaluated diagnostically in addition to being scored as either correct or incorrect. The quality and timing of this feedback is of central importance. For the purpose of supporting learning directly, it makes sense to provide various kinds of help as part of the task performance environment.

Furthermore, the participant benefits from being able to choose which tasks to do in what sequence. Although the collection of tasks available to a participant needs to reflect a full range of content and difficulty, comparability among participants with respect to tasks across participants is not essential.

Again, working through the design process, we identify the salient claims, evidence, and tasks for our purpose and blend these requirements with the constraints described above. The result is a set of models that represents the specifications for this assessment.

- What we want to measure is represented by a student model for Diagnosis. This model is based on some defined set of common speaking and listening skills (e.g., discrimination among tones, recognition of initial and terminal phonetic units, stroke order, recognition of common radical and phonetic components of a character), each of which is represented by a student model variable. We can then accumulate evidence about each of these skills across tasks and report targeted feedback on specific problems the participant exhibits. We can also use this information to assign more tasks that draw on the knowledge and skills with which the participant seems to be having the most trouble. This kind of feedback could be delivered on request as the participant works through the assessment, or it could be delivered at the end of the assessment.

- Evidence to support inferences related to diagnosis is provided by tasks generated from task models designed to fulfill evidentiary requirements for diagnosis. We can reuse the Phonetic Transcription task model as is. We can use a Character Identification task model if we include design specifications for possible responses that reflect the variety of error patterns of interest. For a Reading task we can reuse our Phonetic Transcription task model, but this time request the participant to pronounce the character(s) aloud. The Work product changes, therefore, to be a speech sample. For the Writing task model, we can use the Character Identification task model, but this time request the participant to draw the character. The Work product changes, therefore, to be a picture of a character.

- For this example, we could choose to use support-related variables in our task models to author tasks that give the participant a prompt or help in the form of a phonetic pronunciation guide for the character, or allow the participant to request such help.

- Evidence models appropriate to these student and task models entail evaluation of Work products for identification of specific varieties of problems as well as for correct/incorrect. For the former, specifications for answer keys (evidence rule data) reflect requirements for diagnosis. Each observable will update one or more Diagnosis student model variables. Either human or automated scoring methods could be used, and, in principle, humans could be used for some and automated methods for others. In any case, exactly which features of a response are significant and how they are evaluated should be driven by the nature of the targeted knowledge and skill. This is an example in which automated methods are used to extract basic features of Work products, humans are used to score a pretest sample of performances to provide a criterion evaluation, and an empirical model such as regression or neural networks is used to best approximate human scores in categories of interest.

We cycle through the Delivery Processes as follows:

1. We again begin with the Activity Selection Process. After administrative startup, it selects a task based on the current state of the examinee's student-model variables.

2. The Activity Selection Process sends an instruction to the Presentation Process to start a particular task.

3. The Presentation Process fetches the presentation material from the Task/Evidence Composite Library. It presents it to the participant, either by showing a picture or playing a sound. When the participant finishes, the Presentation Process bundles the response into a Work product and sends it to the Response Scoring Process. For our

four kinds of tasks, the Work products will consist of sound clips, pictures, character strings, and logical identifiers.

4.   The Response Scoring Process for the Reading and Writing tasks requires either human raters or speech and handwriting recognition software. The Response Scoring Process needs to do more work for the student model for Diagnosis than for the Overall Proficiency student model. A single observable with values "right" and "wrong" is no longer sufficient. If the participant is wrong, we want to know what kind of mistake was made: tone confusion, phoneme confusion, mistaking one character with a common radical for another, and so on. The Response Scoring Process for Phonetic Transcription and Character Identification tasks can continue to use key matching algorithms, but these algorithms must set observables to values representing different diagnostic outcomes. In our Lesson Group version, tasks must be scored both as "Correct/Incorrect" and for diagnosis.

5.   The Summary Scoring Process must be more sophisticated as well. Not only must it determine *how much* our beliefs about the participant's abilities should change as a result of our observations, but it must also indicate *which ones* of the variables in the Scoring Record are affected. With the Lesson Group model, this is straightforward: Each task belongs to a Lesson Group, and we assume limited interaction among the groups. However, for the Diagnostic model, the presence of the knowledge, skills, and abilities we are trying to measure is often highly correlated (as is our knowledge about them). Therefore, we use an approach based on multivariate graphical models, a generalization of more familiar psychometric models, for this step (Almond & Mislevy, 1999; Mislevy & Gitomer, 1996).

6.   Finally, the Activity Selection Process would choose the next activity. Selection based on the Diagnostic model would select tasks to focus on identified trouble areas, and would have rules for how and when to shift focus on the basis of the evolving state of knowledge about the values of this examinee's student-model variables.

Although straightforward, this example raises a number of interesting issues for design, scoring, and reporting.

Multimedia.   We need to allow for both audio and pictures as both input and output of tasks. We must choose from among a plethora of potentially useful formats and fonts. Our task model must make it clear to the Presentation Process, Activity Selection Process, and the Response Scoring Process what is expected.

Representational Issues.   Even more basic is our choice for how we represent a character drawing. We could use a static picture (e.g., a bitmap or compressed bitmap format) or describe the character by the series of strokes used to draw it. The former is easier to work with, but the latter is more closely aligned with the principles of Chinese calligraphy. Here we encounter a trade-off between convenience and the quality of evidence of knowledge about certain aspects of writing. Note that the form in which the response is captured as a Work product can have serious implications for automated response scoring, for it determines the nature of the input that will be available to work with.

Input Method. There are several possibilities for inputting characters. These including drawing with a mouse, using a graphics tablet or light pen, or drawing with brush on paper and scanning the result into the computer.

Response Scoring Method. Depending on the optimal granularity of the feedback, we may choose to explore character recognition programs that require the stroke-based representation of the character.

Localization. For use in China, we would like the instructions to be in Chinese. For use in another country, we may want the instructions to be in the language used there.

Reusability. Although we limit this example to teaching reading and writing directly in Chinese, it is easy see how we could extend this tutoring system to include translation tasks. We can also see how we might want to embed tasks of this sort in a high stakes exam that offers placement out of a college course. Standards for interoperability would allow a vendor of such placement exams to purchase and easily incorporate a special purpose Presentation Process for these tasks from a software company whose primary business was making software to support Chinese, Japanese and Korean languages.

CONCLUSION

Automated scoring is an exciting development in the world of assessment. It makes practicable and affordable a wider range of task types, response modes, and student-assessment interactions. Each new technique, however, arrives with its own history, its own terminology, its own protocols and formats—and without a clear understanding of just how the benefits it offers fit in to an assessment system. To capitalize on the potential of automated scoring, it will be of significant benefit to have a shared framework for talking about the roles automated scoring can play in the support of a coherent assessment argument. The framework of evidence-centered design provides such a framework, and can thus prove useful for understanding how automated scoring techniques fit into assessment systems and how to disambiguate issues of assessment design from issues of automated scoring system algorithms.

REFERENCES

Almond, R. G., & Mislevy, R. J. (1999). Graphical models and computerized adaptive testing. *Applied Psychological Measurement, 23*, 223–237.

Almond, R. G., Steinberg, L. S., & Mislevy, R. J. (2002). A four-process architecture for assessment delivery, with connections to assessment design. *Journal of Technology, Learning, and Assessment, 1*(5). Retrieved from: http://www.bc.edu/research/intasc/jtla/journal/v1n5.shtml

Cronbach, L. J. (1989). Construct validation after thirty years. In R. L. Linn (Ed.), *Intelligence: Measurement, theory, and public policy* (pp. 147–171). Urbana, IL: University of Illinois Press.

Embretson, S. (1983). Construct validity: Construct representation versus nomothetic span. *Psychological Bulletin, 93*, 179–197.

Kane, M. T. (1992) An argument-based approach to validity. *Psychological Bulletin*, 112, 527–535.

Messick, S. (1989). Validity. In R.L. Linn (Ed.), *Educational measurement (3rd Ed.)* (pp. 13–103). New York: American Council on Education/Macmillan.

Messick, S. (1994). The interplay of evidence and consequences in the validation of performance assessments. *Educational Researcher, 23*(2), 13–23.

Mislevy, R. J., & Gitomer, D. H. (1996). The role of probability-based inference in an intelligent tutoring system. *User-Modeling and User-Adapted Interaction, 5*, 253–282.

Mislevy, R. J., Sheehan, K. M., & Wingersky, M. S. (1993). How to equate tests with little or no data. *Journal of Educational Measurement, 30*, 55–78.

Mislevy, R. J., Steinberg, L. S., & Almond, R. G. (2003). On the structure of educational assessments. *Measurement: Interdisciplinary Research and Perspectives, 1*, 3–67.

Schum, D. A. (1989). Knowledge, probability, and credibility. *Journal of Behavioral Decision Making, 2*, 39–62.

Wigmore, J. H. (1937). *The science of judicial proof* (3rd ed.). Boston: Little, Brown, & Co.

A GLOSSARY OF EVIDENCE-CENTERED DESIGN TERMS

Activity Selection Process. The Activity Selection Process is the part of the Assessment Cycle that selects a task or other activity for presentation to an examinee.

Administrator. The Administrator is the person responsible for setting up and maintaining the assessment. The Administrator is responsible for starting the process and configuring various choices; for example, whether or not item level feedback will be displayed during the assessment.

Assembly Model. The assembly model, one of a collection of six different types of models that comprise the Conceptual Assessment Framework (CAF), provides the information required to control the selection of tasks for the creation of an assessment.

Assessment. An Assessment is a system (computer, manual, or some combination of the these) that presents examinees, or participants, with work and evaluates the results. This includes high-stakes examinations, diagnostic tests, and coached-practice systems, which include embedded assessment.

Assessment Cycle. The Assessment Cycle is comprised of four basic processes: Activity Selection, Presentation, Response Processing, and Summary Scoring. The Activity Selection Process selects a task or other activity for presentation to an examinee. The Presentation Process displays the task to the examinee and captures the results (or Work products) when the examinee performs the task. The Response Scoring Process identifies the essential features of the response and records these as a series of Observations. The Summary Scoring Process updates the scoring based on the input it receives from the Response Scoring Process. This four-process architecture can work in either synchronous or asynchronous mode.

Claims. Claims are statements about what a student knows or can do, how well, in what circumstances. They are the hypotheses that assessments are meant to support. Tasks and student model variables should be designed so that the student model variables accumulate evidence from task performances, and functions of the final distribution over the student model variables indicate the degree of support for the claims of interest.

Conceptual Assessment Framework (CAF). The Conceptual Assessment Framework builds specific models for use in a particular assessment product (taking into account the specific purposes and requirements of that product). The conceptual assessment framework consists of a collection of six different types of models that define what objects are needed and how an assessment will function for a particular purpose. The models of the CAF are as follows: the Student Model, the Task Model, the Evidence Model, the Assembly Model, the Presentation Model, and the Delivery System Model.

Delivery System Model. The delivery system model, one of a collection of six different types of models that comprise the Conceptual Assessment Framework (CAF), describes which other models will be used, as well as other properties of the assessment that span all four processes, such as platform and security requirements.

Domain Analysis. Domain analysis is the process of marshalling information about the domain of interest, and organizing it in ways that will help inform the design of an assessment. This includes such matters as knowledge that is valued in the domain, features of good performance, situations in which proficiency can be exhibited, and relationships between knowledge and performance.

Domain Model. Domain modeling concerns structuring information about the domain in terms of an evidentiary argument, at a substantive level. This differs from the CAF, which is more akin to specifications for the operational elements and processes used in the actual operation of an assessment.

Evaluation Rules. Evaluation Rules are a type of Evidence Rules that set the values of Observable variables.

Evidence. In educational assessment, Evidence is information or observations that allow inferences to be made about aspects of an examinee's proficiency (which are unobservable) from evaluations of observable behaviors in given performance situations.

Evidence-Centered Design (ECD). Evidence-Centered Design (ECD) is a methodology for designing assessments that underscores the central role of evidentiary reasoning in assessment design. ECD is based on three premises: (1) An assessment must build around the important knowledge in the domain of interest, and an understanding of how that knowledge is acquired and put to use; (2) the chain of reasoning from what participants say and do in assessments to inferences about what they know, can do, or should do next, must be based on the principles of evidentiary reasoning; (3) purpose must be the driving force behind design decisions, which reflect constraints, resources, and conditions of use.

Evidence Model. The evidence model is a set of instructions for interpreting the output of a specific task. It is the bridge between the task model, which describes the task, and the student model, which describes the framework for expressing what is known about the examinee's state of knowledge. The evidence model generally has two parts: (1) A series of Evidence Rules that describe how to identify and characterize essential features of the work product; and (2) a Statistical model that tells how the scoring should be updated given the observed features of the response.

Evidence Rules. Evidence Rules are the rubrics, algorithms, assignment functions, or other methods for evaluating the response (Work product). They specify how values are assigned to Observable variables, and thereby identify those pieces of evidence that can be gleaned from a given response (Work product).

Evidence Rule Data. Evidence Rule Data is data found within the Response Scoring Process. It often takes the form of logical rules.

Examinee. See *Participant*.

Examinee Record. The Examinee Record is a record of tasks to which the participant is exposed, as well as the participant's Work products, Observables, and Scoring Record.

Four Processes. Any assessment must have four different logical processes. The four processes that comprise the Assessment Cycle include the following: (1) The Activity Selection Process: the system responsible for selecting a task from the task library; (2) The Presentation Process: the process responsible for presenting the task to the examinee; (3) The Response Scoring Process: the first step in the scoring process, which identifies the essential features of the response that provide evidence about the examinee's current knowledge, skills, and abilities; (4) The Summary Score Process: the second stage in the scoring process, which updates beliefs about the examinee's knowledge, skills, and abilities based on the evidence provided by the preceding process.

Instructions. Instructions are commands sent by the Activity Selection Process to the Presentation Process.

Measurement Model. The measurement model is that part of the evidence model that explains how the scoring should be updated given the observed features of the response.

Model. A model is a design object in the CAF that provides requirements for one or more of the Four Processes, particularly for the data structures used by those processes (e.g., tasks and Scoring Records). A model describes variables, that appear in data structures used by the Four Processes, whose values are set in the course of authoring the tasks or running the assessment.

Observables / Observable variables. Observables are variables that are produced through the application of Evidence Rules to the task work product. Observables describe characteristics to be evaluated in the work product and/or may represent aggregations of other observables.

Observation. An observation is a specific value for an observable variable for a particular participant.

Parsing Rules. Parsing Rules are a type of Evidence Rules that re-express the work product into a more "convenient" form, where convenient is interpreted to mean the form of the work product required by the Evaluation Rules.

Participant. A participant is the person whose skills are being assessed. A participant directly engages with the assessment for any of a variety of purposes (e.g., certification, tutoring, selection, drill and practice, etc.).

Platform. Platform refers to method that will be used to deliver the presentation materials to the examinees. Platform is defined broadly to include human, computer, paper and pencil, etc.

Presentation Material. Presentation Material is material that is presented to a participant as part of a task (including stimulus, rubric, prompt, possible options for multiple-choice).

Presentation Process. The Presentation Process is the part of the Assessment Cycle that displays the task to the examinee and captures the results (or work products) when the examinee performs the task.

Presentation Material Specification. Presentation Material Specifications are a collection of specifications that describe material that will be presented to the examinee as part of a stimulus, prompt, or instructional program.

Purpose Definition. Assessment is always meant to gather evidence to address some inference, prediction, explanation, diagnosis, instructional guidance, or research issue. Knowing the intended purpose of an assessment is necessary for guiding design decisions, which all impact the amount and kind of evidence they provide for different purposes.

Reporting Rules. Reporting Rules describe how student model variables should be combined or sampled to produce scores, and how those scores should be interpreted.

Response. See *Work Product*.

Response Scoring Process. The Response Scoring Process (which does Response Scoring) is the part of the Assessment Cycle that identifies the essential features of the examinee's response and records these as a series of Observations. At one time referred to as the "Evidence Identification Process," it emphasizes the key observations in the work product that provide evidence.

Response Processing Data. See *Evidence Rule Data*.

Score Reporting. Score reports are summaries of participants' performance that are provided to the user of the assessment information, ideally in terms which are meaningful to that user. Scores are functions of the probability distributions that express knowledge about student model variables. They may take the form of numerical summaries, verbal statement of claims, instructional recommendations, and so on.

Strategy. Strategy refers to the overall method that will be used to select tasks in the assembly model.

Student Model. The student model is a collection of variables representing knowledge, skills, and abilities of an examinee about which inferences will be made. A student model is comprised of the following types of information: (1) student model variables that correspond to aspects of proficiency the assessment is meant to measure; (2) model type that describes the mathematical form of the student model (e.g., univariate IRT, multivariate IRT, or discrete Bayesian Network); (3) Reporting Rules that explain how the student model variables should be combined or sampled to produce scores.

Student Model Variables. Task model variables describe features of the participant that concern knowledge, skills, abilities, propensities toward behavior of certain kinds in certain situations, or other characteristics that are not directly observable. They are the terms in which evidence from participants' performances are synthesized. A student model variable can have a discrete or continuous range. At a given point in time, the assessor's knowledge about the value of a participant's student model variable is expressed as a probability distribution over its range.

Summary Scoring Process. The Summary Scoring Process is the part of the Assessment Cycle that updates the scoring based on the input it receives from Response Scoring Process. At one time referred to as the "Evidence Accumulation Process," the Summary Scoring Process plays an important role in accumulating evidence.

Task. A task is a unit of work requested from an examinee during the course of an assessment. In ECD, a task is a specific instance of a task model.

Task/Evidence Composite Library. The Task/Evidence Composite Library is a database of task objects along with all the information necessary to select and score them. For each such Task/Evidence Composite, the library stores (1) descriptive properties that are used to ensure content coverage and prevent overlap among tasks; (2) specific values of, or references to, Presentation Material and other environmental parameters that are used for delivering the task; (3) specific data that are used to extract the salient characteristics of work products; and (4) Weights of Evidence that are used to update the scoring from performances on this task, specifically, scoring weights, conditional probabilities, or parameters in a psychometric model.

Task Model. A task model is a generic description of a family of tasks that contains (1) a list of variables that are used to describe key features of the tasks, (2) a collection of presentation material specifications that describe material that will be presented to the examinee as part of a stimulus, prompt, or instructional program, and (3) a collection of work product specifications that describe the material that the task will be return to the scoring process.

Task Model Variables. Task model variables describe features of the task that are important for designing, calibrating, selecting, executing, and scoring it. These variables describe features of the task that are important descriptors of the task itself, such as substance, interactivity, size, and complexity, or are descriptors of the task performance environment, such as tools, help, and scaffolding.

Weights of Evidence. Weights of Evidence are parameters that provide information about the size and direction of the contribution an Observable variable makes in updating beliefs about the state of its student model parent(s). The Weights of Evidence provide a way of predicting the performance of an examinee with a given state of the student model variables on a given task. Examples are scoring weights in number-right scoring and item parameters in item response theory models.

Work Product. A work product is the examinee's response a task from a given task model. This could be expressed as a transcript of examinee actions, an artifact created by the examinee and/or other appropriate information. The work product provides an important bridge between the task model and the evidence model. In particular, work products are the input to the Evidence Rules.

3

Human Scoring

Isaac I. Bejar
David M. Williamson
Educational Testing Service

Robert J. Mislevy
University of Maryland

> *The statistical analysis was thought to provide the floor to which the judgment of the experienced clinician could be compared. The floor turned out to be the ceiling.*—Dawes and Corrigan (1974, p. 97)

The formal evaluation of complex performances by expert judges is the most ubiquitous of scoring methods for constructed response tasks. This chapter discusses a range of issues related to evidence identification by means of judges or graders, in other words, human scoring. A chapter on human scoring may seem out of place in a volume taking an evidentiary perspective on *automated* scoring. However, it is naïve to believe that automated scoring can be developed, understood, and deployed in the absence of the contributions of expert human graders. An understanding of the process and outcomes of human scoring is a necessary precondition to meeting the goals of automated scoring systems. In terms of Evidence-Centered Design (ECD), an understanding of human scoring is critical to the development of both the *evidence identification* and the *evidence accumulation* capabilities of automated scoring.

The distinction between evidence identification and evidence accumulation was introduced in chapter 2. Evidence identification is the collection of processes that result in one or more scores from the evaluation of the work product(s) an examinee produces for a single task. Such scores across one or more tasks, in turn, are passed to the evidence accumulation process that uses these values to update the values of student model variables. This distinction between evidence identification and evidence accumulation from the evidence in work products helps to clarify the typical role of graders in assessments that involve constructed responses. Specifically, graders fill the role in which they are most adept at, evidence identification. The scores they produce for a given work product are then typically submitted to a statistical evidence accumulation process, often simple summations, but possibly more advanced treatment. For example, scores obtained by human scoring can be treated as categorical responses that can in turn be analyzed by IRT models to obtain a score based on a set of work products (see Wainer, Brown, Bradlow, Wang, Skorupski, Boulet, & Mislevy, Chap. 6 this volume).

The evaluation of automated methods requires an understanding of the elements that graders attend to when scoring or evaluating essays. Specifically, human scores can serve to evaluate the outcomes of automated scoring (Williamson, Bejar, & Hone, 1999; Williamson, Bejar, & Hone, 2004). Insight into the strengths and limitations of human scoring helps inform an understanding of the strengths and limitations of automated scoring, ultimately resulting in better scoring processes, whether they be completely human, completely automated, or a strategic mixture combining human and automated scoring into some optimal hybrid. The improved understanding of the human scoring processes from an evidentiary perspective is the focus of this chapter. We first present a brief contrast of major aspects of human and automated scoring, as a precursor to understanding the role of human scoring in the validity argument for an assessment. We then review relevant literature from psychological research on judgment, and extract some conclusions relevant to the contrast between human and automated scoring. Recent research and considerations in the context of educational scoring per se are discussed next bringing a cognitive perspective on the grading process into the discussion. This is followed in turn by a discussion of recent extensions of psychometric models to address issues of human scoring. The chapter continues with an empirical study of rater cognition and concludes with a summary and discussion of human scoring as a means of evidence identification.

CONSTRUCT REPRESENTATION AND PRAGMATICS IN HUMAN VERSUS AUTOMATED SCORING

An obvious difference between human and automated scoring is the explicitness, and therefore tractability, of the scoring (evidence identification) instructions. Instructions for human scoring, as part of large-scale assessments, consist of a set of guidelines called a "scoring rubric". Despite training intended to minimize the individual variation in application of this rubric it is likely that each human grader implements the rubric in a slightly different way. (For a readily available tutorial on rubric construction, see Mertler, 2001.) By contrast, automated scoring lacks the interpretive powers of the human scorer. The evidence identification process is far more explicit so that an autonomous automated process can implement it. The implications of this requirement for explicit and concrete evidence rules underlie several other contrasts between automated and human scoring.

An important issue in human scoring is the variability in scoring between raters using identical criteria. In human scoring, this is typically assessed through estimates of inter-rater reliability between similarly qualified and trained human graders on the same work products. This is one of the primary concerns of the human scoring process. The issue has long been recognized, as exemplified by Edgeworth (1888, as cited by Mariano, 2002):

> ... let a number of equally competent critics independently assign a mark to the (work). ... even supposing that the examiners have agreed beforehand as to ... the scale of excellence to be adopted ... there will occur a certain divergence between the verdicts of competent examiners. (p. 2)

That is, a key issue in human scoring is the consistency of interpretation and execution of the scale of excellence or scoring rubric, whereas for automated scoring, the interpretation and execution of a scoring rubric are always identical and replicable. By contrast, for automated scoring a significant issue is whether it is even possible for an automated and computational procedure to identify and extract from a work product the evidence required by the assessment. Because the outcome of evidence identification ultimately finds its way to the student model through the evidence accumulation process, the choice between automated and human scoring could have important implications for the validity of inferences based on test scores. That is, the choice between automated and human scoring in assessment design can have implications for the degree of control that the assessment designers can exert over the *construct representation.*

The term construct representation was introduced by Embretson (1983) to make explicit the distinction between two aspects of validation: *construct representation* and *nomothetic span.* Nomothetic span documents the relationship between scores from a given measure and other construct-relevant measures. This includes much of what we think of as evidential validation, using Messick's (1989) distinction between consequential and evidential validity. Whereas nomothetic span addresses the *external* relationships with other measures and constructs, construct representation addresses the *internal* composition of a measure.

A simple example illustrates the implications of choice of scoring method, either automated or human, on control over construct representation. An assessment of writing ability could address a student model for which spelling proficiency is not an important part of the targeted ability. Human graders might find it difficult to ignore spelling errors, potentially affecting their judgment in scoring. By contrast, an automated scoring system could track spelling errors and either include or exclude these observations during evidence identification, as specified by the assessment design. Thus, automated methods would not only apply a scoring rubric consistently but also enable the assessment designer to more precisely control the meaning of scores (see Powers, Burstein, Chodorow, Fowles, & Kukich, 2002).

The added control over construct representation is possible because of the higher degree of attention to what constitutes evidence and how to capture it. However, in practice, it is an empirical question whether such advantages materialize for any given assessment. For example, the PhonePass system (Bernstein, 2002) is an automated method for assessing certain aspects of speaking proficiency. It does this, however, by means of tasks where the student reads sentences aloud. Responses are scored automatically by means of speech recognition technology. The nomothetic range of the resulting score is impressive (e.g., Jong & Bernstein, 2001), but in an assessment aiming to characterize the communicative competence of test takers (e.g., Butler, Eignor, Jones, McNamara, & Suomi, 2000) it would be fair to say that the construct representation of PhonePass scores is limited. It is not hard to imagine someone performing adequately on a read-aloud task and yet not be able to maintain a conversation, as might be expected of someone who has achieved communicative competence.

In general, construct representation can be shortchanged rather than enhanced by an automated scoring procedure if in the interest of automated scoring the tasks do not elicit the full range of evidence called for by an appropriately broad definition of the construct of interest. Similarly, however, the construct representation of human scores can also be shortchanged by the conditions at a grading session. For example, the volume of responses that needs to be scored can be so large that graders need to operate at a pace that precludes them from exercising their unique capacities to evaluate work products or to accommodate less common responses. According to Cumming, Kantor, and Powers (2002):

> ... a principal criticism has been that the exact nature of the constructs they [raters] assess remains uncertain. For instance, holistic rating scales can conflate many of the complex traits and variables that human judges of students' written compositions perceive (such as fine points of discourse coherence, grammar, lexical usage, or presentation of ideas) into a few simple scale points, rendering the meaning or significance of the judges' assessments in a form that many feel is either superficial or difficult to interpret ...
> (p. 68)

To the extent that an automated scoring system relies solely on such data to build the automated procedure, the construct representation of the resulting scores would be similarly impaired.

In short, from a pragmatic point of view a key goal in any assessment is to maximize construct representation at the least cost. Human scoring might be the way to achieve that goal under some circumstances, but not in others. With these contrasts in mind, we next review the literature on human judgment and human scoring in the context of large-scale educational assessment, which in turn has motivated research on rater cognition. We then present the results of a study of rater cognition that draws significantly from the expert judgment literature as well as the cognitive literature. We draw conclusions about the human scoring from an evidentiary perspective and consider the implications for automated scoring.

EXPERT JUDGMENT

The process of human scoring can be viewed as a form of expert judgment. The literature includes a long standing and particularly relevant debate about whether automated ("statistical") methods of classification based on multiple observations of complex behavior can outperform classifications from the same data by human experts. Much of this work has been inspired by Meehl's (1954) classic book *Clinical Versus Statistical Prediction: A Theoretical Analysis and a Review of the Evidence.* Perhaps the best-known and most frequently cited result from this effort is the finding that a common statistical procedure can often outperform the judgment of expert human practitioners. Specifically, Meehl's literature review found that a simple linear statistical model was more accurate than human experts in predicting outcomes as diverse as parole violations, responses to psychotherapy, and academic success. This work has not only influenced the development of automated scoring efforts, but has also stimulated much work in the field of psychology on the nature of expert judgment. The still-relevant results from a period of intense activity are well presented in Wiggins (1973). Camerer and Johnson (1991) also offered insightful analyses of what underlies the "process-performance paradox in expert judgment".

In a study inspired by the clinical versus statistical prediction debate, Kleinmunz (1963) reported on an attempt to simulate the judgment of expert clinicians using an automated rule-based system. The study asked 10 clinicians to independently classify undergraduate students as "adjusted" or "maladjusted" on the basis of scale scores from a clinical diagnostic assessment called the

Minnesota Multiphasic Personality Inventory, or MMPI (see e.g. Butcher & Rouse, 1996). Measures of the accuracy of these clinician evaluations were determined by comparing their classification with independent criterion classifications derived using multiple methods. The clinician who had the highest agreement between his own classification and the criterion classification was chosen to be the subject of modeling for the logic of the rule-based system. Talk-aloud protocols were used to elicit his reasoning process as he examined additional MMPI profiles. From these, verbalizations on the rationale behind his classifications rules were developed that represented the logic of the clinician's rational evaluation. These logical rules were then implemented as an algorithm in a computer program designed to conduct similar judgments. The resulting algorithm was then applied to a database of 126 cases, and found to outperform the clinician in classifying profiles. Thus, one of the interesting findings of the study was that when an expert's own evaluation logic is used as the basis of an automated judgment system, the system can outperform the very clinician that provided the logic for the evaluation rules!

This finding prompts the question central to all efforts to develop automated scoring or prediction systems: what is it about human judgment that causes it to be both the heart of any automated scoring method and its Achilles' heel? Camerer and Johnson (1991) offered several possibilities that are especially relevant in a clinical setting, such as the tendency of experts to use highly configural rules that, although intuitively appealing, have limited generalizability. Shortly after Meehl published his first work showing the superiority of statistical over clinical prediction, Hammond (1955) published a study of clinical prediction inspired by Brunswick's (1955) Lens Model.

Brunswick's model, as adapted for judgment analysis, is useful in explicitly identifying all the elements of the judgment process and helpful for understanding its fallibility. The Lens Model captures several important aspects of a judgment situation, as represented in Fig. 3.1, adapted from Cooksey (1996, Fig. 1.3). This figure depicts several key concepts. The object about which a judgment is made is called the *stimulus* and can be characterized in terms of a set of *features* that in general are not independent of each other. The right side of the figure depicts the judgment process as consisting of integrating all or a subset of the features into a judgment. The left side of the figure depicts an idealized or "true" integration of all the features into a *criterion*. The

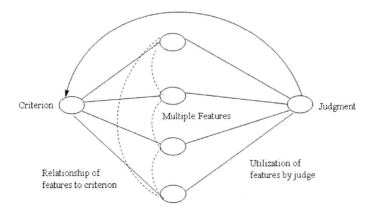

FIG. 3.1. Adaptation of Lens Model to the study of human judgment (adapted from Cooksey, 1996, Fig. 1.3).

performance of the judge is evaluated by the relationship of the judgment to the criterion.

By distinguishing the criterion and the judgment sides, the Lens Model offers a potential explanation of the performance of judges. To maximize the relationship of the judgment to the criterion all features need to be utilized by the judge and weighed in the same manner as they are used for arriving at the criterion. A judge, for a variety of ecological and psychological reasons may not do this and as a result his judgment would not coincide with the criterion. The criterion, for example, might consist of scores arrived at by a deliberate process where all the features are systematically considered and discussed before arriving at the score. By contrast, under a grading situation where a certain level of productivity is expected from judges, time is of the essence and judges might not be as systematic in considering all the different attributes of a response before arriving at a judgment. Moreover, some judges may be more or less sensitive to some of the attributes of the response, which could lead to differences among judges in how highly they score the same responses.

The model can be adapted to cover a range of situations of interest. A distinction is made (Cooksey, 1996) between single-, double-, triple-, and n-systems. The single-system study omits the criterion side. This means the model is usable for the case where the interest is in how a judge integrates the features of a situation to arrive at a judgment. A well-known case of this method is policy capturing. The term *policy capturing* has been used in the past in connection with judgment analysis and even scoring. The term originates in work at Lackland Air Base by Bottenberg and Christal (1961; For some historical notes on this work see notes at http://www.albany.edu/cpr/brunswik/notes/japc.html). The intention of this procedure is to develop a mathematical model (typically linear regression) that would best predict a given judge's policy. The method has been applied recently (Elander & Hardman, 2002) to the scoring of "psychology examinations" by first having graders rate qualitative aspects of responses and then by obtaining a score for each response. The results were not especially informative by their own admission, but the study does illustrate the potential use of policy capturing in scoring in an educational context.

Policy capturing is explicitly an *idiographic* as opposed to a *nomothetic* model. The idiographic–nomothetic distinction was imported into American psychology from German psychology to distinguish models or theories, or analysis of data, meant to apply to individuals or collectives. Several personality theories from the last century, including Gordon Allport's (1937) and George Kelly's (1955), were distinctly idiographic. For example, Kelly's main analytical tool was the Repertory Grid, which can best be described as a form of within-person factor analysis in which the factors extracted from the analysis were unique to the individual not just in terms of dimensionality, but also in terms of their composition because the variables that entered into the analysis were themselves unique to the individual. Kelly interpreted the resulting factors as the filters through which an individual views the world. For clinical purposes, such factors provide a glimpse into the mind of the patient but in a more general context that can provide a set of variables to model an individual's behavior. In particular, such variables could be used to model judgment or rating behavior, as we shall see in a later section. Kelly's theory and methods have found acceptance in cognitive psychology as a method of knowledge elicitation and representation (e.g., Gaines & Shaw, 1993). Moreover, Ford, Bradshaw, Adams-Webber, and Agnew (1993) presented it as a relevant theory for modeling experts in general and specially suited to eliciting their "knowledge," which in the case of graders corresponds to evidence identification expertise. We use the essence of Kelly's elicitation method as part of a study of rater cognition.

To summarize, the literature we have reviewed is useful in introducing the contrast between statistical (or automated) and human scoring in combining information across multiple features of stimuli, and in showing the persistent superiority of the former in predicting criteria. The literature suggests that the criteria experts employ can be modeled algorithmically. From the point of view of construct representation, this means that it is possible to build into an automated scoring procedure the essence of an expert's judging criteria. The evidence shows, however, as illustrated by Kleinmunz (1963) that the clinician may not be the best implementer of an algorithm suggested by his or her own judging behavior. The literature reviewed in this section is equally useful in providing a scientific approach to understanding the judgment process. Potentially, a similar decomposition is useful for the analysis of human scoring in educational contexts. However, Brunswick's model is not a cognitive model in the sense that the mental processes the judge might use to detect and integrate the evidence, that is, the attributes of the object being judged, are not the focus of the theory. In particular, under the Brunswick model, it is not up to the judge to define what constitutes the evidence. In that sense the Brunswick model is of interest primarily for historical and utilitarian reasons. We discuss next cognitively oriented models that emerge from an explicit attempt to understand rating processes, or evidence identification, based on human judgment.

THE EDUCATIONAL ASSESSMENT CONTEXT.

The expert judgment literature provides a number of valuable ideas for studying human scoring by decomposing the judgment task into attributes of the object being rated, and articulating the relationship of those attributes to both the judgment and the overall characteristics of the object being judged. However, the literature is distant from the context in which human scoring occurs most frequently, namely as part of large-scale assessment. In that context, typically, a large number of raters are involved in carrying out the grading. There is a social hierarchy whereby the most senior graders control the process. In addition, a set of more experienced readers are designated as table coordinators, who supervise the raters. Prior to the actual grading, table coordinators, senior graders, and program staff meet to develop or adjust the scoring rubrics associated with each question. In addition, exemplars of responses at each score level are identified. At that point, the graders themselves are trained on the rubric through discussion of the exemplars. Once the graders have been trained, the grading process starts and is monitored closely to identify cases where there is disagreement between two raters. Typically, if any two scores given to a response differ by more than a certain amount, an adjudicator will also grade the particular response. The adjudicator's score is typically either averaged with the other scores for that solution or it is substituted for the score that is thought to be discrepant. Graders are expected to provide a single score to a complex response, such as an essay or drawing, by integrating all of the different qualitative aspects of the response. See Baldwin (2004) for a brief description of the process.

Clearly, a major consideration in these grading sessions is to minimize the disagreement among raters while retaining the relevant variation among the scores of performances of different quality. Training is used to achieve that goal. Training is often based on the grading of "benchmark" cases, that is, cases that have been previously scored by the master graders or chief readers. Ultimately, however, exclusion of judges whose ratings are atypical is a possibility in the interest of maintaining agreement. The emphasis on compliance with the rubric is understandable. Historically, two of the virtues of the multiple-choice item format are its economy and reliability. By contrast, free-response items that require human scoring typically require significantly more response time per question, allowing fewer questions for the assessment as a whole. As a result, score reliability is bound to be low just on account of the lesser number of questions (e.g., Linn & Burton, 1994). Disagreement among judges would erode score reliability further. Thus, it is not surprising that agreement is highly valued. But is it the case that the agreement that is obtained is a function of the rubric being similarly understood by all?

According to Elbow and Yancey (1994), the resulting agreement ".. is purchased at enormous cost: we don't get a picture of how these readers actually read or value these texts ..." (p. 95). Similarly, Huot (1993) argued that the requirements of holistic scoring "seem incongruous to normal reading processes" (p. 207). Important individual differences among raters may remain even after training, as suggested by Elbow and Yancey, because of the fundamentally different value systems of different graders. Similar misgivings had been expressed earlier by Gere (1980).

Studies of the holistic scoring process (e.g., Vaughn, 1991, pp. 112–113) would suggest that the state of affairs described by Elbow and Yancey may be the rule rather than the exception. Vaughn used think-aloud protocols to get a glimpse of the mental processes of raters of English compositions. The results were categorized into predictable categories such as organization, content, and grammar, as well as categories identifying critical attributes that gave an essay a passing or failing grade. Vaughn also categorized the graders into five categories:

- Raters that scrutinize rather than read the solution, searching for a fatal flaw;

- Raters that are primarily influenced by the first impression the papers give them;

- Raters that focus on two major attributes;

- Raters that focus on grammar;

- Raters that take a personal approach.

Vaughn concluded that "raters are not a tabula rasa, and, unlike computers, do not internalize a predetermined grid that they apply uniformly to every essay," (p. 120). If raters are not a tabula rasa, by what methods can we describe what they bring to the grading and how they arrive at scores—in short, their cognition—while grading? Freedman and Calfee (1983) proposed a model of rater cognition consisting of three processes: the reading of the text, the evaluation of the text, and the formulation of a score. They further speculated about extraneous variables that could influence each of these processes. They emphasized the importance of design in the understanding of rater cognition. They used ANOVA to analyze data from experimental designs to help in "untangling the web of variables that influence a person's judgment of a piece of writing." (Freedman & Calfee, 1983, p. 77). Rather than relying on essays as collected, they introduced changes into existing essays to achieve better control of the material to be rated. Specifically, they manipulated four qualitative features of the essays: development, organization, sentence structure, and mechanics. They concluded that the raters in their study were primarily influenced by development and organization.

Wolfe (e.g., 1997) proposed a model that can potentially accommodate the goal of high agreement while maintaining the individuality of the raters. Wolfe acknowledged critics such as Vaughn (1991) by distinguishing hermeneutic and psychometric scoring systems. The goal in a hermeneutic system is not agreement but interpretation. By contrast, he also described a psychometric scoring system as "one that emphasizes maintaining high levels of quantitative indicators of consistency between scorers—a system commonly employed in large-scale writing assessment. ... " (Wolfe, 1997, p. 84). By integrating a hermeneutic and psychometric perspective, Wolfe arrives at a very useful concept, namely scorer proficiency. The concept is useful because there is reason to believe that scoring proficiency is a measurable variable (e.g., Powers & Kubota, 1998). Specifically, Wolfe proposes a cognitive model of scorer cognition consisting of a "framework for scoring" and a "framework for writing". The framework for scoring is the mental processes for representing the object being rated. He bases the framework of scoring on the work of Freedman and Calfee (1983) mentioned earlier, which breaks down the rating process into interpretation, evaluation, and justification. The evaluation subprocess interacts with the framework for writing, which contains the rater's interpretation of the scoring rubric. Under Wolfe's model, the framework for scoring is a nomothetic model, that is, the three processes identified by Freedman and Calfee are assumed to be used by all raters although not necessarily in an equally proficient fashion. The framework of writing is potentially idiographic, meaning that different scorers could have alternative interpretations of the scoring rubric. When raters share a common framework of writing through training, or other means, a high degree of agreement can be expected assuming equal levels of proficiency in applying the framework of scoring. Lack of agreement can be due to raters having different frameworks as well as graders' lack of scoring proficiency.

In summary, the foregoing suggests the value of detailed modeling of raters. The literature reviewed here goes farther cognitively than the expert judgment literature. Although the Brunswick model was a useful conceptual model of the elements of the rating situation from an evidentiary perspective, the literature presented here attempts to deal with the basic conflict between minimizing disagreement and respecting the individual perspectives of each rater. Wolfe's model in particular can be seen as a "student model" for raters consisting of two basic proficiencies: interpretation and application of a rubric. In principle, it is possible to proceed to the next step and define "tasks" that would elicit evidence with respect to these two proficiencies during the course of a grading session or as part of special sessions. It could be especially valuable to chart their development as raters: Do they abandon that initial perspective or do they learn to map from their perspective to the scoring rubric? Is there any evidence for the objections that have been raised against holistic scores, for example, vulnerability to irrelevant attributes such as length and penmanship, the incongruity between grading and reading (Huot, 1993), or the potential vulnerability of the scoring rubric development process to social psychological influences? Understanding these vulnerabilities is important when judges serve as the evidence identification mechanism because such vulnerabilities can ultimately affect construct representation.

PSYCHOMETRIC MODELING

Previous sections argue that human graders, although possessing certain key strengths, are less than perfect examples of ideal scoring mechanisms, even with the various procedures designed to mitigate known weaknesses in human scoring. Moreover, the requirements of operational scoring sessions appear to emphasize the graders' expertise in the scoring process rather than their expertise in the domain of interest. In this section, we briefly examine psychometric approaches, namely Generalizability theory, Facets analysis, and hierarchical rater modeling (HRM), that model the performance characteristics of human graders rather than restricting the analysis solely to the outcomes of scoring.

One psychometric framework that lends itself to human scoring is Generalizability theory (G-theory; Cronbach, Gleser, Nanda, & Rajaratnam, 1972). G-theory was formally proposed in the early 1970s as a general framework that allow the recognition of multiple sources of errors in scores. G-theory lay dormant for several years until the resurgence of performance scoring that rekindled an interest in human graders as part of the assessment landscape. Unlike classical test theory (Gulliksen, 1950), G-theory explicitly attempts to quantify and decompose the multiple sources of error in scores by means of variance component estimation of structured datasets, so called g studies. The outcomes of such studies make it possible to do "what-if" analyses, so called *d-studies*, that estimate the design required to yield scores with a certain degree of generalizability. Under G-theory, raters are treated as a facet of the data collection design, but there is no characterization of specific scorers unless the raters themselves are the focus of analysis. When the focus of analysis is on the examinee (a typical application) graders are treated as a source of error.

A more recent framework is Facets (Linacre, 1989), an extension of the Rasch item response theory (IRT) model to responses scored by raters. Although the Rasch model uses a single parameter for item difficulty, Facets includes an additional parameter for each grader's bias. Unlike G-theory, Facets explicitly allows for differences in severity among graders. That is, both item difficulty and a grader parameter are assumed to jointly determine the probability of an item score. By examining the rater parameters, we can characterize raters with respect to their severity or leniency. A severe rater reduces the probability of a high item score while a lenient rater increases it. Myford and Wolfe (2001) used a Facets approach to analyze data from the Test of Spoken English (TSE) and corroborated the earlier finding by Bejar (1985) of differences among TSE raters in scoring behavior.

Hombo, Donoghue, and Thayer (2001) conducted a simulation study to assess the impact of failing to account for rater severity and leniency, assuming realistic levels of rater leniency/severity. They considered nested designs (where a rater scores all the items for a subset of all examinees) and spiral designs (where raters score all the examinees for a given subset of the items) and concluded:

> Ignoring rater effects in choosing an analysis model can substantially increase the bias in the resulting ability estimates, although this appears to be far less true for the spiral rater designs. These results bode ill for the validity of decisions based on the results of assessments if raters are not modeled. This is especially true when nested rater designs are used. (p. 21)

An important practical question is what to do about unmodeled rater severity in practice. Although monitoring raters is possible, the question of what steps to take when overly lenient or severe raters are identified during the course of grading is a problematic issue, one that has been addressed by Wilson and Case (2000) and Hoskens and Wilson (2001). Wilson and Case emphasized the importance of the timeliness of corrective action during operational scoring. Discovering a severely biased rater necessarily requires time for the evidence to accumulate, and depending on the length of the scoring session it may not be feasible to amend the scores already processed. The increasing availability of online scoring (e.g., Bejar & Whalen, 2001; Romano, Grant, & Farnum, 1999) would seem to ameliorate the problem because the data is available digitally and it is conceivable that analysis to detect rater could be run concurrently with the rating process.

Alternatives to Facets have been proposed (Bock, Brennan, & Muraki, 2002; Patz, Junker, Johnson, & Mariano, 2002)) that make different assumptions about the fundamental mechanism for considering rater effects on scoring. One such difference relates to the assumption of Facets in modeling rater effects as a shift of the IRT item characteristic curve up or down the ability scale (Donoghue & Hombo 2000). That is, the model posits that the effect of the rater is uniform through the range of ability. This is a strong assumption about rater cognition that ideally would be validated. In contrast, a more recent family of models starting with Patz (1996; also see Patz, Junker, Johnson, & Mariano, in press), the hierarchical rater model, (HRM), assumes that a work product has a "true score" expressed as a categorical score, and raters are assumed to differ in how well they can "guess" the score. This assumption, although motivated by technical considerations, might actually be an accurate model of rater cognition under operational scoring conditions. As noted earlier, interrater and benchmark score agreement are highly valued, and graders that do not comply with the rubric are not likely to be invited back. From the point of view of the grader who wished to be invited back, the rating situation psychologically is not unlike anticipating how the table leader would grade the same response. That is, the table leader is the source of the true scores and, in a sense, scoring is about how well the rater can predict predicting how the table leader would have scored the same work product.

Another contrast between Facets and HRM is in the modeling of individual differences in grader bias and with dependence assumptions among graders. In contrast to Facets, which allows for individual differences in grader bias (i.e., leniency–severity), HRM models rate consistency as well. Also, Facets makes the (commonly criticized) assumption of independence of errors of different raters' ratings of the same performance, which leads to the erroneous conclusion that precision of estimating an examinee's proficiency from a fixed number of performances—even one—can increase toward perfection as the number of raters increases. By contrast, HRM recognizes that the number of performances being observed limits the precision of measurement because each performance is itself an imperfect indicator of the examinee's proficiency even if it could be scored without error. In terms of ECD, error-free evidence identification cannot make up for uncertainty that resides in evidence accumulation. A similar correction for use in Facets was proposed by Bock, Brennan, and Muraki (2002), and operates by discounting the information function, that is, attenuating the precision of the estimates of student-model variables when the observables are based on the same fixed set of work products. Wilson and Hoskens (2001) proposed a related solution, namely, treating the multiple raters as a bundle of conditionally dependent variables rather than an independent source of information. Another psychometric model that includes parameters for shared variation among related observations or ratings is Wainer's testlet model, which is discussed more fully in Wainer et al. (chap. 6 this volume).

The addition of covariates to the HRM model (Mariano, 2002) represents a further extension of the arsenal for modeling rater behavior method. The Hierarchy in the HRM model refers to the conception that observed scores, the lowest level of the hierarchy, depend on an ideal rating, which in turn depends on the proficiency of the test takers. At the highest level of the hierarchy is the population of test takers. Mariano (2002, chap. 5) discussed the possibility of introducing covariates at several levels in this hierarchy. For example, a covariate may code for a set of raters belonging to a specific table. However, covariates that are more rater-specific are also possible. For example, how long the rater has been grading is a possible covariate that might be useful in modeling fatigue. In principle, this is a very general scheme. To carry out estimation with such a model requires a sufficient data amount of data. Technically, Mariano dealt with covariates by forming pseudo-raters, which are formed as unique combinations of raters and covariates. For example, if studying the effect of fatigue is of interest a given rater could be modeled as several pseudo-raters where the scores produced during the first hour would constitute one pseudo-rater, the scores from the second hour would constitute another pseudo rater, etcetera. In principle, this scheme could be used to model more cognitive covariates as well.

Because parameter estimation for the HRM requires rating from one or more raters for each item for each examinee, in the statistical model both the evidence identification and evidence accumulation processes are combined. Recall that evidence identification ends at the point of producing a score, an observable variable, for the work product while evidence accumulation is the aggregation of multiple scores on different items or work products to draw a summary conclusion about student model variables describing an examinee. In the case of HRM, this evidence accumulation process is accomplished by means of an IRT model. Moreover, in the case of HRM, there is another layer in between the input to the IRT model, what they call the ideal response, and the actual work product. In HRM that layer is modeled as a signal detection process with each rater having its own "operating characteristic." (See DeCarlo, 2005, for an approach to modeling rater behavior based on signal detection theory.) Fitting a joint model thus permits a characterization of accuracy and biases in evidence identification along with a mechanism for evidence accumulation across tasks. The estimation of all the parameters in the model, including the parameters for raters, is done jointly. Therefore, while evidence identification and accumulation are conceptually distinguishable they are intertwined in the operational implementation of the HRM model.

In summary, psychometricians have risen to the challenge, perhaps first recognized by Edgeworth (1888; see earlier quote), of accommodating the fallibility of judges as a means of evidence identification. G-theory was the first comprehensive psychometric framework to accommodate the variability that raters introduce into the process, but it did not explicitly accommodate modeling individual differences among graders. Subsequent models, starting with Facets, began to accommodate individual difference among raters, initially by modeling simple bias in the case of Facets, and then by adding consistency to the rater model in the case of HRM. HRM has been further expanded to allow a very flexible accommodation of rater covariates. In principle, HRM can be used operationally to analyze data from a scoring session while simultaneously collecting data for modeling rater cognition. Specifically, through the HRM model we can in principle operationalize ideas based on Brunswick's and Wolfe's models of rater cognition by recasting such attributes as rater covariates. As this is written, the parameter estimation of the HRM model is done by Markov Chain Monte Carlo (MCMC) methods, and can take considerable time to estimate. At present, the model does not lend itself to being used interactively as part of a grading session.

AN APPLICATION OF COGNITIVE MODELING FOR HUMAN SCORING[1]

Thus far, discussion has progressed from a consideration of a model for understanding human judgment to the selection of an approach for scoring in educational measurement, and then to psychometric models for understanding human scoring in practice. This section presents a study that illustrates the

---

[1] Parts of this research were presented earlier in Bejar, Yepes-Baraya, & Miller (1997).

process of eliciting, modeling, refining, and empirically assessing the judgment of human graders by making use of constructed response tasks. Specifically, in this study we illustrate a procedure for modeling rater cognition and behavior. It shows a possible approach to modeling graders qualitatively and quantitatively. We use Kelly's Grid Repertory method to identify the qualitative types of evidence each rater uses to characterize responses. Phase I and II of this study are concerned with the elicitation of the types of evidence each judge uses. This approach is idiographic allowing for different judges to adopt different evidentiary schemes. As a desired consequence, the result of this process allows for the possibility that each grader could well be considering the task and aspects of examinee performance very differently, meaning that what they see or look for in a work product is unique to them. Phase III of the study illustrates an approach to quantitative, but still idiographic, modeling of judgment behavior based on classification trees.

Phase I: Undirected Ideographic Evidence Identification Modeling

The objective of Phase I is to elicit from each grader the unique set of attributes (evidence) they deemed relevant to characterize a work product. This study used three teachers with varying degrees of experience. Rater A is a male in his mid-50s and a teacher of AP and honors chemistry in Western New York State with nearly 30 years of teaching experience. Rater B is a female in her late 20s and a teacher of regular chemistry in Central New Jersey with 5 years of teaching experience. Rater C is a male in his mid-50s, a teacher of history and social studies in Central New Jersey with more than 25 years of teaching experience. The three schools where these teachers work are suburban high schools with an academic reputation of excellence.

The three teachers were asked to independently evaluate 180 responses to a constructed-response item (provided in the Appendix found at the end of the chapter) developed for 12th grade science students and used in the Science, Technology and Society content area of the 1990 NAEP science assessment. Specifically, the human graders were each asked to: (a) provide their own answer to the item as though they were an examinee, and (b) classify 180 student responses to the same item "in a number of categories so that all the responses in one category are homogeneous with respect to distinguishable qualitative attributes that are relevant to the grader, as a subject matter expert (SME), for assessment purposes." Teachers were then asked to summarize the criteria they used to make the classifications, thereby indicating the major features of solutions they used to evaluate examinee responses. The resulting sets of scoring criteria for each grader are presented as Table 3.1.

TABLE 3.1
Unidirected Human Scoring Classifications and Criteria

Grader A[*]	Grader B	Grader C
1. Full (2F,2Q) specific	1. Human effects / risk / safety	1. Ethical decision making
2. Pertinent (2F,2Q) vague	2. Cost efficiency / safety	2. Technology
3. Pertinent (2F,2Q) no focus	3. Nuclear waste: storage & location	3. Economic costs of technology
4. Partial (1F,1Q) or (noF, 1Q)	4. Environmental effects / costs	4. Environmental concerns
5. Incomplete (1F,1Q) or (noF, 1Q)	5. Demand for nuclear power	
6. Implied (noF,1Q) or (noF, noQ)		
7. DNR (noF, noQ)		

[*]Note F = factor, Q = questions.

The number of classification categories and the criteria used to arrive at the classifications are substantially different for each of the graders. Grader A arrived at a series of seven ordered groups and indicated the rationale for the order and the classification of responses within each category. The top category consists of responses that mentioned two factors (2F) and two questions (2Q). The lower categories varied in terms of vagueness, specificity, and the number of questions and factors mentioned in the response. Clearly, this is an experienced rater that had participated in many gradings before. Note, however, that the instructions to the rater did not call at this point for construction of a scale, which is what rater A seems to have attempted. Grader B used five categories of student responses based on thematic issues addressed, with overlap in content between categories. Specifically, *Cost* and *Safety* each appear in two of the classification categories. Grader C grouped the responses along clear thematic lines, based on the primary theme of the response.

The results illustrate that in a naturalistic and undirected effort SMEs can indeed bring very different perspectives, and therefore grading models, to a grading session. This variation can be explained in terms of the raters' prior experience with performance assessment and the raters' approaching the task from qualitatively different perspectives. For example, as described earlier, one of the raters developed a scoring scale (Rater A, who was an experienced

Advanced Placement assessment grader) for classification of solutions on a continuum from most appropriate to least appropriate.

The primary finding of interest from this step is that judges indeed can be of different minds and when allowed to do so will bring very different perspectives to a grading session. The example from this study is an extreme one where graders are given complete freedom. As such, the graders were free to implement their assumptions about the most useful classification scheme for the assessment, ranging from the rank ordering scheme based on a quality of response exemplified by Grader A (perhaps as a result of prior experience with this goal from AP assessment scoring), to the classification by kind of qualitative content emphasized in the student response exemplified by Grader C, who is an experienced teacher with a Social Studies background and grouped the responses quite differently than Grader A, and based the groupings on thematic categories of response, such as *ethical decision making*.

Phase II: Application of Repertory Grid to Defining Evidence

A few weeks after the completion of Phase I, a Phase II of ideographic model elicitation was conducted with the same group of three SMEs, using the Repertory Grid methodology (Kelly, 1955) to analyze work products. The Repertory Grid methodology follows a series of steps, illustrated in Fig. 3.2.

The process begins by presenting the SME with responses to the same task from two students (Students 1 and 2). The expert is requested to identify assessment relevant characteristics of responses unique to Student 1, followed by the characteristics of the response unique to Student 2. This is followed by a listing of the assessment relevant characteristics that the responses have in common with each other. This process is then repeated for subsequent pairs of student responses until the responses for all students in the sample have been seen once. For this Phase II study, a subset of 60 responses, selected at random from the original sample of 180 student responses, were formed into 30 pairs for the Repertory Grid method. The goal of this process was to elicit the attributes each rater used in differentiating among paired responses. For each pair of student responses, the raters were asked to identify common and unique characteristics of the paired responses as described above. Once they had done this for the 30 pairs, they listed all the different attributes identified in the 60 student responses, referred to as the *long list*. They were then asked to develop a *short list* of attributes by grouping some of the attributes in the long list under more general headings or categories. Lastly, the raters were instructed to identify which of the attributes from their *short list* were present in each of the remaining 120 (from the original set of 180) responses that had not been used in the identification of attributes.

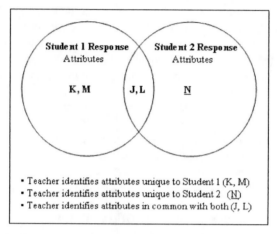

FIG. 3.2. Illustration of the Repertory Grid method.

The resultant short lists of attributes are summarized in Table 3.2. A comparison of Table 3.1 and Table 3.2 suggests a degree of convergence between Grader A and Grader C, with both graders focusing on the specific characteristics of the response independent of some scaling procedure. In addition, both raters make reference to the quality of the student responses, for example, "explicit" versus "implicit" questions, "noncompliance" factors/questions. Grader B's attributes, on the other hand, do not appear to be substantially different from the categories identified in Table 3.1.

TABLE 3.2
Repertory Grid Criteria for Human Scoring

Grader A	Grader B	Grader C
1. Description	1. Cost / production / location	1. Environmental factors
2. Questions Explicit	2. Effectiveness of nuclear power	2. Environmental questions
3. Questions Implicit	3. Nuclear waste: storage & location	3. Economic / health / safety factors
4. Costs	4. Nuclear waste disposal & safety / health concerns	4. Economic / health / safety factors
5. Comparison	5. Demand for nuclear power	5. Noncompliance factors
6. Opinion		6. Noncompliance questions
7. DNR		

Phase III: Empirical Ideographic Evidence Accumulation Modeling

Several weeks after Phase II was completed, the third phase of the study was initiated. During this phase the graders were asked to provide scores for the set of 120 responses for which they had applied the short list of attributes during Phase II. This process required the graders to independently: (a) devise a scale to differentiate between responses that more or less appropriately answered the question, (b) provide a description for each point on the scale to explain the quality level characteristic of that score, and (c) use their scoring system to score each the 120 student responses. The graders used a randomly selected set of 70 responses to develop their scale and to provide descriptions for each point on the scale. As part of this process, they provided a score for each of the 70 responses. Once this scale development was completed, they provided scores according to this scale for the remaining 50 responses. This process enabled us to derive the ideographic models of individual grader judgment behavior on the 70 responses as function of the evidentiary scheme we had elicited for each. We validated the resulting models on data for the 50 responses that had not been used in the development of each judge's model.

We chose to use classification trees as implemented in CART (Salford Systems). The reader is referred to Williamson, Bejar and Hone (2004) for a short introduction to the use of CART in the scoring context. Classification trees were introduced and discussed by Breiman, Friedman, Olshen, and Stone (1984). Given a categorical dependent variable and a set of predictors, CART finds a set of if and then rules that best classifies unseen responses. In the present context, the dependent variable refers to the score assigned by the judges in Phase III. The predictors are the set of attributes used by each judge. Among the many advantages of CART are that it is a nonparametric technique, it is robust to outliers, it allows for the mixture of nominal and numeric variables, it can deal with missing data, and it has a built-in cross-validation process (in certain versions). In the modeling process, CART grows competing trees and ranks them in terms of their accuracy. When CART is able to produce a tree it is an indication of a robust relationship in the data because the analysis includes multiple attempts to grow the tree with different portions of the data. If there is no reliable relationship between the independent variables (qualitative features for scoring) and the dependent variable (scoring outcome) then no classification tree is produced.

Data preparation for CART analyses in these studies included scale-recoding, in which the original scales produced by each rater were recoded to three categories of outcome (dependent) variables yielding approximately equal number of responses in each category for each rater. The CART analyses were conducted using with the CART cross-validation tree-growing procedure using 70 responses for growing the tree and the additional 50 responses were reserved for the cross-validation procedures, so that evaluating tree fit could be evaluated with data that had not been used in growing the classification tree.

Two distinct applications of empirical modeling using CART were employed to analyze rater behavior:

Idiographic Modeling. The goal of this modeling is to derive the individual model for each grader. In the CART analyses, this is achieved by treating an individual grader's holistic scores as the dependent variable and their qualitative features used in judgment as the independent variables. Such an analysis accomplishes two goals: First, if a tree cannot be produced from the data provided it suggests that the grader's holistic scores are not systematically related to the scoring criteria they identified; second, it provides a succinct summary of the judge's approach to scoring based on their evidentiary scheme.

Convergence Modeling. These analyses serve as an empirically based comparison of the similarity between grading models employed by a pair of human graders. This is accomplished using the holistic score of one grader as the dependent variable in CART analysis and the independent variables of a *different* human grader as the independent variables. In this analysis, we are interested in the extent to which the scores from one grader can be understood from the qualitative scoring attributes independently derived by a different grader.

Idiographic Modeling

In the evaluation of within-grader scoring models, the ideographic modeling consisted of CART analyses using a single grader's scoring attributes as the independent variables and the same grader's holistic score as the dependent variables. This analysis produced a CART-induced empirical model of individual grader scoring for Grader A and for Grader C, but not for Grader B. The ability of CART to produce a decision tree for Graders A and C but not for B suggests that Graders A and C consistently provided holistic scores that were a function of the qualitative attributes each had previously identified. Similarly, the lack of a tree for Rater B suggests that this rater did not rate consistently as a function of the qualitative attributes. This inability to produce a tree for Grader B ultimately lead to the conclusion that Grader B, perhaps as a result of being the least experienced teacher in the group, was not systematically using the qualitative scoring features to derive the holistic scores for responses. As a result, no further discussion below is devoted to Grader B.

The scoring model induced by CART for Grader A is presented as Fig. 3.3. This model is represented as a CART classification tree with three terminal nodes and two key attributes: Attributes 3 and 4, *questions explicit* and *costs* respectively (see Table 3.2). When both attributes are present, the resulting holistic score is a 3, the highest possible score. When Attribute 3 is present but Attribute 4 is not present, a score of 2 is obtained. The absence of Attribute 3 results in a score of 1, the lowest possible score. Therefore, Attribute 3 appears to be the most critical attribute in Rater A's model, its presence being a requirement for the highest score and its absence resulting in the lowest score. (Although not included in Fig. 3.3, a surrogate split in Rater A's tree would involve Attribute 6, *opinion*, in place of Attribute 3. According to the model, the presence of Attribute 6 results in a score of 1. This suggests that presence of an opinion rather than evidence in an examinee's response is sufficient to obtain the lowest possible score.) The model fit for this tree is presented as Table 3.3. The upper panel reports the classification accuracy based on the 70 cases used to grow the tree. The lower panel is the classification accuracy based on the application of the tree to the 50 cases that were not used in growing a tree. As is to be expected, there was some degradation in classification accuracy on cross validation with the 50 cases.

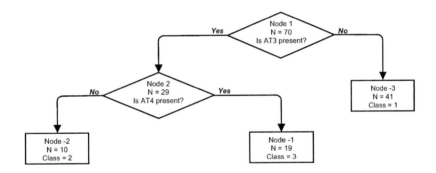

FIG. 3.3. Rater A's classification tree. AT3 and AT4 refer to the third and fourth attributes for Rater A identified in Table 3.2

TABLE 3.3
Rater A Classification Probability Tables

Rater A Calibration sample (N = 70)	Classification Probability Table		
	Predicted Class		
Actual Class	1	2	3
1	0.821	0.071	0.107
2	0.391	0.217	0.391
3	0.263	0.053	0.684

Rater A Cross validation sample (N = 50)	Classification Probability Table		
	Predicted Class		
Actual Class	1	2	3
1	0.941	0.059	0.000
2	0.538	0.192	0.269
3	0.429	0.143	0.429

The scoring model induced by CART for grader C is presented as Fig. 3.4. This model is represented as a CART classification tree with three terminal nodes and two key attributes: Attributes 5 and 6, *noncompliance factors* and *noncompliance questions*, respectively (see Table 3.1). Rater C's scoring rubric included both positive and negative attributes. However, Rater C's model suggests an emphasis on what the responses lacked (Attributes 5 and 6), instead of the presence of positive Attributes 1 through 4. When Attribute 5 is present, the resulting score is 1. When Attribute 5 is not present, but Attribute 6 is present, the resulting score is a 2. When both attributes are missing, the resulting score is a 3. What Rater C's model does not explain is the role of Attributes 1 through 4 in arriving at a score. The fact that Rater C's model assigns a score of 2 when Attribute 6 is present even though it is a *noncompliance question*, suggests that Rater C values questions more highly than factors. The model fit for this tree is presented as Table 3.4.

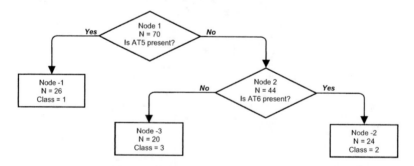

FIG 3.4. Rater C's classification tree. AT5 and AT6 refer to Attributes 5 and 6 for Rater C identified in Table 3.2.

TABLE 3.4
Rater C Classification Probability Tables

Rater C Calibration sample (N = 70)	Classification Probability Table		
	Predicted Class		
Actual Class	1	2	3
1	0.478	0.391	0.130
2	0.355	0.548	0.097
3	0.063	0.000	0.938
Rater C Cross validation sample (N = 50)	Classification Probability Table		
	Predicted Class		
Actual Class	1	2	3
1	0.364	0.591	0.045
2	0.125	0.875	0.000
3	0.000	0.083	0.917

Convergence Modeling

The goal of convergence modeling is to assess the implicit consistency between criteria used by one grader and the criteria used by another grader. These analyses ascertain the degree to which the scoring criteria identified by one grader are consistent with patterns of holistic scoring provided by another grader. This is accomplished by using the holistic score of one grader as the dependent variable in CART analysis and the independent variables of a *different* human grader as the independent variables. The initial analysis uses the holistic scores of Rater A as the dependent variable and the attributes of Rater C as the independent variables while the subsequent analysis uses the holistic scores of Rater C as the dependent variable and the attributes of Rater A as the independent variables. In both cases, we were able to obtain a tree (Figs. 3.5 and 3.6). This suggests that the attributes of each rater can be used to predict the score of the other. From the tree that was grown, all of Rater C's attributes seemed to have predictive value for Rater A's holistic score, except for attribute 3 (economic/health/safety factors). In the case of Rater C's holistic score, two of Rater A's attributes have predictive value: Attributes 1 and 7, *description* and *Does Not Respond (DNR)*, respectively. When *description* is present, the score is 2. When *description* and *DNR* are not present, the score is 3. When *description* is not present and *DNR* is present, the score is 1.

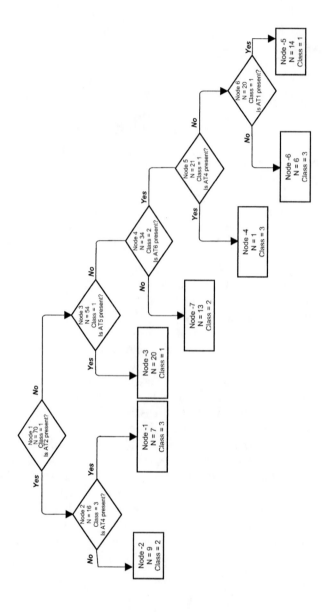

FIG. 3.5. Regression of Rater A's holistic scores on Rater C's attributes. The attributes mentioned in each diamond refer to the attributes for Rater C in Table 3.2.

74

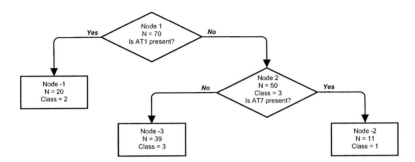

FIG 3.6. Regression of Rater C's holistic scores on Rater A's attributes. The attributes identified in each diamond refer to the attributes for Rater A identified in Table 3.2.

In summary, this exploration applied tree regression to obtain idiographic models of rater cognition by first eliciting from raters the distinguishing features among open-ended responses to a NAEP science problem by means of a structured procedure, Kelly's Grid Repertory Method. Subsequently, the graders were asked to assess the global quality of a set of responses. CART was used to infer the cross-validated classification tree for each rater separately. For the least experienced rater, Rater B, no classification tree was estimated and it was hypothesized that the teacher had not developed sufficiently as an assessor in order to characterize responses at the feature level or globally in a consistent manner. For the more experienced raters, it was possible to generate a classification tree for which there was substantial agreement with a qualitative analysis of each rater's behavior.

In addition to within-rater analyses, we carried out convergence analyses to further explore the utility of CART as a methodology to study rater cognition. This effort found that it was possible to fit a model for the holistic scores of Rater A based on the attributes of Rater C and vice versa. This suggested the feasibility of analyses aimed at understanding one rater's behavior in terms of the attributes of a second rater.

These analyses suggest that the CART methodology may be a valuable tool in helping to understand and control the characteristics of human scoring. This application may include facilitating the elicitation and model construction for ideographic human scoring models, as well as understanding a judge's judgments in terms of the evidentiary scheme from a different judge.

SUMMARY AND CONCLUSIONS

Regardless of whether an assessment is scored by human graders or by some automated mechanism, a goal of any assessment is to ensure that the construct is appropriately represented in the final scores, or outcomes, of the assessment process. This chapter examined human scoring with that goal in mind. Specifically, we examined the strengths and weaknesses of human scorers in evidence identification for operational human scoring of complex response data. The judgment literature was useful in introducing a competition of sorts between human and algorithmic approaches to judgment, thus beginning to raise the question of the relative merit of expert judges for evidence identification. In addition, this literature introduced the Lens Model, for understanding human judgment. The model can be viewed as juxtaposing two competing means of arriving at a judgment. In that sense, not only is it potentially useful to model human judgment, but also useful as a means of understanding differences among judges or, in general, alternative evidence identification procedures.

The literature related to large scale testing was also useful in addressing the question of the effectiveness of human scorers in the evidence identification process. It highlighted the fact that the conditions under which large-scale assessment scoring takes place essentially precludes the raters from operating as SMEs because of the emphasis on inter rater agreement, perhaps at the expense of construct representation. In effect, the process reduces human raters to mechanical means of evidence identification. This discussion suggests the possibility of a scoring proficiency of human graders that relates to the ability of domain experts to apply their expertise under the constraints of a scoring rubric. That is, graders who are equally proficient in their domains of expertise may not be equally proficient in the rubric-guided evaluation of domain-relevant responses submitted as part of an operational testing program.

The psychometric literature we reviewed has been characterized by an emphasis on individual differences among raters primarily in terms of rater bias and consistency. The Hierarchical Rater Model (HRM) offered by far the most general framework for taking into account individual differences among raters. Under this model, it is possible to incorporate covariates at different levels of the hierarchy to enable modeling of rater behavior. Also, under the HRM the rater's task is seen as predicting an ideal score, which matches the reality that in large scale assessment scoring the table leaders have the last word in determining the score that a work product deserves. Also, conceptually, there is a good fit of the HRM with the Lens Model if we equate the ideal with the "criterion."

The empirical analyses in this chapter presented the results of a rater cognition study using regression trees (CART) for modeling a rater's scores as a function of a previously established idiographic evidentiary scheme. The essence of the approach is to first elicit the criteria from expert judges and then model their judgments as a function of those criteria. We demonstrated the feasibility of the approach by showing that we were able to model the judgment of the most experienced teachers. It was not possible to obtain a valid empirical model of the grading characteristics of the least experienced teacher, suggesting that expertise in judging work products is an ability not perfectly correlated with subject matter expertise. The study was useful as a means of illustrating an approach to better understanding judgments. From studies such as these we gain a better understanding of the judgments and, and perhaps, are able to suggest covariates that could be tested at a larger scale through psychometric models such as the HRM. However, as noted previously, what to do in the middle of a grading with raters that are not behaving as expected can be a logistical problem.

All in all, expert judges used as a means for evidence identification pose significant challenges. It is appropriate to mention, because this is a volume on automated scoring, that the infrastructure required to adequately support scoring in large-scale assessment is quite complex. In addition to a complex model like HRM to fully deal with the variability among raters and their possible biases, there are also the logistics of the grading session and the expense of housing and feeding large number of scorers, all of which are repeated on a periodic basis. As noted earlier, from a pragmatic perspective a reasonable goal of any assessment is to maximize construct representation at the least cost. At some point, it is not unreasonable to raise the question of whether automated scoring provides a practical alternative to human scoring in achieving that goal. By raising this question we are not endorsing the use of automated scoring in every case, of course. Rather, we propose that the decision to choose automated or human scoring should be a conscious one where the primary goal is to maximize construct representation in the least costly fashion at the time the decision must be made.

ACKNOWLEDGMENTS

The authors are grateful to colleagues Doug Baldwin, Michal Beller, Dan Eignor, Mary Fowles, and Kathy Sheehan for helping to improve the manuscript.

REFERENCES

Allport, G. W. (1937). *Personality: A psychological interpretation.* New York: Holt.

Baldwin, D. (2004) A guide to standardized writing assessment. *Educational Leadership, 62* (2), 72–75.

Bejar, I. I. (1985). *A preliminary study of raters for the Test of Spoken English* (TOEFL Research Report No. 18). Princeton, NJ: Educational Testing Service.

Bejar, I. I., & Whalen, S. J. (2001). *Methods and systems for presentation and evaluation of constructed responses assessed by human evaluators.* U.S. Patent No. 6,526,258. Washington, DC: U.S. Patent and Trademark Office.

Bejar, I. I., Yepes-Baraya, M., & Miller, S. J. (1997). *Characterization of complex performance: from qualitative features to scores and decisions.* Presented at the National Council on Measurement in Education, Chicago, IL.

Bernstein, J. (2002). *Method and apparatus for estimating fitness to perform tasks based on linguistic and other aspects of spoken responses in constrained interactions.* U.S. Patent No. 6,157,913. Washington, DC: U.S. Patent and Trademark Office.

Bock, R. D., Brennan, R. L. & Muraki, E. (2002). The information in multiple ratings. *Applied Psychological Measurement, 26* (4), 364–375.

Bottenberg, R. A., & Christal, R. E. (1961). *An iterative technique for clustering criteria which retains optimum predictive efficiency.* Report WADD-TN-61-30. Lackland AFB, Tex.: Personnel Research Laboratory, Wright Air Development Division.

Breiman, L., Friedman, J. H., Olshen, R. A., & Stone, C. J. (1984). *Classification and regression trees.* Belmont, CA: Wadsworth.

Brunswick, E. (1955). Representative design and probabilistic theory. *Psychological Review, 62,* 236–242.

Butcher, J. N., & Rouse, S. (1996). Clinical personality assessment. *Annual Review of Psychology, 47,* 87–111.

Butler, F., Eignor, D., Jones, S., McNamara, T. F., & Suomi, B. (2000). *TOEFL 2000 speaking framework: A working paper* (TOEFL Monograph Series, Report No. 20). Princeton, NJ: Educational Testing Service.

Camerer, C. F., & Johnson, E. J. (1991). The process performance paradox in expert judgment: How can experts know so much and predict so badly? In K. A. Ericsson & J. Smith (Eds.), *Toward a general theory of expertise: Prospects and limits* (pp. 195–217). New York: Cambridge University Press.

Cooksey, R. W. (1996). *Judgment analysis: Theory, methods, and applications.* New York: Academic Press.

Cronbach, L. J., Gleser, G. C., Nanda, H., & Rajaratnam, N. (1972). *The dependability of behavioral measurements: Theory of generalizability for scores and profiles.* New York: Wiley.

Cumming, A., Kantor, R., & Powers, D.E. (2002). Decision making while rating ESL/EFL writing tasks: A descriptive framework. *The Modern Language Journal,* 67–96.

Dawes, R. M., & Corrigan, B. (1979). Linear models in decision making. *Psychological Bulletin, 81,* 95–106.

DeCarlo, L. T. (2005). A model of rater behavior in essay grading based on signal detection theory. *Journal of Educational Measurement, 42,* 53-76.

Donoghue, J. R., & Hombo, C. M. (2000, April). *A comparison of different model assumptions about rater effects.* Paper presented at the Annual Meeting of the National Council on Measurement in Education, New Orleans, LA.

Edgeworth, F. Y. (1888). The statistics of examinations. *Journal of the Royal Statistical Society, 51*, 599–635.

Elander, J., & Hardman, D. (2002). An application of judgment analysis to examination marking in psychology. *British Journal of Psychology, 93*, 303–328.

Elbow, P., & Yancey, K. B. (1994). On the nature of holistic scoring: An inquiry composed on e-mail. *Assessing Writing, 1* (1), 91–107.

Embretson, S. (1983). Construct validity: Construct representation versus nomothetic span. *Psychological Bulletin, 93*, 179–197.

Ford, K. M., Bradshaw, J. M., Adams-Webber, J. R., & Agnew, N. M. (1993). Knowledge acquisition as a constructive modeling activity. *International Journal of Intelligent Systems, 8* (1) 9–32.

Freedman, S. W., & Calfee, R. C. (1983). Holistic assessment of writing: Experimental design and cognitive theory. In P. Mosenthal, L. Tamor, & S. A. Walmsley (Eds.), *Research on writing: Principles and methods.* (pp. 75-98). NY: Longman.

Gaines, B., & Shaw, M. (1993). Knowledge acquisition tools based on personal construct psychology. *The Knowledge Engineering Review, 8* (1), 1–43

Gere, A. R. (1980). Written composition: Toward a theory of evaluation. *College English, 42,* 44–48.

Gulliksen, H. (1950). *Theory of mental tests.* New York: Wiley.

Hammond, K. R. (1955). Probabilistic functioning and the clinical method. *Psychological Review, 62*, 255–262.

Hombo, C. M., Donoghue, J. R., & Thayer, D. T. (2001). *A simulation study of the effect of rater designs on ability estimation* (Research Report 01-05). Princeton, NJ: Educational Testing Service

Hoskens, M. & Wilson, M. (2001). Real-time feedback on rater drift in constructed response items: An example from the Golden Sate Examination. *Journal of Educational Measurement, 38,* 121–145.

Huot, B. (1993). The influence of holistic scoring procedures on reading and rating student essays. In M. Williamson & B. Huot (Eds.), *Validating holistic scoring for writing assessment: Theoretical and empirical foundations* (pp. 206–236). Cresskill, NJ: Hampton Press.

Jong, J. H. A. L. D., & Bernstein, J. (2001). *Relating PhonePass overall scores to the Council of Europe framework level descriptors.* Technology in Language Education: Meeting the Challenges of Research and Practice, Hong Kong. (Downloaded from http://lc.ust.hk/~centre/conf2001/proceed/dejong.pdf, on January 8, 2006).

Kelly, G. A. (1955). *The psychology of personal constructs.* New York: Norton.

Kleinmuntz, B. (1963). MMPI decision rules for the identification of college maladjustment: a digital computer approach. *Psychological Monographs, 77,* (14, Whole No. 477.)

Linacre, J. M. (1989). *Many-faceted Rasch Measurement.* Chicago: MESA Press.

Linn, R. L., & Burton, E. (1994). Performance-based assessment: Implications of task specificity. *Educational Measurement: Issues and Practice, 13* (1), 5– 8, 15.

Mariano, L. T. (2002). Information accumulation, model selection and rater behavior in constructed response assessments. Unpublished PhD thesis, Carnegie Mellon University, Pittsburgh, PA.

Meehl, P. E. (1954). *Clinical versus statistical prediction: A theoretical analysis and a review of the evidence.* Minneapolis, MN: University of Minnesota Press.

Mertler, C. A. (2001). Designing scoring rubrics for your classroom. *Practical Assessment, Research & Evaluation, 7* (25). Retrieved November 16, 2003 from http://ericae.net/pare/getvn.asp?v=7&n=25.

Messick, S. (1989). Validity. In R. Linn (Ed.), *Educational Measurement* (3rd ed.). pp. 13-103. New York: American Council on Education and Macmillan.

Myford, C. M., & Wolfe, E. W. (2001). *Detecting and measuring rater effects using many-facet Rasch measurement: An instructional module.* Manuscript submitted for publication.

Patz, R. J. (1996). *Markov Chain Monte Carlo methods for item response theory models with applications for the National Assessment of Educational Progress.* Doctoral dissertation, Department of Statistics, Carnegie Mellon University.

Patz, R. J., Junker, B. W., Johnson, M. S., & Mariano, L. T. (in press). The Hierarchical Rater Model for rated test items and its application to large scale educational assessment data. *Journal of Educational and Behavioral Statistics.*

Powers, D., & Kubota, M. (1998). *Qualifying essay readers for an online scoring network (OSN).* (RR 98-20). Princeton, NJ: Educational Testing Service.

Powers, D. E., Burstein, J. C., Chodorow, M. S., Fowles, M. E., & Kukich, K. (2002). Comparing the validity of automated and human scoring of essays. *Journal of Educational Computing Research 26* (4), 407–425.

Romano, F. J., Grant, M., & Farnum, M. D. (1999). *Computerized system for scoring constructed responses and methods for training, monitoring, and evaluating human rater's scoring of constructed responses.* U.S. Patent No. 5,991,595. Washington, DC: U. S. Patent and Trademark Office.

Vaughan, C. (1991). Holistic assessment: What goes on in the rater's mind? In L. Hamp-Lyons (Ed.), *Second language writing in academic contexts* (pp. 111–125). Norwood, NJ: Ablex.

Wiggins, J. S. (1973). *Personality and prediction: Principles of personality assessment.* Reading, MA: Addison-Wesley.

Williamson, D. M., Bejar, I. I., & Hone, A. S. (1999). Mental Model comparison of computerized and human scoring. *Journal of Educational Measurement 36*(2), 158-184.

Williamson, D. M., Bejar, I. I., & Hone, A. S. (2004). Automated tools for subject matter expert evaluation of automated scoring. *Applied Measurement in Education 17*(4), 323-357.

Wilson, M., & Case, H. (2000). An examination of variation in rater severity over time: A study of rater drift. In M. Wilson & G. Engelhard (Eds.) *Objective measurement: Theory into practice* (Vol. V, pp. 113–133). Stamford, CT: Ablex.

Wilson, M. & Hoskens, M. (2001). The Rater Bundle Model. *Journal of Educational and Behavioral Statistics, 26,* 283–306.

Wolfe, E. (1997). The relationship between essay reading style and scoring proficiency in a psychometric scoring system. *Assessing Writing 4* (1), 83–106.

APPENDIX. NAEP ITEM[2]

Question 13. Nuclear power generation is a method of producing electricity using the energy released from radioactive fuels.

People who oppose nuclear power generation assert that ...

STATEMENT: Nuclear power is more harmful to the environment than are fossil-fuel burning plants.

Write a paragraph describing the *factors* that need to be considered in calculating the environmental costs of nuclear power plants compared to those of fossil fuel plants.
What *questions* would you ask to gather data to support or refute the statement above? For example, you might consider dust or debris a factor and ask whether nuclear plants are cleaner than fossil-fueled plants.

Responses were scored into the following categories:

> 5—The student describes aspects or poses questions about *three issues that relate to environmental effects* of either nuclear power plants or fossil-fuel burning plants, other than "dust or debris" or "Are nuclear power plants cleaner than fossil-fuel fueled plants?" as given in the example.

> 4—The student describes aspects or poses questions about two issues that relate to environmental effects of either nuclear power plants or fossil-fuel burning plants, other than "dust or debris" or "Are nuclear power plants cleaner than fossil-fuel fueled plants?" as given in the example.

> 3—The student describes aspects or poses questions about one issue that relate to environmental effects of either nuclear power plants or fossil-fuel burning plants, other than "dust or debris" or "Are nuclear power plants cleaner than fossil-fuel fueled plants?" as given in the example.

> 2—Incorrect response.

> 1—No response.

---

[2] These data were reported previously in Bejar, Yepes-Baraya, & Miller (1997).

4

Rule-Based Methods for Automated Scoring: Application in a Licensing Context

Henry Braun
Isaac I. Bejar
David M. Williamson
Educational Testing Service

> *How can intelligence emerge from non-intelligence? We'll show that you can build a mind from many little parts, each mindless by itself.*—Marvin Minsky (1985, p. 17)

> *Hence to the extent that the mind is unable to juxtapose consciously a large number of ideas, each coherent group of detailed constituent ideas must be reduced in consciousness to a single idea; until the mind can consciously juxtapose them with due attention to each, so as to produce a its single final idea.*—Wigmore (1913; 2nd Edition, 1931, p. 109; cited in Schum, 2003, p. 4)

It is fitting that this chapter follows one on human scoring since a rule-based approach to scoring essentially attempts to embody the reasoning of experts, conceived as a combination of logical evaluations. It is also appropriate that it appears early in the volume because, in comparison to some of the methods discussed in subsequent chapters, logical rules are conceptually straightforward and one of the earliest approaches to representing expert decision-making. A by-product of this conceptual simplicity is that the relationship between programmed rules and outcomes are directly inspectable. In this chapter, we demonstrate how relatively simple rules can be harnessed to execute the equivalent of what would generally be considered higher order reasoning. In this case, the higher order reasoning involves the expert evaluation of solutions to complex constructed response tasks, submitted as part of a nationwide licensure examination.

Although this presentation of rule-based systems is grounded in a particular application, the approach and methodology described is quite general and could be used in many different settings. Indeed, we argue that such systems are generally capable of yielding valid judgments so long as the rules are elicited through a design process that is mindful of the goals of the assessment and are refined through a rigorously planned and carefully executed series of studies. While the assessment design effort for the case study we present in this chapter preceded the formal development of evidence-centered design (ECD), the design effort was consistent with many of the principles of ECD. Indeed, the issues encountered—and addressed—in this effort influenced some of the thinking that ultimately resulted in the ECD methodology. (See Mislevy et al., Chap. 2, this volume.)

The chapter begins with some background on rule-based scoring systems and the specific licensure-related assessment to which it was applied. We then introduce the student, evidence and task models and include a detailed description of the rules used to score a particular complex work product. The remaining sections contain an extended discussion of a number of validity considerations, along with some concluding thoughts.

BACKGROUND

Rule-based Systems

In the introduction to this volume, we noted that the rapid advance of different technologies—and the desire to put them to good use in the context of assessment—is the impetus for exciting innovations in assessment design, development and administration. But, as a distinguished writer on engineering design has noted,

> The concept of failure is central to the design process, and it is by thinking in terms of obviating failure that successful designs are achieved. (Petrosky, 1994, p. 1)

Petrosky's insight is highly relevant. In this chapter, as well as the rest of the volume, we approach assessment as a design discipline (Braun, 2000). Our goal is to share our hard-won knowledge to preclude "design failures." There is a direct parallel between Petrosky's perspective on the design process and the view that good design in scientific work (including assessment design) should be driven by the need to counter expected threats to the validity of the intended inferences (Shadish, Cook, & Campbell, 2002). Of course, we are using the term *assessment* here to refer to all components of the system, including the scoring.

In the present context, assessment design choices can be broadly described as either retrospective or prospective. A retrospective approach can be considered when there is an ongoing assessment for which traditional scoring methods have been employed and where now automated scoring is viewed as both desirable and feasible. The prospective design approach is called for when automated scoring is to be incorporated either into an entirely new assessment or the radical redesign of an existing assessment.[1]

A major practical difference between the two is that in the retrospective approach the development process can be informed by both extant tasks (prompts, design problems, etc.) and the data consisting of candidate responses, along with the corresponding scores assigned by human judges. It is natural, then, to take advantage of the existing data and aim to develop a system that explicitly emulates or predicts the criterion judgments that are at hand. This case is best exemplified by the automated scoring of writing (e.g., Deane, Chap. 9, this volume; Shermis and Bernstein 2003; Valenti, Neri & Cucchiarelli, 2003; Yang, Buckendahl, Juszkiewicz, & Bhola, 2004), where the criterion scores provided by judges are used in developing a scoring algorithm and also serve as the target for the output of that algorithm. The intention is that the score produced by the algorithm essentially emulate the outcome of the human rating process.

For this approach to be consistent with ECD principles, it is necessary that (a) the criterion scores produced by human scorers adequately reflect the evidence relevant to the goals of the assessment and, (b) the automated scoring predictions of the criterion scores are based on response characteristics constituting evidence consonant with a construct validity argument. The review of human scoring in chapter 3 suggests that, in general, we cannot assume (a). The retrospective approach, therefore, is not necessarily the best approach to follow.

When a prospective approach is called for, an ECD perspective is especially helpful because the evidentiary trail required for the design of the assessment becomes the specification for the evidence models to be executed by automated procedures. This evidentiary trail consists of identifiable response attributes that inform both the student and task models. One possible strategy, although by no means the only one, for combining and summarizing the evidence is through rules.

The use of rule-based systems in automated scoring is a direct attempt to apply ideas of expert systems in an assessment context. At the time the

---

[1] The distinction between retrospective and prospective "approaches" is somewhat arbitrary and for that reason it may be better to think of them as phases. For example, the validation of a prospectively developed system could well involve human experts independently scoring work products after scores have been produced by automated means. This is illustrated in Williamson, Bejar, and Hone (1999).

assessment described in the next section was under development, expert systems were quite popular (Buchanan & Smith, 1989) and had been built for a wide variety of applications. Buchanan and Smith distinguished between expert systems dealing with "interpretation" problems, such as data interpretation (Smith & Young, 1984); and "construction" problems, such as system configuration (e.g., Rauch-Hindin, 1986). Applications in medical diagnosis have been numerous. For example, MYCIN (Shortliffe, 1976) was an expert system built to diagnose infectious diseases.

Buchanan and Smith (1989) listed the following as important characteristics of an expert system:

1. The system reasons with domain specific knowledge that is symbolic and numeric.

2. The system uses domain specific algorithmic and heuristic methods

3. The system performs well

4. The system is capable of explaining its reasoning

5. The system retains flexibility.

The first two attributes highlight the domain specific nature of expert systems and constitute a departure from more generic approaches, such as policy capturing, discussed in chapter 3. The implementation of expert systems requires a detailed representation of the domain of application and the objects that exist in that domain. It is this detailed representation that makes the system capable of "explaining its reasoning." Finally, the ability of the system to perform well and flexibly are attributes typical of experts. Indeed, it should be possible to apply an expert system successfully across many problems within the domain. This last requirement is usually necessary for the implementation of expert systems to be economically practicable. In the extended example we present, automated procedures were developed to accommodate entire classes of problems, rather than only specific instances of a class. Such an approach was necessary both to protect the integrity of the scores and to avoid the costly process of customizing a procedure for each specific problem (Bejar, 2002).

In short, an expert system or rule-based approach is a natural extension of human scoring. It is founded on the assumption that it is possible to glean from a pool of domain experts knowledge and practices sufficient to implement a logical, reproducible and domain expertise-based system for scoring. Ideally, these experts should be both seasoned practitioners and experienced judges of candidates' responses to the kinds of tasks intended to elicit their competence. Not surprisingly, the development of an expert system generally requires intense interactions with domain experts over an extended period of time.

THE COMPUTERIZED ARCHITECT REGISTRATION EXAMINATION

Our approach to the development of a rule-based system for automated scoring will be illustrated by our work on the Architectural Registration Examination (ARE), an assessment battery that is sponsored by the National Council of Architectural Registration Boards (NCARB). The ARE is a critical component of architectural registration, the process by which each state and Canadian province licenses individuals to practice architecture. There is an explicit expectation that candidates who have passed the relevant set of examinations will consistently generate designs that "obviate failure," especially with respect to the health, safety and welfare of the client and of the public. Thus, the design of such an assessment should be focused on assisting the authorities in making correct decisions about the relevant competencies of the candidates. The stakes are especially high because the outcome affects not only the life of the candidate but also the lives of many others.

In 1997, the ARE became the first fully computerized licensure test to incorporate automated scoring of complex constructed responses in operational testing. Given the high stakes of this assessment, this was a bold move on the part of the profession and the licensing authorities—especially since there were no examples of successful implementations to guide the effort. It should also be noted that the structure and format of the design problems in the new battery differed substantially from those in the paper-and-pencil ARE. In particular, a single twelve hour design problem was replaced by a set of more modular tasks.[2]

The computerized ARE consists of nine divisions, with six divisions consisting of multiple-choice items and three consisting of vignettes, or open-

---

[2] During the 35 years prior to 1997, the ARE took the form of a set of paper-and-pencil examinations (called divisions) that included both multiple-choice divisions and "graphic" divisions. For the latter, candidates had to execute various drawings that were then graded by expert architects assembled for the purpose by NCARB and the testing contractor. The most challenging division consisted of a single problem requiring the candidate to design a two-story building and to execute four drawings (two floor plans, an elevation and a cross-section). Twelve hours were allotted for the problem. In the late 1980s, the NCARB began to plan for a transition to computer delivery. One impetus was the cost of scoring the graphic divisions, an amount approaching one million dollars per year—even though the graders volunteered their time! Of course, it was also the case that the profession was increasingly turning to technology, especially computer-aided design (CAD), and there was recognition that the ARE could not lag too far behind if it was to maintain its credibility. Accordingly, in the fall of 1987 NCARB asked ETS to generate a plan for developing a computerized ARE. The plan was accepted in the spring of 1988 and work began immediately. NCARB made available to ETS a number of expert architects/graders whose contributions were essential to the success of the project. The last administration of the old ARE took place in the fall of 1996 and the new examination began operation in February 1997. See Bejar and Braun (1999).

ended graphic design problems. Divisions may be taken in any order, each one targeting a different area of professional competence. Because passing a division requires significant preparation, candidates typically complete the full battery of nine divisions over an extended period of time. The vignettes in the three graphic divisions are solved by the candidate with the aid of a primitive (by commercial standards) CAD interface. The submitted designs are evaluated by a set of rule-based automated scoring algorithms to determine the degree to which the design requirements of the vignette and general professional standards are met. More information on the graphic design vignettes can be found in Braun, Brittingham, Bejar, Chalifour, DeVore, and Hone (2000).

Each of the graphic divisions comprises several vignettes, with each vignette drawn from a different class of problems, called a *vignette type*. Each vignette type was considered a separate subdomain of the division and a scoring system was built to score solutions to any vignette of that type. Although it is possible, in principle, to design a single scoring system to accommodate a number of vignette types, this was not the case here. The domain specificity alluded to by Buchanan and Smith (1989) was very strong and made it necessary to treat each vignette type separately.

We captured the expertise of the architects through an iterative cycle of intense group discussions, which included statisticians, programmers and test developers. The experts were selected to represent a variety of perspectives. The expert committee membership rotated periodically and ranged in number from 6 to 10. The fact that the specifications for the vignette types and the test administration protocols were developed concurrently made the process particularly demanding, as there was no candidate data available for discussion or testing. On the other hand, the simultaneous development of the delivery interface and the scoring algorithms made it possible to insure their coordination. In retrospect, this process was consistent with the principles of ECD, embodying an emphasis on the development of an evidential structure for drawing inferences based on a set of generalized task models incorporating critical design challenges.

As we shall see, the scoring rules can be represented by hierarchical trees. The end nodes of these trees are design solution attributes, or features, that are extracted directly from a candidate's work product. We will not devote much time to feature extraction, which is necessarily domain specific. The interested reader is referred to Reid-Green (1995a, 1995b, 1996a, 1996b) and Oltman, Bejar, & Kim (1993). The scoring rules govern the evaluation of the features, as well as the combination of those evaluations at higher levels of the tree.

There are many other considerations that informed the design of the test administration environment and had a bearing on the development of the scoring algorithms, as well as the overall validity argument for the assessment (Bejar & Braun, 1994; Bennett & Bejar, 1998). These are not the main focus of this chapter. A detailed description of the ARE effort is contained in the project technical report (Bejar & Braun, 1999), and the interested reader is referred to that publication for further information.

To make the subsequent discussion more concrete, we present an example of the interface and the task presentation environment for a particular vignette type, called "Block Diagram." It calls for the candidate to generate a schematic floor plan for a single story building. Figure 4.1 presents the program, which provides the candidate with the information needed to begin the design work. This includes a site description, the number of rooms in the building, desired circulation patterns, internal constraints (e.g., required adjacencies and non-adjacencies), and external constraints (e.g., the location of the main entrance and required views). Figure 4.2 displays the base drawing, further design information and icons representing the various design tools and resources available to the candidate. Figure 4.3 shows a solution to the design

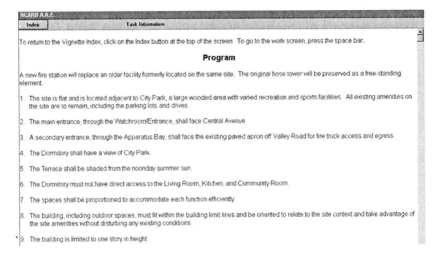

FIG. 4.1. An example of a task prompt for the ARE. Figure reprinted from Williamson, Bejar, and Hone (1999), by permission of Blackwell Publishing.

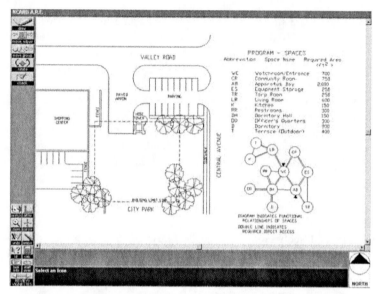

FIG. 4.2. An illustrative base diagram for an ARE task. Figure reprinted from
Williamson, Bejar, and Hone (1999), by permission of Blackwell Publishing.

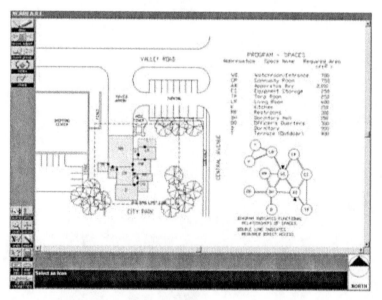

FIG. 4.3. A sample solution to an ARE task.

problem superimposed on Fig. 4.2. Note that the color monitors employed in practice permit better distinctions among various tools, drawing and solution elements than do these black and white figures. (More information on the administration and scoring of the ARE may be found in Bejar & Braun, 1994; Bejar & Braun, 1999; Kenney, 1997).

STUDENT, EVIDENCE, AND TASK MODELS IN A LICENSING CONTEXT

As noted earlier, the development of the computerized ARE preceded the formulation of ECD. Nonetheless, in this section, we consider some design decisions from an ECD perspective, illustrating the applicability of ECD methodology in this setting, as well as the general consistency of ECD methods with the development process. For a discussion of another licensure assessment designed from an ECD perspective, see Mislevy, Steinberg, Breyer, Almond, and Johnson (2002).

Student Model

The key claim to be made about an individual who successfully completes the ARE battery concerns his or her competence to practice architecture in a manner that protects the interests of the clients of architectural services and, especially, the health, safety and welfare of the public. Figure 4.4 presents a differentiated model of architectural competence that displays nine branches, each corresponding to a specific subcompetency. Of course, a full, fine-grained student model would expand each branch to represent the relevant proficiencies. An example for the Site Planning branch of the student model is displayed in Fig. 4.5.

Site Planning involves the ability to integrate programmatic requirements (i.e., the intended site use) with environmental requirements and constraints (related to geography, topography, climate and vegetation), along with the legal and regulatory aspects of site development. A successful outcome is a coherent and workable plan for the placement of buildings and/or other improvements on the site. The ability to generate such a plan involves several sub-skills, including:

- Site Design—the ability to employ general principles of site planning

- Site Zoning—the ability to design with due regard to the limitations determined by zoning and setback restrictions

- Site Parking—the ability to design and layout vehicular parking and traffic patterns that respect site requirements, principles of vehicular circulation and relevant regulations

- Site Analysis—the ability to identify and delineate land subdivisions that are appropriate for the construction of various types of structures and other surface improvements

- Site Section—the ability to understand how the site design requirements, such as site features, grading, building placement, and solar, wind or view restrictions, impact site sections and profiles

- Site Grading—the ability to modify a site's topographical characteristics to meet programmatic and regulatory requirements

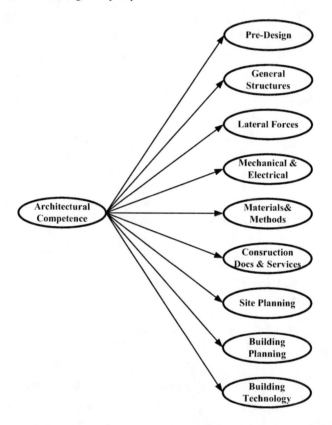

FIG. 4.4.   Course-grained student model for the ARE showing the nine proficiencies that define architectural competence.

In the development of job-related assessments, a job analysis is mandated (e.g., Uniform Employee Selection Guidelines) to identify the knowledge, skills, and abilities, (KSAs) that are the constituent elements of professional competence. Development of the new ARE was informed by an existing job analysis (Stecher, 1989), as well as a subsequent one (National Council of Architectural Registration Boards, 1994) that was carried out, in part, to take account of the rapidly evolving role of computers in architectural practice. Figure 4.5 also shows schematically the interplay of subskills and KSAs. In fact, to arrive at the final set of subskills associated with a given division, a table of subskills by KSAs was maintained. By postulating which KSAs a particular subskill depends on, the table can be filled in; how well a given collection of subskills covers all the KSAs can then be determined.

The final design of the ARE is isomorphic to the student model. That is, each branch in Fig. 4.4 corresponds to a division of the ARE battery, with the last three branches mapping into the three graphic divisions. Each graphic division follows the patterns of Fig. 4.5. Each subskill, such as Site Design, corresponds to a vignette type in the division. (See Bejar, 2002, for further discussion.)

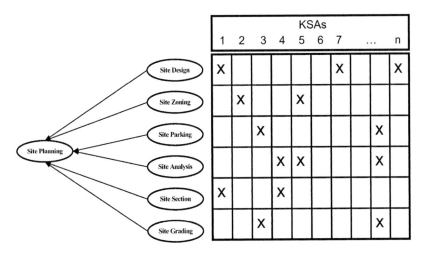

FIG. 4.5. Fine-grained representation of one proficiency (site planning) consisting of six subskills.

Explicating proficiencies at the grain size detailed in this section was necessary both to delineate the proficiencies targeted by the assessment and to inform the development of tasks that would elicit those proficiencies. It remains, however, to determine what grain size is appropriate for accumulating information with a (probability-based) measurement model. The same model of proficiency can support a very fine-grained measurement model, such as that used in an intelligent tutoring system, or a coarse-grained model of overall proficiency across the entire domain of tasks. A decision should be based on the purpose of the assessment, and that decision is then reflected in the specific nature of the evidence identification and evidence accumulation processes embedded in the evidence model, as described in the following section.

Evidence Models

Inasmuch as the primary purpose of the ARE is to contribute to the certification of an individual for professional practice, its evidentiary requirements are narrowly focused on discriminating between candidates who are capable of competent practice and those who are not. The evidence models are expected neither to support making fine distinctions between different levels of competent practice nor to distinguish examinees grossly deficient in the KSAs required for competent practice from those who are close to reaching competence. Moreover, in view of the critical role of the assessment in the certification process, it was decided (in consultation with NCARB officials) that a judgment of competence for practice would be a conjunctive determination based on the results in the nine branches displayed in Fig. 4 4.

The evidence models for the ARE differ somewhat from the nature of evidence models commonly discussed in ECD. In large part, these differences reflect the fact that ARE scoring development predated development of the ECD methodology. In most applications of ECD, the evidence model consists of two distinct components: evidence identification and evidence accumulation. Evidence identification is essentially a data reduction process in which student work products (whether multiple-choice selections or complex constructed responses) are summarized in one or more new variables, called observables. As such, evidence identification makes no direct inferences about examinees, but is oriented toward providing convenient descriptions of task performance in a manner suitable for subsequent inferences. By contrast, evidence accumulation is the process of drawing explicit inferences about ability attributes of individuals or groups on the basis of these observables. The true values of proficiency are not verifiable but are inferred from the pattern of values represented by observables. Typically, this requires some probabilistic estimate of the proficiency.

ECD emphasizes the path from data to inference. In contrast, much of traditional test development treats the evidence identification process and the evidence accumulation process as only implicitly related, rather than as explicit stages in a validity argument. For example, typical test blueprints take a content (evidence identification) orientation and focus on describing a matrix of relationships between item content and content identified as important in the domain. It also inventories the anticipated range and depth of evidence identified in the test administration.

The evidence accumulation phase of traditional test development processes is instantiated in the final stages of assessment design through such processes as IRT calibration and scaling and/or cut score studies. Evidence accumulation in terms of total scores or IRT ability estimation is tantamount to measuring proficiency at carrying out tasks in the domain, treating as given whatever decisions have been made to define the domain, the tasks, the work products, and the evidence identification procedures. In summary, traditional test design includes both the evidence identification and the evidence accumulation processes, but typically as separate activities that are connected only through the final step of calibration or cut-score determination.

A similar observation can be made about scoring development for the ARE. Although the demands of the automated scoring algorithms shifted the development toward a more ECD-like process, the overall design had its roots in standard conceptions of assessment design. Development began with a research-based investigation of the domain of interest, ultimately resulting in a student model of domain performance (described in the previous section). Evidence model development was treated much like blueprint development for traditional assessment design, with an emphasis on obtaining evidence with respect to the variety of skills represented in the student model, rather than on inferences with respect to the ability levels of examinees at each sub-proficiency. The skills identified in the student model were built in to the evidence model (and ultimately the tasks themselves) as aspects of the assessment task design and scoring rule structure, rather than treated explicitly as subproficiencies to be estimated individually from the data.

With respect to evidence identification, the challenge confronting the working group, then, was to specify the evidential basis for making a judgment of minimal competence in the three general areas addressed by the graphic divisions of the ARE. With a multiple-choice format, it is conceivable that one can directly link individual items to specific KSAs and base the evidence identification process explicitly on those KSAs. (In fact, this is often done in tests used in K–12 settings where, instead of KSAs, one deals with content standards (e.g., Linn, 2001). In the ARE, the evidence identification process is not based on single linkages between observations and proficiencies, but instead builds a chain of evidential steps, beginning at the data level and progressing through a series of increasingly coarse-grained summaries of performance, culminating in the determination of solution adequacy. In effect, there are two sets of linkages for ARE scoring: An explicit set of evidence identification rules as just described and an implicit linkage of each of these series of summary variables to one or more proficiency variables targeted by the assessment.

The major distinction between traditional approaches and the ECD approach to assessment design is how explicit the linkages between evidence and proficiencies are, and at what stage in the design process are they developed. The ARE reflects an ECD approach to explicit chains of reasoning: It incorporates this logical argument into the scoring, based on guidelines developed by a panel of experts[3] through an iterative process. Experts generally do not focus on specific KSAs in evaluating a work product. Rather, they reason on the basis of implicit KSAs in evaluating the functionality and appropriateness of the response in the context of the purpose of the assessment task. The evidence identification process embodied in the scoring rules shares this characteristic of expert human graders.

To properly reflect the extent to which the processes employed by expert human graders were studied and incorporated into the design of the scoring rules, we refer to the scoring strategy used in the ARE as a "mental modeling" approach, following Johnson-Laird's (1983) usage of the term:

> A model makes explicit those objects, properties, and relations, that are relevant to potential actions, that is, it makes them available to inference and decision-making without the need for further processing. (Johnson-Laird, 1993, p. 16)

A key component of the automated scoring design involved the elicitation of the relevant "objects, properties, and relations" of the universe of design solutions from expert architects. This proved to be critical to the success of the project because the universe of potential designs satisfying key requirements was sufficiently large and complex to preclude scoring strategies based on

---

[3] It should be noted that for a different type of assessment it may be quite appropriate to formulate evidence models designed to report at the level of individual KSAs. For diagnostic purposes, for example, it would be essential to report to a student what skills were not demonstrated adequately.

template matching. From a practical point of view, success required that the committee reach agreement on the *process* of evidence identification; that is, on the appropriate standards and criteria to be used in evaluating submitted work rather than on summarily evaluating the work itself. Because ARE consists almost entirely of evidence identification rules, it is useful to distinguish between two qualitatively different stages of this process: feature extraction and evidence synthesis. These are discussed in following sections.

Feature Extraction. To illustrate the scoring process, we use the Site Planning area of competence. As illustrated in Fig. 4.5, Site Planning consists of six architectural proficiencies (Design, Zoning, Parking, Analysis, Section, and Grading). The first phase in the evidence identification process is *feature extraction*, which is the selection and quantification of those aspects (features) of a design solution that will serve as the basis of an evaluative judgment of the work product. In many ways, it is the most technically challenging portion of algorithm development. In the ARE, features are functions of the objects, properties and relations contained in a solution. Features can take various forms: The presence or absence of a certain design object, counts of a class of objects, measures of objects or types of relationships among objects. Some examples of features relevant to site planning include:

- Setbacks—Whether the candidate respected property line setbacks by placing a building footprint sufficiently inside the property line.

- Accessibility—Whether a building provides sufficient hallway width and doorway placement to allow access to individuals in wheelchairs.

- Parking—Whether the correct number of parking slots has been included.

- Water flow—Whether a site is graded to properly direct the flow of water.

Once the desired scoring features are unambiguously defined (often not a trivial task—even for a committee of experts), the next step is to develop computer algorithms that are able to implement selection and quantification. Usually this is quite straightforward. For example, it is relatively simple to determine whether any of the building objects in the (CAD-developed) blueprint infringe on the property setback line or whether the correct number of parking slots has been designed. In other cases, however, the programming challenges can be significant. Examples include determining accessibility or analyzing the flow of water across a site (see Bejar, 1991; Reid-Green, 1995b).

In principle, all the information required for feature extraction can be found in the solution itself. However, in practice, the characteristics of the CAD interface can strongly influence the ease with which a feature extraction algorithm can be implemented. Similarly, the conventions for representing the location and orientation of digital objects, their boundary conditions, their grain size, their spatial relationships to other digital objects, and even their method of selection and manipulation, all have a bearing on feature extraction. Thus, the software underlying the feature extraction algorithms and the software enabling the design process employed by the candidate must co-evolve during the assessment development process. This is the basis of the admonition that "it's not only the scoring!" (Bennett & Bejar, 1998; Bennett, Chap. 11, this volume). Indeed, assessment design is an essential aspect of automated scoring development, and explains why the concepts and organizational structure of ECD can be so helpful.

Once a feature has been extracted and quantified (presence/absence, count, measurement, etc.), it has to be evaluated for quality or appropriateness with respect to one or more relevant criteria. In the case of the ARE, the criteria were set by the committee of architects, after considerable deliberation and extensive review of sample solutions. In addition, the committee had to determine how many categories would be needed to code the results of the evaluation of each feature. The number of categories—and how they are defined—determines how much information is carried forward at each succeeding stage of evidence identification.[4]

A particular implementation of a feature extraction and evaluation algorithm can have significant implications for the capability of the system to reflect the reasoning followed by expert human graders. For example, a human grader may disregard (rightly or wrongly) a relatively minor infraction of a scoring rule, indicating that a dichotomous categorization is not sufficient for modeling human graders. Alternatively, it may suggest that in a dichotomous categorization, very minor infractions should be considered "appropriate" rather than "inappropriate." On other occasions, a human grader may accord minor infractions great weight, as when the violations are repeated frequently, with apparent disregard of the relevant regulations or standards of practice.

In point of fact, a recurring challenge concerned the treatment of ambiguous evidence of competence. Considerations of data sufficiency suggest propagating the uncertainty through the evaluation process until a clear decision can, or

---

[4] There is substantial similarity between the goals, processes and outcomes of the committee's work on feature extraction rules and those commonly applied in cut score studies. The extent and nature of the discussion on appropriate standards to apply to the task, the emphasis on a performance meeting agreed upon standards given the intent of the design, and the deliberation over borderline cases, are all hallmarks of both types of activities.

must, be made. There are theories of evidence (e.g., belief theory; Shafer, 1976) that constitute generalizations of the Bayesian decision-making paradigm in that they permit some of the mass of the subjective probability distribution to be left unallocated until further data are available. These theories served as inspiration for deciding on a trichotomous categorization of feature evaluations. Under this scheme, the outcome of an evaluation can take one of three values: Clearly "acceptable" (denoted as "A"), clearly "unacceptable" (denoted as "U"), or "indeterminate" (denoted as "I").

An assignment of "A" is made when there is a strong consensus among expert human graders that the value or quality of the feature is at least minimally adequate. This includes, therefore, not only perfect implementations but also those that are flawed but judged to exceed an appropriate threshold. For example, counts or measurements that fall within a certain range might all be assigned an "A." More complex features can be treated in a similar manner. In addition, allowance can be made for the characteristics of the interface. By way of illustration, the slight movement of the cursor as the mouse button is released can cause some small displacement of a design object that could be easily overlooked by the candidate. Finally, some latitude may be accorded to the candidate if there is a consensus among the graders that the feature is "difficult" to implement.

The assignment of "U" signifies a strong consensus that a solution incorporates an incorrect implementation of the feature or even fails to adhere to the feature requirements altogether. Finally, the designation of "I" can reflect a lack of consensus, with some graders arguing for "A" and others arguing for "U." In other cases, the "I" signifies that the feature implementation may be minimally sufficient, but that there are significant deficiencies. The "I," like the other classifications, is carried forward into the subsequent (evidence synthesis) stages of evidence identification process (see the following section), where it contributes to the summary evaluation. Note that for some features there is no possibility of disagreement or ambiguity, and only the designations of "A" or "U" are employed.

An ongoing concern of the committee was how well the rules governing the assignment of "A," "I," and "U" designations would generalize to other tasks and to the universe of candidate solutions generated during operational testing. As a result, many features engendered considerable discussion among the graders about how to define the thresholds for the "A," "I," and "U" categories.

To convey our approach to both feature extraction and evidence synthesis, we turn to a particular vignette type, concerned with the design and furnishing of a public restroom that is wheelchair accessible. Although this is one of the simpler vignette types, and actually is not used in the ARE, it is sufficient to illustrate key aspects of vignette scoring.

As we indicated earlier, feature extraction can be straightforward or challenging. Consider a composite feature called Room Occurrences (feature code F19), consisting of several features. (These labels will be helpful in subsequent figures representing the logic of evidence synthesis.) The evaluation criterion associated with F19 is that all prescribed toilet rooms be designed and present in the solution; a criterion that can be readily addressed in the scoring algorithm. The criterion for a feature called Width (feature code F1) requires the measurement of the width of each entry door—again a simple computation. On the other hand, the feature called View (feature code F15) requires the analysis of the view of a passerby looking into the room. This cannot be obtained by direct inspection but can be determined using some basic geometry. This vignette and its scoring features will be revisited in greater detail in a subsequent section.

In other vignette types, extraction of certain features required extensive analysis and creative solutions. Some examples are provided in Reid-Green (1995a, 1995b, 1996a, & 1996b). In most instances, these efforts resulted in algorithms that were successful. In others, it was necessary to strike a balance between the idealized characteristics of the KSAs of interest and what was technically feasible given the constraints of the interface, the limits of what could be asked of the candidate and the software available for scoring. In only a few instances was substantial compromise necessary. Naturally, these decisions were also influenced by the cost, time and effort that would be required for the development and implementation of the algorithm, as well as by the degree to which the targeted scoring feature related to the ARE's purpose of protecting the public's health, safety and welfare. In every case, however, the algorithm development was the result of committee consideration of the construct representation argument embodied in the algorithm.

For each vignette type, draft algorithms were evaluated on data obtained from field trials, representing examples of typical implementations, as well as on solutions generated by the committee, constituting "stress testing" or limit cases. On the basis of these evaluations, algorithms were revised and tested on additional field trial data and reviewed by a new committee of architects. Further discipline was imposed on the process by the requirement that the evidence identification algorithms had to be equally successful with all solutions regardless of the particular vignette administered.

Evidence Synthesis. The previous section described some of the issues that arise in feature extraction and evaluation. The categorization of each feature as A, I, or U constitutes the evidential summary that serves as the basis for the overall judgment of the quality of the design solution. The transition from the evaluation of anywhere from 15 to 40 features (depending on the vignette type) to that overall judgment is referred to as evidence synthesis. This process is unavoidably complex because the tasks are so open-ended. There are an effectively infinite number of acceptable design solutions and a similar number of unacceptable ones. Accordingly, a principled approach to scoring must involve a general characterization of the solutions that belong to each category, whereas the scoring engine must be able to apply that characterization to any conceivable work product and classify it correctly.

Although it is theoretically possible for a scoring engine to map a vector of feature scores directly into a vignette score, this did not correspond to the mental processes used by the expert architects. When expert architects grade, they used various mechanisms to help represent and manage their evaluation strategy. Scoring algorithm development focused on representing the intermediate clusters of related features that could be scored and then combined with other clusters for yet further evaluation. This feature clustering approach mimics the kind of groupings of similar features that expert human graders use. The creation of clusters and combinations of clusters results in a hierarchical structure that can be easily represented, as illustrated in Fig. 4.6.

The hierarchy in Fig. 4.6 is represented as a tree with labeled boxes at each node. The topmost box, labeled "Accessibility Toilet" represents both an aspect of student proficiency and the name of the vignette that explicitly targets that ability. The six boxes at the next level, marked "Entry Door" through "Room Placement," constitute a convenient synthesis of the evidence from the point of view of expert architects. Note that this representation does not necessarily correspond to particular student model variables—it is about aspects of work products, not aspects of proficiency by means of which that work may have been done. The structure of the tree was derived from discussions with the architects and was strongly influenced by the "chunking" process they use in the visual inspection of a solution to assess its appropriateness and functionality.

Typically, these clusters contained a modest number of features and the architects were asked to evaluate a cluster based on the component feature evaluations. This process was facilitated by a matrix representation (described later), which also very easily accommodated assigning differential importance

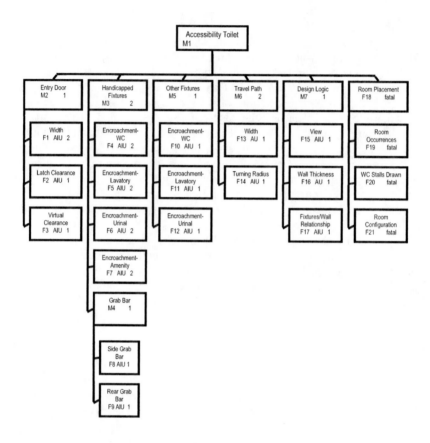

FIG. 4.6 An example evidence synthesis scoring tree.

to various features. Empirically, we found that trained judges could comfortably and reliably consider the interactions among as many as five or so features.

Typically, these clusters contained a modest number of features and the architects were asked to evaluate a cluster based on the component feature evaluations. This process was facilitated by a matrix representation (described later), which also very easily accommodated assigning differential importance to various features. Empirically, we found that trained judges could comfortably and reliably consider the interactions among as many as five or so features.

At the next level are intermediate clusters (labeled with an "M" and an identification number, e.g. M2) and/or features extracted directly from the candidate's solution (labeled with an "F" and an identification number, e.g., F3). Each box also contains the feature name, the score categories associated with the feature (either AIU, to indicate that "A," "I," and "U" are all possible outcomes or AU to indicate that only the score of "A" and "U" are possible outcomes) and the relative importance weighting (either "1" or "2") for the feature (described in the following section).

In this example, the six high-level components of the vignette are: "Entry Door," "Handicapped Fixtures," "Other Fixtures," "Travel Path," "Design Logic," and "Room Placement." The first four are specific to this vignette type, while the other two are rather more general and can be found, *mutatis mutandis*, in a number of vignette types. With the exception of Handicapped Fixtures, each branch of the hierarchy has depth two: The particular high-level component and the observable features associated with that component. The branch for Handicapped Fixtures has depth three since one of the features, "Grab Bar," associated directly with that component is itself composed of two features: "Side Grab Bar" and "Rear Grab Bar." It should be noted that more complex vignette types have hierarchies with greater maximal depths and as many as 60 features. Before describing some of the details of the evidence synthesis process, a few points are in order:

1.   The utilization of the A, I, and U categories is a type of data compression. In using these categories in the evidence synthesis process, we are implicitly assuming that the actual values of the features do not contain much useful information, beyond the categories, at least with respect to the vignette score and the goals of the assessment.

2.   The introduction of the Indeterminate or I category adds useful flexibility to the feature evaluation process. In effect, it allows the judges (and, therefore, the scoring engine) to defer judgment, as it were, about a feature, or a cluster of features, until evidence from other features is available. As we will see later, too many "I's," especially when they are associated with critical features, leads to a designation of U for the solution as a whole. This seems entirely appropriate: The purpose of the examination is to provide an opportunity for the candidate to demonstrate competence and a surfeit of "I's" means the candidate's performance on the vignette has been unconvincing, at best.

3.   The evidence synthesis process begins at the bottom of the tree with feature scoring. Once the lower level features have been categorized as A, I, or U, they can, in turn, be combined with other clusters or features for further evaluation. The process continues until the high-level components have been evaluated and their scores combined to yield an A, I, or U designation for the vignette as a whole.

4.   Some features are considered so critical to the integrity of the solution that a score of U is designated a "fatal flaw" (labeled "F") and results in a score of U for the

solution, irrespective of the scores on the other features. In our illustrative vignette type, there are three such features: Room Occurrences (F19), WC Stalls Drawn (F20), and Room Configuration (F21). In F19, for example, all prescribed toilet rooms must be designed; otherwise the feature is assigned an F. The reasoning is quite straightforward: By failing to design one or more of the rooms, the candidate has so changed the problem that the solution offered has to be considered nonresponsive.

Returning to our illustration, we note that the simplest cluster occurs when F8 and F9 (Side Grab Bar and Rear Grab Bar) are combined to form the composite feature M4 (Grab Bar). Each feature can take three values (A/I/U), so a full matrix representation of these combinations consists of nine cells. Because the features are compensatory and weighted equally, there are only six unique scoring combinations and these can be conveniently represented by a two dimensional matrix, which is displayed in Fig. 4.7. The two axes represent the number of I's and the number of U's, totaled over the two component features. (Note that the number of A's can be deduced from the number of features and the counts of I's and U's.) The cell in the upper left-hand corner corresponds to the situation in which both features have been awarded an A. The standard setting process must associate with each possible cell an A, I, or U representing the judgment of the value of the composite feature, given the values of its constituents. As the figure shows, M4 is designated A only if both F8 and F9 are A. If one of the features is A and the other I, then M4 is designated I. Otherwise, M4 is designated U.

FIG. 4.7.　Evidence synthesis for two low level features.

A more complex situation is illustrated by the evaluation of Handicapped Features (M3), which comprises four extracted features (F4, F5, F6, F7) and the composite feature M4 treated just above. The judges agreed that the extracted features should be weighted equally but more than M4. Accordingly, in what follows each extracted feature is assigned a multiplier of 2 and M4, a multiplier of 1. The process of synthesis is represented by a matrix (M3), which is displayed in Fig. 4.8. Now the axes represent the (weighted) numbers of I's and U's. That is, if one of the features assigned a multiplier of 2 is designated an I (U), then it is counted as 2I (2U) in the accumulation process.

Thus, if the 5-tuple (F4, F5, F6, F7, M4) takes the values (A, A, I, I, U), then it is classified as belonging in the cell corresponding to (4I, U) in M3. That is, the I's for F6 and F7 are each multiplied by 2 and added, whereas the U for M4 is left unchanged. Again the standard-setting process for M3 requires associating with each cell of the matrix an A, I, or U. Note that because of the specific number of features and weights, certain combinations of I's and U's are not possible. For example, it is impossible to have one I and one U, because only a single feature has multiplier 1.

M3: Handicapped Fixtures

Composed of:	Matrices/features	Multiplier	Possible Values
	F4 Encroachment - WC	2	AIU
	F5 Encroachement - Lavatory	2	AIU
	F6 Encroachment - Urinal	2	AIU
	F7 Encroachment - Amenity	2	AIU
	M4 Grab Bar	1	AIU

U's

M3	0	1	2	3	4	5	6	7	8	9	10
0	A	A	I	I	U						
1	A		I		U						
2	A	I	I	I	U						
3	I		I		U						
4	I	I	U								
5	I	U									
6	I	U									
7	U										
8											
9											
10											

(I's — row axis label)

FIG. 4.8. Evidence synthesis for a combination of low and higher level features.

To complete the analysis, we present in Fig. 4.9 the matrix for evaluating the vignette as a whole, combining the scores for the high level components. Aside from Room Placement (F18), where anything less than an A is a fatal flaw, there are five such components, three with multiplier 1 and two with multiplier 2. Again the cell entries represent the score for the solution based on the weighted counts of I's and U's. For example, if the 5-tuple (M2, M3, M5, M6, M7) takes the value (A, I, A, A, U), then the solution falls in the (2I, U) cell and is scored I.

The process described here is sufficiently flexible to accommodate a wide range of vignette types. Indeed, in developing scoring systems for more than 20 vignette types, no difficulties were ever encountered in building an appropriate hierarchical structure to guide evidence synthesis. Moreover, the tree-like hierarchical structure provides an explicit framework to guide evidence synthesis. It both reflects and encourages the "chunking" that experts engage in as they evaluate increasingly complex aspects of the ensemble of potential solutions. The transparency of the representation assists in establishing the credibility of the system among various stakeholders. It also enhances the efficiency of the process of revision that is characteristic of such efforts.

M1: Master

Composed of:	Matrices/features	Multiplier	Possible Values
	M2 Entry Door	1	AIU
	M3 Handicapped Features	2	AIU
	M5 Other Fixtures	1	AIU
	M6 Travel Path	2	AIU
	M7 Design Logic	1	AIU

U's

M1	0	1	2	3	4	5	6	7	8	9	10
0	A	A	I	I	U						
1	A	A	I	U							
2	A	I	I	U							
3	A	I	I	U							
4	I	I	U	U							
5	I	U	U								
6	U										
7											
8											
9											
10											

(I's along the left vertical axis)

FIG. 4.9. Evidence synthesis for highest level features.

In fact, each successive version of the tree structure was subjected to repeated examination and recalibration on the basis of field trial data and committee discussion. The ultimate goal of this process of "tree tweaking" was to obtain scores (A, I, or U) produced by the algorithm that were as close as possible to the consensus scores of the human graders, when such scores could be defended by the human graders who produced them, for all solutions to all instantiations of the vignette type. Discrepancies in the scores were carefully examined and often resulted in various modifications to the tree. These included: (a) Reorganizing the tree structure to better reflect the mental models employed by expert human graders; (b) Revising the thresholds for the A, I, and U categories; (c) Varying the weights associated with different nodes in the tree structure. Revision continued until the committee was satisfied both that the scores generated were construct valid and that the tree was sufficiently robust for operational use.[5]

EVIDENCE ACCUMULATION

Distinguishing between evidence identification (describing and summarizing aspects of the work submitted) and evidence accumulation (representing an inference about the examinees based on that evidence) can be a point of confusion. For some testing programs, the transition from evidence identification to evidence accumulation is signaled by a shift in methodology. One example is the transition from the if–then logic of evidence rules for evidence identification to the statistical inference engine of item response theory. An example of such a distinction appears in Williamson et. al. (Chap. 7, this volume), which describes Bayesian networks as an evidence accumulation engine for evidence derived and summarized from work products via a rule-based evidence identification process.

In the case of ARE, the distinction between evidence identification and evidence accumulation is more subtle, due in part to the use of similar rule-based method for both processes. Figure 4.10 illustrates the full scoring process, including both evidence identification and evidence accumulation, for an ARE division score. The rightmost part of the figure represents a raw work product from a vignette. The arrows emerging from this work product to the variables

---

[5] Interestingly, relatively few instances of "I" have been observed for the overall vignette scores operationally, with some having an occurrence rate of less than 1% and the maximum rate still only 23% (Williamson, 2000).

labeled f_1 through f_{11} represent feature extraction; that is, the computation of 11 hypothetical scoring features derived from the work product. At this point, the evidence synthesis process begins; the 11 features are used in the successive determination of the scoring matrices, labeled M_1 through M_4. The combination of these matrices ultimately results in a vignette score, labeled V_1. This vignette score is considered in conjunction with the scores of the other vignettes in the division, designated V_2 and V_3, to yield the division pass/fail decision, labeled D_1. The division score is meant to indicate the presence or absence of sufficient ability for practicing as a licensed architect. In the ARE context, then, the evidence accumulation process simply involves the determination of the division pass/fail decision from the scores on the component vignettes.

Because the automated scoring mechanism relies on the same process from work product to summary division score reporting, one may wonder how the point of transition from evidence identification to evidence accumulation can be identified. Formally, the transition occurs at the point when a probabilistic model is invoked; that is, when the process enters the realm of statistical inference. For example, in a multiple-choice exam, combining the responses to estimate ability constitutes evidence accumulation because the result of the accumulation is thought of, both in classical test theory and in IRT, as being the realization of a stochastic process.

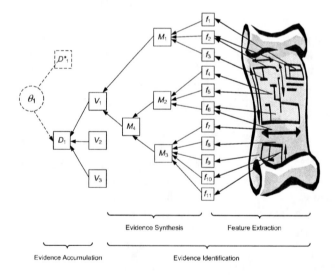

FIG. 4.10. Relationship among feature extraction, evidence synthesis, evidence identification, and evidence accumulation.

In fact, statistical analysis of operational data can clarify the distinction between evidence identification and evidence accumulation. The determination of the appropriate level for estimating score reliability signals the introduction of statistical inference and consequently that the scores at that level are generated by an evidence accumulation process. In the case of the ARE, the reliability estimates are computed at the division pass/fail level, implying that the transition from individual vignette scores to the summary pass/fail determination for the division constitutes the evidence accumulation process. The underlying proficiency is represented in Fig. 4.10 as θ_I. Its relation to the observed pass/fail score is represented by the dotted arrow to D_I. From a true score theory perspective, the criterion of interest is the "true" pass/fail status of an examinee, represented in Fig. 4.10 as D^*_I, which is also related to θ_I.

TASK MODEL

The purpose of the task model for a vignette type is to guide the development of assessment tasks that can elicit the evidence called for by the evidence model (see chap. 2). The specification of a task model (i.e., the aspects of the task to be controlled and the level of detail required) depends on the goals of the assessment. For the ARE, a task model comprises such elements as the format and content of the stimulus materials, the resources available to the candidate and the format of the work product. A well-designed task model should support the generation of multiple instantiations of the vignette type having sufficiently equivalent or predictable psychometric characteristics for the purpose of the assessment. It should also facilitate the development of a scoring system that can accurately evaluate the work products associated with any of those instantiations with few, if any, modifications needed.

The use of complex constructed response tasks in a high-stakes assessment presents multiple challenges not typically encountered in multiple-choice or low-stakes assessments. One stems from the extended period of time typically needed for examinees to complete complex domain tasks. It is not unusual for complex assessment tasks to require more than 30 minutes, and even as much as 2 hours, to complete. The extended time requirements prevent the administration of many such tasks in a single assessment session. This can severely limit the opportunity to pretest additional tasks and the feasibility of employing equating techniques that rely on multiple items and imbedded equating blocks. Moreover, when such tasks are computer-administered at secure testing sites, any time allocated for additional tasks, such as pretesting, also incurs a nontrivial expense that must typically be passed on to the examinee.

Another challenge in an environment in which traditional equating is infeasible, is safeguarding task security while simultaneously maintaining a uniform standard of evaluation. For assessments that provide continuous testing, repeated use of the same tasks enables even casual sharing of assessment experiences to provide unfair advantage to examinees who receive such knowledge in advance of their session. The consequences of such a disclosure to a testing program can be severe (e.g., Swan, Forte, Rochon, & Rymniak, 2001). One mechanism for dealing with that risk is to pre-assemble several forms and rotate them so that the content at any given point in time is less predictable. An alternative approach, used for the ARE, is through disciplined construction of vignette *isomorphs* (Bejar & Yocom, 1991; Simon & Hays, 1976); that is, a set of vignettes that demand performance of the same domain tasks, use identical features in scoring, have highly similar statistical characteristics, and measure the same knowledge and skills, but appear to be substantively different. The goal in generating such isomorphs is to have a pool of interchangeable vignettes that can be drawn at random to create alternate test forms. For assessments that use automated scoring to evaluate the work products from complex constructed response tasks, the production of isomorphs is further constrained by the requirement that each vignette be scorable using an identical algorithm. On the other hand, this constraint, if grounded in well-defined criteria and pre-programmed expectations about the nature of the work product, contributes to the rigor of the process and, ultimately, the validity of the assessment.

In practice, each candidate sitting for a division assessment receives a form consisting of vignettes drawn randomly at the time of administration from multiple pools of isomorphs. Specifically, the generated test form must include one task from each of the major areas of competence identified in the student model. The success of this approach in addressing the comparability and fairness issues that arise in on-demand testing depends on the validity of the assumption of psychometric equivalence of the vignettes in the pool corresponding to a vignette type. At the least, the vignettes should be roughly equal in difficulty; more precisely, they should be sufficiently similar so that the outcome of testing would be the same if the examinee were presented an alternative set of vignettes drawn from the pool. Traditionally, test forms composed of multiple-choice items are equated in order to enhance their psychometric equivalence. (Kolen & Brennan, 1995.) Unfortunately, the equating of tests composed exclusively of complex tasks is not a well-understood process and, in any case, would be highly infeasible with forms administered to relatively few candidates. The strategy chosen for ARE was to invest substantial effort, both theoretical and empirical, in refining the task models so that vignettes generated according to the task model specifications would be psychometrically equivalent.

Accordingly, the specifications for each vignette type included precise guidelines for the setting and complexity of the vignettes to be generated, the cognitive processes required, the scoring criteria, and interface considerations. The purpose of this level of detail was to insure that additional instances of each vignette type would tap the same constructs, be similar in difficulty and could be efficiently produced. To minimize the possibility of reverse engineering the vignette pool, slight variations were introduced in the generation of the isomorphs based on the same set of background materials (e.g., site plans or building designs). The intended (approximate) psychometric equivalence of a set of vignette isomorphs was tested incrementally, first through cognitive analyses, then through several rounds of field trials and, finally, through the national field test.

An extensive cognitive analysis was conducted (Akin, 1994).[6] Additional cognitive analyses were carried out at ETS (Katz, 1994a, 1994b; Katz, Martinez, Sheehan, & Tatsuoka, 1993; Martinez, 1993; Martinez & Katz, 1992). Of special interest were the expert–novice analyses of the block diagram vignette type, which shed light on the nature of vignette difficulty. Bridgeman, Bejar and Friedman (1999) analyzed difficulty equivalence, as well as equivalence with respect to timing and the presence of practice effects. The results were consistent with the cognitive analyses of Akin (1994). However, some vignette types exhibited considerably more variability in difficulty among isomorphs. This was attributed to the fact that there was little experience in creating sets of isomorphs for vignette types that had not been used in the paper and pencil format. However, it was noted by Bridgeman et al. (1999) that the architects who graded the solutions usually were able to advance an explanation for the lack of isomorphicity, whenever it occurred. Their conjectures were corroborated from another perspective by Bejar and Oltman (1999), who used a generalizability framework to estimate the relative contribution to measurement error of differences in difficulty among isomorphs.

A key issue in the design of performance tasks for high-stakes assessment is the tradeoff between achieving real-world fidelity and efficiently eliciting sufficient evidence to inform decision making. Another is balancing time and cost against standards of psychometric quality. A third, of great salience to the

---

[6] Akin was uniquely qualified to carry out the analyses since he is both a psychologist and an architect and, as a student of Herb Simon, was very familiar with problem isomorphs and equivalence.

ARE, is the tension between allowing candidates maximal flexibility in designing their solutions and maintaining the feasibility of employing a single automated scoring system for each vignette type. These issues shaped the design discussions and their satisfactory resolution was greatly aided by the simultaneous development of the task models and the automated scoring system. Indeed, from the outset, the goal of the design team was not simply to computerize the existing paper-and-pencil tasks, but to reconsider the evidential needs of the assessment with respect to student model variables and the new delivery and scoring capabilities.

As a case in point, previous versions of the ARE included tasks that achieved high real-world fidelity but possessed less than satisfactory psychometric properties. For example, as noted earlier, the building design division consisted of a single 12-hour task that posed the challenge of designing a two-story building that met a number of programmatic requirements. It was recognized by some that, despite its "authenticity," this division was problematic in view of the complexity of the task in a time-constrained, high-stakes testing situation. In particular, given the amount of design work demanded and the sequential dependencies in the drafting process, it was difficult for candidates to recover from an error made in the design process, even when such an error was discovered fairly early on. Moreover, the reliability and generalizability of the score on a single problem, however "authentic," is generally lower than that of a set of component problems requiring a comparable amount of time, especially if the component problems are embedded in different practice settings.

Decisions to change the structure of a division were not made lightly. They were the product of ongoing discussions regarding how best to elicit evidence about the key KSAs contained in the student model and the nature of domain tasks that must be represented in the assessment. Of course, there was great weight given to the findings of the job analysis, as well as the obvious relationships between many elements of practice and the characteristics of task models that allow for their observation. Typically, a consensus on the general characteristics of a vignette type was achieved without great debate. The real challenge was to develop an elaborated task model for each vignette type to precisely establish the parameters within which different instantiations of the vignette would be generated.

Throughout the process of delineating task models, there was an effort to balance considerations of the time/cost of development and administration against those related to the evidential value of the resulting work products with respect to the targeted student model variables. Occasionally, conflicts arose between the ideal level of specificity and grain size in a work product (from the point of view of facilitating accurate scoring) and the constraints of time and cost. In some cases, that conflict could not be settled until empirical evidence was collected.

Such an issue appeared in the development of the Block Diagram task model (see Figs. 4.1 through 4.3) with respect to a KSA labeled "design logic." This is a rather nebulous term employed by architects to describe higher order design requirements, which are usually implicit rather than explicit. The question became: What is the minimal number of rooms and constraints required to elicit relevant evidence about the candidate's level of design logic? Clearly, three rooms and two constraints would be insufficient whereas 20 rooms and 30 constraints would be impractical. But how should the parameters of the task model be set in order to obtain evidence sufficient to satisfy a diverse group of experts, while respecting the very real constraints on testing time? Such issues could only be resolved through discussion, careful review of candidate solutions and consideration of the function of the vignette type in the division as a whole.

Finally, as we indicated earlier, another important consideration was managing the tension between allowing flexibility of task performance and the feasibility of developing automated scoring algorithms that could correctly evaluate any submitted solution. Successful development of an automated scoring system was more likely if the required candidate solutions were bounded in their complexity. Even so, the broad range of architectural tasks, coupled with the realization that scoring algorithms would require much more than straightforward template matching, strongly suggested that implementing automated scoring would be very challenging. Resolving the tradeoff between task model characteristics and scoring development also influenced interface design, tutorial needs, as well as other aspects of the administration and delivery infrastructure. Lessons learned in this process contributed to a better understanding of the variety of factors that can influence automated scoring development (Bennett & Bejar, 1998).

The reader is referred to Bejar (2002) for additional information on the task modeling approach in ARE. Moreover, the scoring algorithms have been shown to be sufficiently robust to be able to accurately score not only the original pool of vignettes but also those generated subsequently during the operational phase of the ARE.

VALIDITY

Any assessment system, particularly one used for high stakes purposes, must be subjected to rigorous validation. The standard treatment of validity can be found in Messick (1989), where validity is defined as

> ... an integrated evaluative judgment of the degree to which empirical evidence and theoretical rationales support the adequacy and appropriateness of inferences and actions based on test scores or other modes of assessment. (p. 13)

It is important to recognize that it is not the instrument itself that is validated but the "inferences and actions," in a particular context, that are based on scores obtained from the instrument. The two main threats to validity are construct underrepresentation and construct irrelevant variance. The former refers to an assessment that does not fully or appropriately capture the different aspects of the construct that it targets. (For example, one must examine whether all the KSAs are adequately tapped and whether the evaluation of work products is consistent with the goals of the assessment.) The latter refers to sources of score variance that are unrelated to the intended construct. Establishing validity is a demanding enterprise and, as Cronbach (1988) pointed out, should be seen as a continuing activity involving the accumulation of many different kinds of evidence. This is especially the case for an operational testing program.

A useful distinction among types of validity evidence is provided by Embretson (1983), who distinguished between construct representation and nomothetic span. Nomothetic span is the degree of association between the scores or related results obtained from the assessment and the outcomes of other, independent measures. The analysis of patterns of association can include both expected convergent evidence (i.e. high positive correlations among measures of conceptually similar constructs) and discriminant evidence (i.e., low positive or even negative correlations among measures of conceptually dissimilar constructs). For further details, see Campbell and Fisk (1959). The acceptance by both measurement experts and the general public of a validity claim concerning an assessment and, *inter alia*, the appropriateness of automated scoring algorithms, depends on adequate evidence for construct representation, nomothetic span, and lack of construct irrelevant variance. .

Evidence Identification and Validity

Our intention in this section is not to provide a comprehensive treatment of the validity of the ARE but, rather, to focus on those issues that are directly concerned with the use of automated scoring. It bears mentioning, though, that an ECD approach to task design and the development of rules to implement evidence models is conceptually consistent with Messick's elaborated notion of validity and should increase the likelihood that the final product will meet the various criteria for validity. Furthermore, adopting a mental modeling approach to scoring also should contribute to the construct validity of the final system.

Nonetheless, no matter how rigorously the ECD process has been followed, a serious validation effort must still be mounted.

In particular, if we think of evidence identification as a series of steps in a process of data selection and data compression, then we must justify the discarding of some amount of information at each step. This can be especially difficult when the development effort is undertaken in what we have termed the "prospective mode", where there is a paucity of relevant data. These difficulties are exacerbated in a licensure setting because of the lack of generally accepted external criteria (Kane, 1992; 1994).

The implications of automated scoring for validity can be somewhat crudely categorized as indirect and direct. By indirect, we mean how the intention to employ some version of automated scoring influences the student and task models, while by direct we mean how the implementation of automated scoring affects the development of the evidence model. Both categories can include positive and negative effects. We turn our attention first to the indirect implications.

We have argued elsewhere (Bejar & Braun, 1994; Braun, 1994) that the introduction of automated scoring imposes a stringent discipline on the task construction process. Task developers must strictly satisfy the requirements of the task model in order to ensure that the scoring system can accommodate all instances of a particular class of problems (a vignette type in the present context.) When the task model itself has been developed from an evidentiary perspective, the consistency of the resulting set of instances greatly reduces the effects of one common source of construct irrelevant variance.

On the other hand, attempting to implement automated scoring can threaten validity. Rejecting certain vignette types because it proves infeasible to score the resulting work products could lead to construct underrepresentation. Indeed, more vignette types were developed than were ultimately included in the three graphic divisions. In all cases but one, vignette types were discarded because it was decided that the overlap in KSAs with other vignette types was too great, given the constraints on testing time. There was one vignette type, however, that probably would have been retained had it proven feasible to score all the relevant features. Even in that case, there was sufficient coverage of the relevant KSAs so that the committee felt comfortable with the decision. Obviously, such a positive outcome is not a forgone conclusion in any setting. We also note that automated scoring systems are both more precise and more consistent than human raters. Because variation among raters and even within raters over time is a source of construct irrelevant variance, the use of such systems essentially eliminates this worry. (Of course, this does not eliminate concerns about accuracy of scoring, which must be dealt with as well.)

In considering how a commitment to automated scoring shapes the evidence model, we acknowledge that there are many approaches to automated scoring, varying both in how they draw upon human knowledge and how they accumulate evidence. Although almost all approaches establish validity arguments to address issues related to construct representation and to nomothetic span, they often differ in their relative emphasis. Those that favor construct representation tend to rely on the logic of the design process. Those that favor nomothetic span tend to focus on empirical methods using the "gold standard" represented by scores from expert human graders working under ideal conditions.

For the ARE, scoring development focused on maintaining construct representation and, consequently, required extended study of expert human graders' cognitions as they engaged in the evidence identification. That is, we attempted to understand the processes by which graders select and evaluate relevant features, then combine those evaluations and, eventually, reach a summative judgment. The instantiation of that understanding in a system of rules constitutes what we have termed a "mental model" approach to automated scoring.

Developing such a mental model involved extensive knowledge elicitation from the graders and other experts, embedded in an iterative process of construction, critique and revision. This effort was facilitated by the fact that, at every stage, there was an explicit representation of the current model and that its operations could be studied at the desired level of granularity. This transparency facilitated the explicit tracing of the scoring rationale, thereby allowing for "… the specific reasoning behind every score [to] be inspected, critiqued, and directly manipulated" (Williamson, Bejar, & Hone, 1999, p. 159). At the same time, this work was complicated by the challenge of explicating and reconciling, to the extent possible, the natural variations among expert human graders. Consequently, the final system is the instantiation of a mental model that represents the best aspects of various graders' cognitive processes and strategies, rather than those of any single grader or of a "typical" grader.

Evidence Accumulation and Validity

Although our emphasis has been on feature extraction and evidence synthesis (i.e., scoring at the vignette level), ultimately, a critical element in the validity argument for the ARE concerns the appropriateness of the rules generating pass/fail decisions for each division of the ARE. We use the term evidence accumulation to refer to the process of combining the scores of the different vignettes comprising the division into a pass/fail decision for the division.

The ARE effort represented a departure from the conventional practice of formulating the cut score or standard *after* the assessment has been designed. (See Cizek, 2001, for a review of concepts and methods.) From an ECD perspective, the principal outcome of the assessment is a decision as to whether the candidate has demonstrated sufficiently mastery of the field to merit licensure. Therefore, the entire assessment design and development effort should embody a standard setting process, rather than treating standard setting as an afterthought.

It may not be obvious how to set a cut score for a test that has not yet been administered. Fortunately, our approach to design proved very helpful in this regard. In particular, in formulating a task model, the architects considered what evidence was consistent with someone being "above the cut" (the A vignette score), when the evidence was inconclusive (the I vignette score), and when the evidence was consistent with someone "below the cut" (the U vignette score). Essentially the same process that was applied at the vignette level can be applied at the division level, with the vignette types comprising a division playing the role of basic elements that are evaluated and evidence accumulated to the division level. Again, a matrix representation can facilitate the process. Because this form of standard setting is done in the absence of data, we refer to it as setting *competence standards*.

Although response data may not be available, it does not mean the process cannot be rigorous. To set the competence standards the committee was divided into two groups. Each group independently examined all the different combinations of vignette type scores, organized in a partially ordered tree. One group started at the top of the tree (0 I's and 0 U's) and the other at the bottom of the tree (all U's) and worked its way toward the center of the tree. Remarkably, the two groups decided on essentially the same boundary, differing perhaps on only one combination—a discrepancy that was relatively easily resolved. For each graphic division, the consistency and reasonableness of the resulting standard was checked by employing an entirely different, quantitative approach. For more details, consult Bejar, Braun, and Lewis (1997a, 1997b)

Of course, competence standards may be either too harsh or too lenient. Therefore, the final step in the standard setting process is to examine the competence standards in light of test data and make any necessary adjustments. We refer to the (possibly) modified competence standards as *performance standards*. As Bejar et al. (1997b) put it:

Competence standards can be thought of as defining the level of performance required to pass when the candidate is performing under idealized conditions. Competence standards are set by design, taking into account all that is known about the constructs under measurement, and the tasks that have been designed to measure those constructs. By contrast, performance standards refer to the level of performance required to pass when the candidate is performing under normal test taking circumstances. Whereas competence standards can be set in the abstract, performance standards require the empirical analysis of actual performance by candidates under operational test taking conditions. (p. 8)

Notwithstanding the extensive efforts to develop a valid automated scoring system, it is certainly possible for subtle flaws to surface once the test becomes operational: There is no substitute for processing hundreds or even thousands of solutions obtained under realistic examination conditions. Unfortunately, it is costly and difficult (if not impossible) to obtain such a broad sampling of student work prior to going "live" with the final version of the system. Thus, ongoing monitoring of scoring during the operational phase is not only a prudent step in support of test validity, but also serves as a mechanism for continuous improvement. At the same time, proposed changes to the algorithms must be carefully thought through and tested to make sure that consistency with previous results is maintained (where appropriate) and that new flaws are not inadvertently introduced.

Ongoing monitoring can also lead to better understanding of the underlying constructs and their links to the ensemble of assessment tasks (Williamson et al., 1999). This is especially important when one considers that, over time, new vignettes or even new vignette types must be introduced into the assessment battery, often with only minimal pretesting. This raises the potential for "validity drift"; that is, the inadvertent reduction in emphasis of important aspects of proficiency, leading to construct underrepresentation. A strong evidentiary approach to the design, development and improvement of automated scoring can both stimulate and facilitate consideration by test designers of the relevant issues. Thus, design decisions are made in full cognizance of their implications for the "mental models" instantiated in the current system of scoring rules and for the validity of the scores generated by the new system. Methods for monitoring the validity of automated scoring systems have been discussed by Williamson, Bejar, and Hone (2004).

SUMMARY

In this chapter, we have described the development of a set of rule-based scoring systems to score complex work products. The presentation was organized to be consistent with the ECD framework and emphasized the power of an evidentiary perspective in unifying task design and scoring. The process was illustrated in the context of a demanding, high-stakes assessment, the evaluation of architectural competence for purposes of licensure. With respect to the development process, the presentation highlighted both the interdisciplinary nature of the work and the critical contributions of domain experts, appropriately mediated by project staff, throughout the process. It also provided a realistic picture of the kinds of design decisions that must be made, as well as the scope of effort required, to obtain working systems yielding valid scores.

Our methodology was inspired by the expert system literature and incorporates a number of innovations for eliciting and characterizing the knowledge of experts. Most importantly, perhaps, we have demonstrated that it is possible to successfully emulate complex human performance by concatenating a large number of simple rules representing both the explicit and implicit reasoning of experts. Notwithstanding the specialized arena in which we carried out our work, we believe that this approach can be readily adapted to new domains, different symbol systems and a variety of purposes.

REFERENCES

Akin, O. (1994, May). *Calibration of problem difficulty: In architectural design problems designed for the automated licensing examination system in the United States of America.* Unpublished Manuscript, Princeton, NJ.

Bejar, I. I. (1991). A methodology for scoring open-ended architectural design problems. *Journal of Applied Psychology, 76*(4), 522–532.

Bejar, I. I. (1993, June). *Optimization approach to the design of tests consisting of complex tasks.* Paper presented at a meeting of the Psychometric Society, Barcelona, Spain.

Bejar, I. I. (2002). Generative testing: From conception to implementation. In S. Irvine, & P. C. Kyllonen (Eds.), *Generating items from cognitive tests: Theory and practice,* (pp. 199–217). Mahwah, NJ: Lawrence Erlbaum Associates.

Bejar, I. I., & Braun, H. (1994). On the synergy between assessment and instruction: Early lessons from computer-based simulations. *Machine-Mediated Learning, 4*(1), 5–25.

Bejar, I. I., & Braun, H. I. (1999). Architectural simulations: From research to implementation. *Final Report to the National Council of Architectural Registration Boards.* (ETS RM-99-02). Princeton, NJ: Educational Testing Service.

Bejar, I. I., & Oltman, P. K. (1999). *Generalizability analyses of architectural design performance.* Unpublished report; Educational Testing Service, Princeton, NJ.

Bejar, I. I., & Yocom, P. (1991). A generative approach to the modeling of isomorphic hidden-figure items. *Applied Psychological Measurement, 15*(2), 129–137.

Bejar, I. I., Braun, H. I., & Lewis, C. (1997a, April). *Background documentation for recommending pass/fail criteria for the NCARB standard setting: Approach, results, and recommendation.* Unpublished paper, Educational Testing Service, Princeton, NJ.

Bejar, I. I., Braun, H. I., & Lewis, C. (1997b, April). *Standard setting procedures and results for the open-ended ARE 97 divisions: Final report.* Princeton, NJ: Educational Testing Service.

Bennett, R. E., & Bejar, I. I. (1998). Validity and automated scoring: It's not only the scoring. *Educational Measurement Issues and Practice, 17*, 9–17.

Braun, H. I. (1994). Assessing technology in assessment. In E. L. Baker & H. F. O'Neill, Jr. (Eds.), *Technology assessment in education and training* (pp. 231–246). Hillsdale, NJ: Lawrence Erlbaum Associates.

Braun, H. I. (2000). A post-modern view of the problem of language assessment. In A. J. Kunnan (Ed.), *Studies in language testing 9: Fairness and validation in language assessment. Selected papers from the 19th Language Testing Research Colloquium* (pp 263–272). Cambridge, UK: University of Cambridge, Local Examinations Syndicate.

Braun, H. I., Brittingham, P. D., Bejar, I. I., Chalifour, C. L., Devore, R. N., & Hone, A. S. (2000). *U.S. Patent No. 6,056,556.* Washington, DC: U.S. Patent and Trademark Office.

Bridgeman, B., Bejar, I., & Friedman, D. (1999). Fairness issues in a computer-based architectural licensure examination. *Computers in Human Behavior, 15*, 419–440.

Buchanan, B. G., & and Smith, R. J. (1989) Fundamentals of Expert Systems. In A. Barr, P. R. Cohen, & E. A. Feigenbaum (Eds.), *The handbook of artificial intelligence* (Vol. IV; pp. 149–192). NY: Addison Wesley.

Campbell, D. T., & Fisk, D. W. (1959). Convergent and discriminant validation by the multitrait-multimethod matrix. *Psychological Bulletin, 56*, 81–105.

Cizek, G. J. (Ed.) (2001) *Setting performance standards: Concepts, methods and perspectives.* Mahwah, NJ: Lawrence Erlbaum Associates.

Cronbach, L. J. (1988). Five perspectives on validity argument. In H. Wainer and H. I. Braun (Eds.), *Test Validity* (pp. 3–17). Hillsdale, NJ: Lawrence Erlbaum Associates.

Embretson, S. (1983). Construct validity: Construct representation versus nomothetic span. *American Psychologist, 93*, 179–197.

Higgins, D., Burstein, J., Marcu, D., & Gentile, C. (2004). Evaluating multiple aspects of coherence in student essays. *HLT-NAACL 2004: Proceedings of the Main Conference*, 185–192.

Johnson-Laird, P. N. (1983) *Mental models.* Cambridge, MA: Harvard University Press.

Johnson-Laird, P. N. (1993) *Human and machine thinking.* Hillsdale, NJ: Lawrence Erlbaum Associates.

Kane, M. T. (1992). An argument-based approach to validity. *Psychological Bulletin, 112*, 527–535.

Kane, M. (1994). Validating interpretive arguments for licensure and certification examinations. *Evaluation & The Health Professions, 17*, 133–159.

Katz, I. R. (1994a, April). *From laboratory to test booklet: Using expert-novice comparisons to guide design of performance assessments.* Paper presented at the annual meeting of the American Educational Research Association, New Orleans, LA.

Katz, I. R. (1994b, May). Coping with the complexity of design: Avoiding conflicts and prioritizing constraints. In A. Ram & K. Eiselt (Eds.), *Proceedings of the 16th annual conference of the Cognitive Science Society* (pp. 485–489). Hillsdale, NJ: Lawrence Erlbaum Associates.

Katz, I. R., Martinez, M. E., Sheehan, K. M, & Tatsuoka, K. K. (1993). *Extending: the rule space model to a semantically-rich domain: Diagnostic assessment in architecture* (Research Report No. RR-93-42-ONR). Princeton, NJ: Educational Testing Service.

Kenney, J. F. (1997). New testing methodologies for the architect registration examination. *CLEAR Exam Review, 8*(2), 23–29.

Kolen, M. J., & Brennan, R. L. (1995). *Test equating: Methods and practices.* New York, NY: Springer.

Linn, R. L. (2001). Assessments and accountability (condensed version). *Practical Assessment, Research & Evaluation, 7*(11). Retrieved July 26, 2004 from http://PAREonline.net/getvn.asp?v=7&n=11.

Martinez, M. E. (1993). Problem solving correlates of new assessment forms in architecture. *Applied Measurement in Education, 6*(3), 167–180.

Martinez, M. E., & Katz, I. R. (1992). Cognitive processing requirements of constructed figural response and multiple-choice items in architecture assessment. *Educational Assessment. 3*(l), 83–98.

Messick, S. (1989). Validity. In R. L. Linn (Ed.), *Educational measurement* (pp. 13–103). New York: American Council on Education.

Minsky, M. (1985). *The society of mind.* New York: Simon & Schuster.

Mislevy, R. J., Steinberg, L. S., Breyer, F. J., Almond, R. G., & Johnson, L. (2002). Making sense of data from complex assessments. *Applied Measurement in Education, 15*, 363–378.

National Council of Architectural Registration Boards. (1994). *National council of architectural registration boards: Comprehensive task analysis report.* Monterey, CA: CTB/McGraw-Hill.

Oltman, P. K., Bejar, I. I., & Kim, S. H. (1993). An approach to automated scoring of architectural designs. In U. Flemming & S. van Wyk (Eds.), *CAAD Futures 93* (pp. 215–224). Pittsburgh, PA: Elsevier Science Publishers.

Petrosky, H. (1994) *Design paradigms: Case histories of error and judgment in engineering.* New York: Cambridge University Press.

Rauch-Hindin, W. B. (1986). *Artificial intelligence in business, science, and industry: Volume I-Fundamentals, Volume II-Applications.* Englewood Cliffs, NJ: Prentice-Hall

Reid-Green, K. S. (1995a). *An algorithm for determining if an object can be viewed from another object* (Research Memorandum No. RM-95-3). Princeton, NJ: Educational Testing Service.

Reid-Green, K. S. (1995b). *An algorithm for converting contours to elevation grids* (Research Report No. RR-95-7). Princeton, NJ: Educational Testing Service.

Reid-Green, K. S. (1996a). *A computer method for verification of wheelchair accessibility in an office* (Research Memorandum No. RM-96-1). Princeton, NJ: Educational Testing Service.

Reid-Green, K. S. (1996b). *Insolation and shadow* (Research Report No. RR-96-18). Princeton, NJ: Educational Testing Service.

Shadish, W. R., Cook, T. D., & Campbell, D. T. (2002). *Experimental and quasi-experimental designs for generalized causal inference.* Boston, MA: Houghton Mifflin.

Shafer, G. (1976). *A Mathematical Theory of Evidence.* Princeton, NJ: Princeton University Press.

Shermis, M. D & Burstein J. (2003) *Automated essay scoring: A cross-disciplinary perspective.* Mahwah, NJ: Lawrence Erlbaum Associates.

Shortliffe, E. H. (1976). *Computer-based medical consultation: MYCIN.* New York: American Elsevier.

Shum, B. S. (2003). The roots of computer supported argument visualization. In P. A. Kirscher, S. J. Buckingham Shum, & C. S. Carr (Eds.), *Visualizing argumentation: Software tools for collaborative and educational sense-making* (pp. 3–24). New York, NY: Springer.

Simon, H. A. & Hayes, J. R. (1976). The understanding process: Problem isomorphs. *Cognitive Psychology 8*(2), 165–190.

Smith, R. G., & Young, R. L., (1984). The design of the dipmeter advisor system. *Proceedings of the ACM Annual Conference*, 15-23.

Stecher, B. (1989, February). A national study of activities and knowledge/skills requirements of architects. Unpublished report; Educational Testing Service, Pasadena, CA.

Swan, P., Forte, K., Rochon, T., & Rymniak, M., (2001). Testing in China: Memo. Council of Graduate Schools (Retrieved on August 4, 2004, from http://www.cgsnet.org/HotTopics/memo.htm

Valenti, S., Neri, F. & Cucchiarelli, A. (2003) An overview of current research on automated essay grading. *Journal of Information Technology Education, 2*, 319–330.

Wigmore, H. J. A. (1913). *The principles of judicial proof as given by logic, psychology and general experience and illustrated in judicial trials* (2nd Ed.). Boston: Little Brown.

Williamson, D. M. (1997, May). *NCARB performance cutscore implementation plan*. Unpublished manuscript, Educational Testing Service, Princeton, NJ.

Williamson, D. M. (2000). *Statistical summary report*. Unpublished report, Chauncey Group International.

Williamson, D. M., Bejar, I. I., & Hone, A. (1999). 'Mental model' comparison of automated and human scoring. *Journal of Educational Measurement, 36*(2), 158–184.

Williamson, D. M., Bejar, I. I., & Hone, A. S. (2004). Automated tools for subject matter expert evaluation of automated scoring. *Applied Measurement in Education, 17*(4), 323–357.

Yang, Y., Buckendahl, C. W., Juszkiewicz, P. J., & Bhola, D. S. (2004). A review of strategies for validating computer-automated scoring. *Applied Measurement in Education, 15*(4), 391–412.

5

A Regression-Based Procedure for Automated Scoring of a Complex Medical Performance Assessment

Melissa J. Margolis
Brian E. Clauser
National Board of Medical Examiners

> *A proposition deserves some degree of trust only when it has survived serious attempts to falsify it.*—L. J. Cronbach (1980, p. 3)

This chapter describes the application of a regression-based, automated scoring procedure to a complex, high-stakes, computer-delivered performance assessment used in medical licensure testing. Although the scoring procedure is described in the context of this specific assessment, the results are of more general interest because variations on the procedure described in this chapter have applications for scoring a wide range of complex computer-delivered test items.

The chapter begins with a review of the history behind the development of the performance assessment of interest. This assessment is described in detail and information about the types of evidence about examinee proficiency that the assessment is intended to elicit and capture is presented. The framework for producing scores that approximate expert ratings is then described, beginning with a brief history of the use of regression-based procedures to approximate expert judgments and continuing with a discussion of the technical issues associated with such applications. The chapter continues with a summary of empirical evaluations of the regression-based scoring procedure as applied to the present assessment. Finally, a discussion of advantages and disadvantages of this approach for scoring performance assessments and a consideration of possible variations and modifications of the general model that is described in the following pages concludes the chapter.

AN OVERVIEW OF THE ASSESSMENT

History and Context

Throughout its 95-year history, the main focus of the National Board of Medical Examiners® (NBME®) has been the development and administration of tests for physician licensure in the United States. During that period, the structure of these tests has varied. From 1922 until the early 1950s, the National Board examination process consisted of three examinations taken at different points during medical training. Part I was a 3-day essay examination in the basic sciences, and it was generally taken after completion of the second year of medical school. Part II, a 2-day written examination in the clinical sciences, was taken around the time of graduation from medical school. Part III was taken toward the end of the first year of postgraduate training, and it consisted of a "1-day practical oral examination on clinical and laboratory problems, conducted at the bedside" (Hubbard & Levit, 1985).

In the early 1950s, the NBME responded to the increasing use of fixed-format, multiple-choice test items and undertook a study (along with the Educational Testing Service) comparing the relative merits of essay and multiple-choice items. This study, done using the Part I and II examinations, indicated that the multiple-choice scores corresponded much more closely with an external criterion (instructor evaluations) than did essay grades. The multiple-choice tests were also found to be more reliable; both of these factors led to the decision by the NBME to discontinue essay testing. Although the format of Parts I and II had changed, the format of Part III remained the same. In the 1960s, however, psychometric examination of this component of the test yielded concerns about standardization; for example, scores on this test were often a factor of the specific examiner providing the evaluation. In addition, practical considerations such as the required number of examiners and patients led to concerns about the feasibility of continued administration. The combination of these two critical factors led to the ultimate decision to drop the bedside oral component of the examination.

Despite the elimination of the bedside oral examination, experts still believed that fully adequate evaluation for physician licensure could not be based solely on multiple-choice items. Patient management requires the ability to integrate and respond to new information such as changes in the patient's condition and the results of laboratory tests; it was widely believed that multiple-choice items were not well suited to the evaluation of this ability. Figure 5.1 illustrates the taxonomy of physician competencies described by Miller (1990). In this taxonomy, knowledge is the foundation upon which all subsequent skills and competencies are built. The second level of the hierarchy requires that physicians advance from simply having knowledge to having the ability to integrate that knowledge within a theoretical framework. Multiple-choice exams represent an efficient means of assessing physician proficiency at both of these levels. At the two higher levels in this taxonomy, the physician must move beyond the theoretical framework and effectively apply knowledge in practical settings. The highest level requires assessment of how the physician

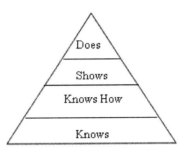

FIG. 5.1. Miller's Taxonomy of Physician Competencies.

actually performs in practice on a daily basis. By necessity, this type of assessment depends on direct evaluation of the physician's performance in a practice setting either through on-site observation or chart audits. In contrast, the third level of the hierarchy in which the physician "shows how" requires assessment formats that simulate important components of the practice environment. Because multiple-choice examinations were originally viewed as addressing the knowledge component only, test developers constructed complex paper-and-pencil tasks known as Patient Management Problems (PMPs) to more closely approximate the challenges that face physicians in actual practice settings. In this format, examinees would "manage" a patient by choosing from a list of possible courses of action. When the desired course of action was selected, a latent image pen was used to reveal the results of that particular action (Hubbard & Levit, 1985). Based on the obtained results, new options were provided as the examinee moved through the case

The fact that a substantial proportion of testing time for Part III was allocated to this format suggests that PMPs were viewed as an important addition to licensure testing. Unfortunately, careful examination of the format led to the conclusion that it was seriously flawed (Webster, Shea, Norcini, Grosso, & Swanson, 1988). Two issues proved to be particularly problematic. First, the format was presented in a printed test booklet and it was therefore possible for examinees to page ahead and review the available options as the case unfolded. This potential source of prompting created an unfair advantage for the test-savvy examinee and therefore was a serious threat to test validity. In addition to problems with the format, scoring issues created additional threats to validity. Some scoring procedures were shown to favor the thorough novice over the more efficient and adept expert. Others were limited by the fact that an examinee could achieve an adequate score simply by avoiding potentially dangerous or intrusive options. The combined impact of these limitations led to a decision by the National Board of Medical Examiners (NBME) to discontinue use of this testing format (National Board of Medical Examiners, 1987, 1988). This decision was subsequently adopted by most other medically oriented licensure and certification organizations.

Interest in the use of bedside oral examinations and PMPs reflected a focus on the importance of assessing the examinee's ability to formulate questions in a relatively undefined problem space and to integrate information over changing conditions. At least at the time that these formats were used, it was believed that multiple-choice questions were unable to assess these higher level cognitive skills. The bedside oral examination (when presented skillfully) required examinees to display these skills. Although PMPs required some level of prompt because of the fixed-response format, this item type similarly pushed the examinee to display the desired skills.

Although the factors motivating the use of these two assessment procedures may have been quite similar, the procedures differed in important ways. The bedside oral examination required examinees to provide evidence that they could formulate the problem and integrate evolving information. The limitation of this approach was the lack of standardization. By contrast, the evidence collected using PMPs was standardized, but the format constrained the responses and therefore limited the extent to which the resulting evidence could support inferences of interest. Dissatisfaction with these limitations combined with the ongoing desire/need for a standardized format to assess these critical aspects of physician behavior motivated the development of computer-based case simulations (CCSs).

Computer-Based Case Simulations

The idea for the CCS format was conceived in the late 1960s, and from the outset the intention was to create an unprompted interface that would allow examinees to manage patients in a dynamic, simulated, patient-care environment (Hubbard & Levit, 1985; Melnick, 1990; Melnick & Clyman, 1988). As one might imagine, the format has evolved substantially during its years of development.

In 1992, the medical licensure process was streamlined in order to create a single pathway to licensure in the United States for allopathic physicians. The components of the test became known as Step 1, Step 2, and Step 3, and the entire three-part examination process became known as the United States

Medical Licensing Examination™ (USMLE™). In 1999, the USMLE system moved from paper and pencil to a computerized administration format; this change allowed for the inclusion of the CCS component in the licensure process. In the current form of the CCS assessment, each examinee completes nine cases as part of the 2-day Step 3 examination. (The full test includes approximately 500 multiple-choice items as well as tutorials and an end-of-examination survey.) Each CCS case begins with a short opening scenario describing the patient's appearance and location (see Fig. 5.2 for an example). Examinees are then provided with initial vital signs and information about the patient's history. Following presentation of this initial information, examinees are left unprompted and must choose from four main categories of actions. They can: (a) request more comprehensive history information or specific physical examination information (see Fig. 5.3); (b) go to an order sheet where they can order tests, treatments, and consultations using free-text entry (see Fig. 5.4); (c) advance the case through simulated time (using the interface shown in Fig 5.5); or (d) make decisions about changing the patient's location (e.g., move the patient from the emergency department to the intensive care unit). Results of ordered tests become available after the passage of a realistic duration of simulated time, and the patient's condition also changes over time based on both the underlying problem and the examinee's actions.

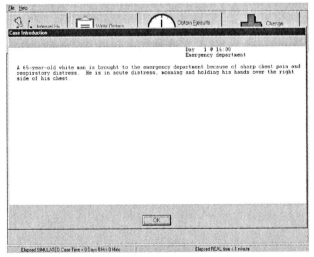

FIG. 5.2. CCS interface showing sample opening scenario Primum® Computer-based Case Simulation. Copyright © 1988–2004 by the National Board of Medical Examiners®. Reprinted by permission. All rights reserved.

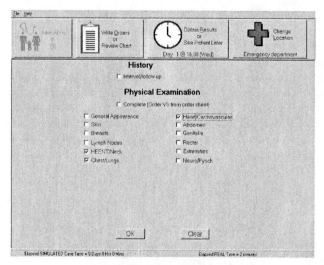

FIG. 5.3. CCS interface showing sample History and Physical Examination screen. Primum® Computer-based Case Simulation. Copyright © 1988–2004 by the National Board of Medical Examiners®. Reprinted by permission. All rights reserved.

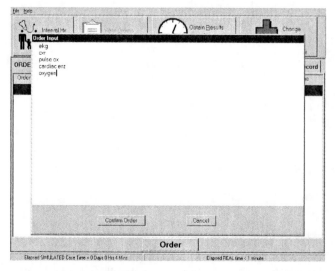

FIG. 5.4. CCS interface showing order screen. Primum® Computer-based Case Simulation. Copyright © 1988–2004 by the National Board of Medical Examiners®. Reprinted by permission. All rights reserved.

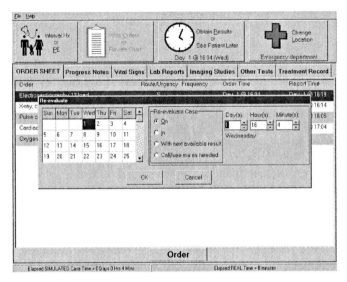

FIG. 5. 5. CCS interface showing calendar/clock screen. Primum® Computer-based Case Simulation. Copyright © 1988–2004 by the National Board of Medical Examiners®. Reprinted by permission. All rights reserved.

In terms of information produced about examinee proficiency, the intention in using case simulations is similar to that discussed for the bedside oral examination. The focus is on requiring the examinee to formulate the problem and collect and integrate new information about the patient. The collected evidence shares in common with PMPs that it is standardized. Unlike the evidence associated with PMPs, however, the evidence produced when an examinee manages a case simulation is unconstrained in that actions are not selected from a list and orders can be entered in any sequence that an examinee chooses. The result is a complete listing of everything that an examinee does while managing a simulated case; this "transaction" list is used for scoring and it includes not only the orders that were entered on the sheet but also the sequence of the orders, the simulated time at which each action was ordered, and the simulated time at which results were seen or the orders were carried out. To enhance the fidelity of the simulation, once a test or treatment is ordered there will be a realistic delay before results become available to the examinee. In addition to the information recorded for scoring, the system has the capacity to record complete information on examinee actions including a record of every keystroke, the real time at which the keystroke was entered, and the state of the system at that time. (This information can be used to examine test-taking behavior.)

CCS Delivery

The delivery model supporting CCS assessment is unavoidably complex, though it is hoped that this complexity functions to support valid assessment and is largely transparent to examinees. Both multiple-choice items and CCS cases are selected from banks of pretested items. Task selection is designed to produce a balanced assessment that meets complex content specifications so that examinees taking different forms have an equivalent assessment.

The CCS case presentation process includes links to a complex database that supports each case; this database contains more than 10,000 actions available to the examinee (comprising several thousand unique tests, treatments, consultations, etc.). Because the examinee makes free-text entries to order specific actions, the system must be flexible enough to recognize a range of alternatives for requesting any given action; these alternatives include abbreviations, generic and brand names, and acronyms. If an entry is not recognized by the system, the examinee is presented with a list of options that are alphabetically similar to the term that was entered.

As described previously, the patient's condition changes over simulated time based on both the patient's underlying problem and the examinee's actions. This requires that the database contain information that accurately reflects the patient's condition at the simulated time at which the results were requested. The system also provides examinees with realistic updates that mimic the input that a physician might receive from the nursing staff in a hospital or from the patient's family.

Development of Scoring Categories

Allowing open-ended examinee responses results in the possibility of thousands of actions being requested at any time and in any sequence; the process of identifying and accumulating evidence about examinee proficiency is therefore necessarily complex. Guided by clinical expertise and empirical information about examinee performance, experts develop scoring keys that allow the system to identify aspects of the performance that provide essential evidence. This requires a consideration of each of the several thousand unique actions that an examinee might order and making a judgment about whether that action should be considered appropriate in the context of the case. For actions that are considered appropriate (or potentially beneficial), additional consideration is given to the level of importance of the action. Three levels of beneficial actions typically have been used: actions considered essential for adequate treatment, actions considered important for optimal treatment, and actions considered desirable for optimal treatment. On a case-specific basis, certain actions are considered neutral because they do not provide useful evidence about proficiency in that particular case scenario. Finally, actions that are non-indicated for a case must be categorized by the associated level of risk or intrusiveness. As with the beneficial actions, three levels of non-indicated actions typically are used.

The complexity of the problem dictates that the classification of items is not simply a matter of identifying those items that should be considered appropriate and those that should be considered inappropriate. For some actions, this classification may change because of issues related to timing or sequence. For example, a bacterial culture may be a desirable diagnostic step if taken prior to beginning antibiotics. The same culture ordered after initiation of antibiotics may be of no value. Similarly, an appropriate treatment ordered after diagnostic steps are completed may be highly desirable. The same treatment ordered before confirmation of the diagnosis may be risky, even if the patient outcome likely would be positive. The complexity of the key development process is still further complicated by the fact that an action ordered early in a case may reflect greater proficiency than the same action ordered later in the case when deterioration in the patient's condition may make the diagnosis more obvious.

Examinee performance on each case is quantified by combining the individual pieces of evidence (e.g., beneficial and non-indicated actions) that have been captured and identified into a numeric score. In CCS, the process by which evidence is accumulated to produce a score is based on a linear regression model. The motivation in using this approach was to create a score that closely approximated that which would have been produced if the performance had been reviewed and rated by a group of experts. The first step in producing scores based on expert ratings is to recruit experts to provide those ratings. This rating process is described in the next section.

Development of the Rating System

An important requirement in recruiting experts to provide ratings on CCS cases is to select individuals from a wide range of specialty areas. After this representative group is recruited, the members are oriented to the CCS system and are presented with a case to manage just as an examinee would (i.e., without prior knowledge of the correct diagnosis). When they are satisfied that they are sufficiently familiar with the way that the case unfolds, the experts then develop rating criteria. To do so, they first identify the action, sequence, and timing requirements for optimal performance; this performance is given the highest score. They then reach agreement about a framework for defining sub-optimal scores by identifying the beneficial actions that might be missing or the types of risky or intrusive actions that could be present to achieve each score level.

After defining their rating criteria, the experts then independently rate a sample of transaction lists. Again, these lists provide a complete performance record that shows (a) each action ordered by the examinee, in sequence, along with (b) the simulated time at which the action was ordered, and (c) other supporting information such as the time at which the results of laboratory tests became available to the examinee. After rating the sample transaction lists, the experts discuss their ratings. They are not required to reach consensus; the main purpose of this practice activity is to get an idea of the way that the other raters are rating. Once they have reviewed the sample transaction lists, the raters proceed with the actual transaction lists. The ratings that result from the main rating session are averaged across raters, and the mean rating is used as the dependent measure in a regression equation.

The specifics of the independent measures used in the regression equation may vary from case to case. In the simplest form of the model, seven independent variables are used. Three of these variables represent counts of beneficial actions ordered by the examinee; specifically, they are counts of actions within each of the three levels of beneficial actions (those considered essential for adequate treatment, those considered important for optimal treatment, and those considered desirable for optimal treatment). Similarly, three of the variables represent counts of actions within each of three levels of non-indicated actions. These levels are defined as: (a) those actions which are non-indicated but non-intrusive and associated with little risk to the patient; (b) those actions that are non-indicated and intrusive or associated with moderate risk; and (c) those actions which are associated with significant risk. The seventh variable represents the timeliness of treatment by numerically accounting for the timeframe in which the examinee completed the last of the essential actions. More complicated variations on this basic theme may include individual variables for each of the essential actions or other composite variables (such as all diagnostic actions, all treatment actions, etc.).

The results of numerous empirical evaluations of these modeling procedures are summarized in a later section of this chapter. In general, it can be said that this regression-based procedure has been successful in providing a score that correlates with expert ratings approximately as well as does a score produced by averaging the ratings of two experts (Clauser, Margolis, Clyman, & Ross, 1997). The next section will provide more detailed information regarding the history of regression-based approaches for approximating expert judgments.

THE REGRESSION-BASED SCORING PROCEDURE

History of the Use of Linear Regression for Modeling Expert Judgments

The history of linear regression as a means of capturing expert judgment policy precedes direct applications to testing and measurement by several decades. Shortly after the turn of the 20th century, Pearson (1915) suggested that statistical models should be able to outperform humans in making complex decisions. As with much of Pearson's work, his interest at this time was with biometrics. His suggestion was that the sex of individuals whose bones were being examined could better be determined by parametric tests than by expert judgment.

A few years later, Thorndike (1918) made a similar suggestion about assessing the fitness of men for a specified task. Pearson and Thorndike have an obvious lineage among experts in educational assessment, but the use of statistical methods for predicting or approximating human judgments has a much broader history. For example, in 1923, Henry Wallace (Secretary of Agriculture, later to become Vice-President under Franklin Roosevelt) suggested that such models could be used in place of expert judgments of the quality of corn (Dawes & Corrigan, 1974).

In the middle of the 20th century, Meehl (1954) published a classic monograph presenting evidence that statistical procedures could be superior to expert judgments in producing diagnostic decisions. This theme was continued by Dawes and Corrigan (1974) in a paper in which they presented various examples of the robust performance of linear models for decision making. Beyond arguing for the general usefulness of these models, Dawes and Corrigan (1974) made the point that the models tend to be robust even if the weights assigned to the independent variables are poorly estimated. They noted that, under many conditions, unit weighting of variables is effective. In a subsequent paper, Dawes, Faust and Meehl (1989) suggested that one important reason for the superiority of these models over expert judgments is that experts tend to be influenced by irrelevant variables (ones that should have a weight of zero). Wainer (1976) similarly considered the potential usefulness of unit weighting and demonstrated algebraically that, under a variety of conditions, the specific choice of the weights was of limited importance. Simply put, unit weights can be shown to be as useful as specifically estimated weights when the variables are correlated and the actual differences between the magnitude of the true weights is modest.

The body of work contributed by Paul Meehl is central to the literature on the use of linear models to approximate expert judgments, but he is far from the only contributor to the field (see Camerer & Johnson, 1991, for a review of this literature). The extensive work in this area led Meehl to conclude (three decades after publication of his book) that "there is no controversy in the social sciences that shows such a large body of qualitatively diverse studies coming out so uniformly in the same direction" (Meehl, 1986, p. 373). The reader should be aware that although the literature on the use of linear models to predict expert judgment is uniform in its conclusions, the broader study of expertise can claim no such unanimity. Technical problems with the analytic procedures have created difficulty with interpretation of results (Cronbach, 1955; Cronbach & Gleser, 1953), and in general the study of how experts make decisions has been much less productive than the study of how to approximate expert judgments (Camerer & Johnson, 1991).

Given the history of the use of statistical models (linear regression in particular) as a means of approximating or replacing expert judgment, it is not surprising that these procedures have found applications in optimizing test scores. In 1923, Kelley described multiple regression as a basis for assigning weights to components of an examination when a criterion score is available. Kelley's assumption was that an assessment produced individual component scores in the form of item scores, subscores, or possibly individual test scores from components of a battery. These subscores could then be used as the independent variables and the criterion score as the dependent variable. The resulting regression weights would provide a means of weighting the component subscores so that the composite score approximated the criterion.

This combined history made regression an obvious procedure for use in automated scoring approaches for complex task formats. In the 1960s, Page (1966) began developing computerized procedures for scoring essays. He first identified quantifiable characteristics of the essay that correlated with expert ratings. These characteristics might include various counts such as the average number of words per sentence, total length of the essay, average number of letters per word, number of commas in the essay, and number of semicolons, and these counts could then be used as the independent variables in a regression with expert ratings acting as the dependent variable. Page (1966; 1995) demonstrated that this approach could produce a score that correlated with an expert rating approximately as well as two expert ratings would correlate with each other.

An interesting feature of Page's approach is that there is no requirement that the characteristics included as independent variables are the same characteristics that the experts attend to when rating an essay. The independent variables may be proxies for variables of direct interest that simply correlate with those characteristics. Continuing with the previous example, although it may be true that in general an essay with more commas is probably better than one with fewer commas, experts would be unlikely to say that more commas was a direct indicator of writing quality.

These proxies have the desirable characteristic that they may be more easily identified or quantified than are the actual characteristics of interest. This suggests a significant potential advantage in key development for this approach. The advantage, however, does not come without cost. Collecting proxy information may be simpler and more efficient, but these variables also may introduce construct-irrelevant variance to the resulting scores (Clauser, Kane, & Swanson, 2002). To continue with the previous example, although the use of commas may be associated with superior essays, it does not follow that an essay with more commas is a superior essay. Some examinees may tend to overuse commas. In such cases, reducing the number of commas actually would improve the quality of the writing. This potential problem is exacerbated when the characteristic is one that can be manipulated easily; examinees could be coached to increase the number of commas in their writing, and this could result in systematically biasing those scores.

Technical Issues in the Use of Regression-Based Procedures

The statistical methodologies that support regression-based procedures are well known (e.g., see Kelley, 1947, and Tabachnick & Fidell, 1996). The simplest and possibly most widely used procedure is linear regression based on ordinary least squares. The principle is that the weights in the linear model are estimated so that the sum of the squared difference between the estimated dependent measure and the observed value of the dependent measure are minimized. Equation 1 provides an example of the type of regression model that is used in scoring CCS:

$$y = \beta_0 + \beta_1 X_1 + \beta_2 X_2 + \beta_3 X_3 + \beta_4 X_4 + \beta_5 X_5 + \beta_6 X_6 + \beta_7 X_7 \tag{1}$$

In equation 1, β_0 represents the intercept. β_1 through β_7 represent the weights associated with the variables X_1 through X_7. In a typical model for a CCS case, these variables might represent the counts of actions ordered for the three levels of appropriate actions, counts of actions ordered for the three levels of non-indicated actions, and timing.

Estimating the βs allows the equation to be used to produce $\hat{y}$ as an estimate of the rating of performances for which the Xs are available but ratings are not. The procedure is trivial to implement in commonly available statistical packages (e.g., SPSS, SAS). Table 5.1 provides descriptive statistics for variables taken from a sample case. Table 5.2 presents the results of the regression analysis for

TABLE 5.1.
Descriptive Information for Variables from a Sample CCS Case

Variable	Mean	SD	Minimum	Maximum
Most Important Benefits	5.86	2.22	0	7
More Important Benefits	2.67	1.30	0	4
Least Important Benefits	4.03	1.63	0	7
Timing	9.55	3.09	0	12
Detractor1	.13	.43	0	4
Detractor2	.19	.43	0	2
Detractor3	.01	.06	0	1
Rating	4.95	1.95	1	9
Predicted Rating	4.95	1.68	−.66	6.96

TABLE 5.2
Regression Results for Variables from a Sample CCS Case

Variable	B	SE B	Beta
Most Important Benefits	.491	.037	.560
More Important Benefits	.087	.061	.059
Least Important Benefits	.357	.045	.301
Timing	.067	.027	.106
Detractor1	−.009	.158	−.002
Detractor2	−.531	.156	−.118
Detractor3	−1.777	.999	−.059

this data set. The ratings were on a scale from 1 to 9, and the mean value is near the midpoint of that scale. Within the linear regression framework, it is necessarily the case that the mean of the predicted scores will be equal to the mean value of the dependent measure (in this case the mean rating). The distribution of the predicted scores will not be equivalent to that for the dependent measure unless the multiple correlation coefficient equals 1.0 (i.e., unless the independent measures completely account for the variance in the dependent measure). In this example, $R = .86$. This value reflects the ratio of the standard deviation of the predicted score to that of the dependent measure (1.68/1.95). The square of this value represents the proportion of variance in the dependent measure that is accounted for by the independent measures.

This shrinkage in the score scale that occurs when moving from the dependent measure to the predicted score has important implications for use and interpretation of scores produced using these procedures. One important issue is the meaning of values associated with the dependent measure. If the rating scale is defined in terms of the adequacy of the performance (e.g., a "3" is considered "minimally acceptable performance for an examinee entering unsupervised practice"), the same value on the predicted score scale will not have the same interpretation. This would be an important issue if a cut-score were established based on these definitions. Similarly, the accuracy of the predicted scores cannot be assessed based on the direct correspondence between ratings and predicted scores for the same performance. At a minimum, it would be necessary to rescale the predicted scores before making such a comparison.

Throughout the pages that follow, the examples of application of the regression models to score computer-based case simulations use a dependent measure that represents expert ratings of an actual examinee performance. It should be noted that the expertise literature includes discussion of the potential advantages of creating artificial performance profiles for use as the stimulus material (Naylor & Wherry, 1965; Wherry, Naylor, Wherry, & Fallis, 1965). The usefulness of such simulated material is likely to depend on its complexity. The two papers just cited suggest that such material may be an efficient and effective basis for modeling expert policies. In an unpublished study completed by the NBME that used simulated performance profiles, however, the results were less satisfactory. It is likely that the critical factor distinguishing these settings is that the context examined in the Naylor and Wherry (1965) and Wherry, Naylor, Wherry, & Fallis (1965) studies required judgments about score profiles in which the relationships could satisfactorily be accounted for in a variance-covariance matrix. The performances to be judged in scoring CCS require a more complex arrangement of information that would include not only intercorrelations among the set of actions being ordered but consideration of factors such as timing and sequence of actions as well.

EMPIRICAL INVESTIGATIONS OF REGRESSION-BASED SCORING FOR CCS

This section provides a review of research that investigates the performance of the regression-based scoring system applied to computer-based case simulations. Correlational evidence will be reported first and is intended to illuminate the nature of the relationship between computer-generated scores and expert ratings of the same performances. This will be followed by the results of comparing the regression-based procedure to a rule-based scoring system that is conceptually similar to the mental-model approach described in chapter 6. Work describing the reliability or generalizability of the computer-generated scores and comparing the results to those from an alternative procedure will then be presented. True-score or universe-score correlations will also be presented as evidence of the correspondence between the proficiency measured by the regression-based scoring system and that assessed by the ratings of experts. Similar correlations will be provided for the aforementioned rule-based system.

Finally, results will be reported that describe the performance of CCS in operational testing. The reported studies describe the relationship between the CCS scores and those from the MCQ-based component of the examination. Information is also provided on the performance of subgroups of examinees defined by demographic characteristics such as gender and native versus non-native English language status.

Correlational Evidence

Early research into using a regression-based scoring system to score computer-based case simulations focused entirely on the correlations between scores and expert ratings for a sample of performances. The first investigation of this methodology applied the regression procedure at the test level (Clauser, Subhiyah, Piemme, Greenberg, Clyman, et al., 1993). With this application, counts of examinee actions in various scoring categories were used as the independent measures and case-level ratings were combined to produce a test-level rating that was used as the dependent measure. On cross validation, the correlation between the ratings and the predicted score based on the regression was approximately 0.1 higher than the correlation between the ratings and an unweighted score.

This initial encouraging result motivated follow-up work in which the regressions were applied at the case rather than the test level. This allowed for the possibility that the optimal weights for actions in given categories would vary substantially from case to case. Results for this procedure demonstrated that applying the regression at the case level was advantageous and again suggested that scores produced using the regression weights were substantially more highly correlated to the ratings than were the raw (unweighted) scores (Clauser, Subhiyah, Nungester, Ripkey, Clyman, et al., 1995).

At this point in the research and development process, there was general agreement that the regression-based procedure was promising. However, concern was expressed about the discontinuity between the logical/cognitive process used by the content experts and the logic underlying the regression equation. This led to a considerable effort to develop a scoring system that more directly approximated the rules that experts applied when rating examinee performances. The resulting system used the same scorable units that were aggregated using the regression-based procedure but incorporated these units within lengthy arguments based on Boolean logic (Clauser, Ross, Clyman, Rose, Margolis, et al., 1997).

Figure 5.6 (reproduced from Clauser, Margolis, Clyman, & Ross, 1997) provides an example of these logical arguments for a sample case. Production of this rule-based scoring algorithm is a three-step process. A committee of experts is oriented to the specifics of the case presentation and completes the case as the examinee would (i.e., without prior knowledge of the correct diagnosis). Discussion follows in which alternative management strategies, questions are asked about what results examinees would see if they ordered specific tests at specified times during the progress of the case, and problems that may arise for the less competent physician are considered. The group then discusses what specific actions (laboratory tests, treatments, consultations) are required in what sequence (if any) and in what time frame to warrant a given score on a scale from one to nine. The second step in developing the algorithm requires codifying the discussion into rule statements that represent scorable units (producing code like that in Fig. 5.6). The code is then used to score a group of performances that have been also rated by experts. The final step in the development process is refinement of the code. Performances that have significant discrepancies between the rating and the score (large residuals) are identified and in consultation with experts the code is modified to account for these discrepancies as appropriate.

```
COMPUTE SC=1

IF (B8 > 0 AND B9 > 0) SC = 2

IF (B4 > 0  AND B6 > 0) OR
   (B4 > 0 AND B7 > 0 AND B8 > 0) OR
   (B6 > 0 AND B7 > 0 AND B8 > 0)  SC = 2.5

IF (B10 > 0 OR B12 > 0)  SC = 3

IF (B4 > 0 AND B6 > 0 AND B7 > 0) OR
   (B4 > 0 AND (B10 > 0  OR B12 > 0)) OR
   (B6 > 0 AND (B10 > 0 OR B12 > 0)) OR
   (B4 > 0 AND B6 > 0 AND B7 > 0 AND B8 > 0) SC = 3.5

IF ((B4 > 0 AND B6 > 0 AND B7 > 0 AND (B10 ≥ 1 OR B12 ≥ 1)) OR
   (B3 > 0 AND B4 > 0 AND B5 > 0 AND B6 > 0 AND B7 > 0 AND B8 > 0) OR
   (B4 > 0 AND B7 > 0 AND (B10 > 0 OR B12 > 0)) OR
   (B6 > 0 AND B7 > 0 AND (B10 > 0 OR B12 > 0)) OR
   (B2 > 0 AND B4 > 0 AND B12 > 0) OR
   (B2 > 0 AND B6 > 0 AND B12 > 0)) SC = 4

IF (B4 > 0 AND B6 > 0 AND B7 > 0 AND (B10 ≥ 2 OR B12 ≥ 2)) SC = 4.5

IF (B3 > 0 AND B4 > 0 AND B5 > 0 AND B6 > 0 AND B7 > 0 AND
   (B10 ≥ 3 OR B12 ≥ 3) AND B11 ≥ 2) SC = 5

IF ((B4 > 0 AND B5 > 0 AND B6 > 0 AND
   B7 > 0 AND B8 > 0 AND B9 > 0 AND (B10 > 0 OR B12 > 0)) OR
   (B1 > 0 AND B2 > 0 AND B4 > 0 AND B5 > 0 AND
   B7 > 0 AND B8 > 0 AND B9 > 0 AND (B10 > 0 OR B12 > 0)) OR
   (B4 > 0 AND B5 > 0 AND B7 > 0 AND B8 > 0 AND B10 > 0
   AND B12 > 0 AND B14 > 0) OR
   (B1 > 0 AND B2 > 0 AND B4 ≥ 2 AND B5 ≥ 2 AND
   B6 > 0 AND B7 > 0 AND B10 ≥ 3 AND
   B11 ≥ 2 AND B12 ≥ 2)) SC = 6
```

IF (B1 > 0 AND B2 > 0 AND B4 ≥ 2 AND B5 ≥ 2 AND
  B6 > 0 AND B8 ≥ 2 AND B9 ≥ 2 AND B10 ≥ 3 AND
  B11 ≥ 2 AND B12 ≥ 2 AND B13 > 0) SC = 6.5

IF (B4 ≥ 2 AND B5 ≥ 2 AND
  B6 > 0 AND B7 > 0 AND B8 ≥ 2 AND B9 > 0 AND B10 ≥ 2) OR
  (B1 > 0 AND B2 > 0 AND B4 ≥ 2 AND B5 ≥ 2 AND B6 > 0 AND B8 ≥ 2 AND
  B9 ≥ 2 AND B10 ≥ 3 AND B11 ≥ 2 AND B12 ≥ 2 AND B13 > 0 AND B14 > 0) OR
  (B4 ≥ 2 AND B5 ≥ 2 AND B6 > 0 AND B7 > 0 AND B8 ≥ 2 AND
  B10 ≥ 2 AND B14 > 0) SC = 7

IF (B1 > 0 AND B2 > 0 AND B4 ≥ 2 AND B5 ≥ 2 AND B6 > 0 AND B8 ≥ 2 AND
  B9 ≥ 2 AND B10 ≥ 3 AND B11 ≥ 2 AND B12 ≥ 2 AND B13 > 0
  AND B14 > 0) SC = 7.5

IF ((B4 > 0 AND B5 > 0 AND B6 > 0 AND B7 > 0 AND B8 > 0 AND B9 > 0 AND
  B10 > 0 AND B11 > 0 AND B12 > 0 AND B13 > 0 AND B14 > 0) OR
  (B4 ≥ 2 AND B5 ≥ 2 AND B7 > 0 AND
  B8 ≥ 2 AND B9 ≥ 2 AND B10 ≥ 3 AND
  B11 ≥ 2 AND B14 > 0)) SC = 8

IF (B1 > 0 AND B2 > 0 AND B4 ≥ 2 AND B5 ≥ 2 AND
  B6 > 0 AND B7 > 0 AND B8 ≥ 2 AND B9 ≥ 2 AND B10 ≥ 3 AND
  B11 ≥ 2 AND B12 ≥ 2 AND B13 > 0 AND B14 > 0) SC = 9

IF (RCOUNT = 1) SC1 = (SC - 1)
IF (RCOUNT = 2) SC1 = (SC - 2)
IF (RCOUNT > 2) SC1 = (SC - 4)

IF (ICOUNT = 2) SC2 = (SC1 - 1)
IF (ICOUNT > 2) SC2 = (SC1 - 2)

VARIABLE LABELS:
 B1 History
 B2 Physical examination
 B3 Gonococcal culture (ordered before antibiotic)
 B4 Gonococcal culture (time of order)
 B5 Gonococcal culture (type of culture)
 B6 Chlamydia culture
 B7 Pregnancy test
 B8 Blood analysis
 B9 Urinalysis
 B10 Antibiotic
 B11 Antibiotic (time of order)
 B12 Gonococcal culture followed by antibiotic
 B13 Repeat abdominal examination
 B14 Ferrous sulfate
 RCOUNT Number of nonindicated risky actions ordered
 ICOUNT Number of nonindicated non-risky actions ordered

FIG. 5.6: Sample logical statements used to produce rule-based scores for a single computer-based case simulation. Copyright © (1997) by the National Council on Measurement in Education; reproduced with permission from the publisher.

The initial research examining this procedure indicated that, like the regression-based procedure, this rule-based approach provided scores that were more highly correlated with the ratings than were the raw scores produced by counting the appropriate actions and removing points for inappropriate actions (Clauser, Margolis, et al., 1997; Clauser, Ross, et al., 1997). However, a direct comparison with the regression-based procedure indicated that this alternative approach failed to account for as great a proportion of the variance associated with the ratings as did the regression-based procedure. Table 5.3 presents the correlations between the ratings of case performance for a sample of examinees and the scores produced using three different procedures: raw score, regression-based score, and rule-based score (Clauser, Margolis, et al., 1997). Based on these data, the mean correlation between the raw scores and the ratings was .72, suggesting that the scores account for approximately 53% of the variance in the ratings. The mean correlation between the regression-based scores and ratings was .87 (accounting for 75% of the variance), and the mean correlation between the rule-based scores and the ratings was .82 (accounting for approximately 67% of the variance).

These results suggest that the relationship between the ratings and the regression-based score is stronger than that same relationship for the raw and rule-based scores. The original paper also reports cross-validated results for both the regression-based and rule-based scores that indicate that the results change relatively little on cross-validation. The correlations reported in the previous paragraph are between the scores and ratings produced by the group whose policies were modeled to produce those scores. It is sensible to imagine that the results would have been different if a different set of raters had been involved. The question then becomes one of how strongly these scores would have correlated to ratings from a different group of experts. Table 5.4 (reproduced from Clauser, Margolis, et al, 1997) provides such correlations.

TABLE 5.3
Correlations Between Ratings of Case Performance and Scores Produced with
Raw, Regression-Based, and Rule-Based Scoring Procedures.[*]

Case	Raw Score	Regression-Based Score	Rule-Based Score
1	.76	.81	.77
2	.66	.91	.85
3	.78	.89	.87
4	.80	.88	.84
5	.77	.84	.69
6	.71	.86	.87
7	.54	.79	.79
8	.78	.95	.86

Note. [*]Copyright © (1997) by the National Council on Measurement in Education; reproduced with permission from the publisher.

TABLE 5.4
Correlations Between Ratings from a Second Group of Raters and
(1) An Original Set of Ratings; (2) Scores Produced Using the Regression-
based Scoring Procedure; and (3) Scores Produced Using the Rule-Based
Scoring Procedure.[*]

Case	Raw Score	Regression-Based Score	Rule-Based Score
1	.78	.76	.71
2	.92	.89	.86
3	.88	.82	.80
4	.89	.86	.87
5	.87	.76	.65
6	.80	.69	.67
7	.63	.56	.60
8	.93	.89	.78

Note. [*]Copyright © (1997) by the National Council on Measurement in
Education; reproduced with permission from the publisher.

The first column shows the relationship between the original ratings and
those from the independent group. The second column presents the ratings
between the regression-based scores (modeled on ratings from the first group of
raters) and the ratings of the independent group. The third column of
correlations reflects the relationship between the rule-based scores (based on the
policies of the first group) and the ratings of the second, independent group.
The means for these three columns are .84, .78, and .74, respectively. These
latter two values are lower than the equivalent correlations with the ratings used
to model the scores, but considering that the two sets of ratings correlate at only
.84, these values seem impressive.

Overall, the results indicate that the regression-based scores are consistently
more strongly related to the expert ratings than are unweighted scores and, on
average, that they are more strongly related to the ratings than are the rule-based
scores. Additionally, the regression-based scores correlate at least as highly with
the ratings on which they were modeled as do the ratings of an independent
group of experts. The average correlation between the regression-based scores
and the ratings across the eight cases studied was .87. On cross validation, this
value dropped less than .01. The average correlation between groups of raters
was only .84. Together, these results provided strong evidence for the usefulness
of the regression-based procedure.

Generalizability of the Scores

The results reported to this point have focused on relationships that exist at the case level. Given that the scores are likely to be interpreted at the test level, it is a matter of interest to know how scores produced with this procedure generalize across cases. Clauser, Swanson, and Clyman (1999) examined the generalizability of ratings, regression-based scores, and rule-based scores for a sample of 200 examinees who had completed 16 case simulations. Each examinee performance was independently rated by the same four experts, yielding a fully crossed person-by-case-by-rater design. Generalizability analyses for the two scores were conducted separately. Each analysis used a person-by-case design applied to the scores for the 200 examinees for each of the 16 cases. With the person-by-case-by-rater design, generalizability theory breaks down the total score variance into seven score effects: persons, cases, raters, three 2-way interactions and one 3-way interaction. The person variance is often referred to as universe score variance and is conceptually similar to true-score variance in classical test theory. The remaining six score effects potentially contribute to measurement error. Which of these sources of variance contributes to error depends on the intended interpretation of the scores. For relative decisions about examinees, if all examinees complete the same set of cases and are scored by the same raters, the person by case, person by rater, and person by case by rater terms will contribute to error variance. In generalizability theory terms, this is referred to as relative error. When scores are to be interpreted in terms of an examinee's mastery of a domain rather than in comparison to other examinees or when examinees are compared using scores based on different sets of raters and/or cases, all six of these score effects contribute to error variance. See Brennan (2001) for a more complete explanation. These estimated error variances provide a basis for estimating a standard error of measurement for scores under conditions in which the tests vary in length. In the case of ratings, the estimated error variances provide a basis for estimating a standard error of measurement under conditions in which the number of raters per case also varies.

In the case of the scores produced with these three procedures, the score scales vary considerably. The universe score variance for the ratings is .52, for the regression-based score it is .34, and for the rule-based score it is .65. Given this variability, a direct comparison of the estimated standard errors or error variances is inappropriate. One sensible alternative is to compare generalizability coefficients or dependability coefficients. The generalizability coefficient is defined as the ratio of the universe score variance to the sum of the universe score variance and the relative error variance. This is equivalent to coefficient alpha for the fully crossed person by case design. The dependability coefficient is defined as the ratio of the universe score variance to the sum of the universe score variance and the absolute error variance. (As just suggested, these values change as the number of cases and raters change.) With one rater and one case, the relative error variance for ratings is 2.55 and the absolute error is 2.99. For the regression-based scores, the relative error is 1.46 and the absolute error is 1.90. The analogous values for the rule-based score are 3.52 and 4.12. If the test length is increased from a single case to 10 cases, these error variances decrease by a factor of ten.

Based on these values, the generalizability coefficient for a 10-case test scored by a single rater is approximately .67. The generalizability coefficient for a 10-case test scored using the regression-based procedure is similar—approximately .70. The analogous value for the rule-based procedure is .65. The dependability coefficients for the same three testing conditions are .63, .64, and .61 for the ratings, regression-based scores, and rule-based scores, respectively. This suggests that scores produced using the regression-based procedure are (a) as generalizable as those produced using a single expert rater; and (b) more generalizable than those produced using the rule-based procedure. Although these results indicate that the regression-based scores are more generalizable than the ratings, these scores are not as generalizable as those produced by the group of four raters. The generalizability coefficient for a 10-case test scored by four raters is .72; the equivalent dependability coefficient is .65.

In addition to allowing inferences about the generalizability of scores, examining results at the test rather than the case level allows for the potential of examining true-score or universe-score correlations between the various scores. This analysis provides insight into the extent to which the ratings and the automated scores measure the same underlying proficiency. This correlation is of particular importance if a comparison is to be made between the generalizability of two scoring systems. If, for example, the regression-based procedure achieves a higher generalizability at the expense of a lower true-score correlation with the ratings, the advantage of the increased generalizability would be called into question. The implication would be that the algorithm was sensitive to some aspect of examinee performance that was consistent across cases but was unrelated to the proficiency measured by the ratings. Clauser, Swanson, and Clyman (1999) presented a procedure for estimating this true-score correlation (within a classical test theory framework) based on a set of scores and ratings for a single test form. The results indicate that both automated scoring procedures have true-score correlations with the ratings that are approximately unity.

The use of automated scoring systems has the important feature that once an algorithm is developed for a specific case or task, it can be implemented with perfect consistency. If the same performance is scored twice, it will necessarily receive the same score on each occasion. To the extent that the resulting score represents the intended policy of the expert raters, this consistency is certainly a desirable characteristic of the scoring procedure. However, to the extent that the procedure operationalizes the policy of a particular group of experts at a particular moment, the use of such a procedure raises the question of how different scores might have been if they had been based on the judgments of a different (but equivalent) group of experts. The results presented in the previous paragraphs provide important information about the generalizability of scores across cases. A subsequent study examined the generalizability of these scores across groups of raters (Clauser, Harik, & Clyman, 2000).

For this study, 12 content experts were recruited and given common orientation to the simulation, the regression-based scoring procedure, and the rating process. They were then divided into three groups of four. The three groups each went through the rating process for the same set of four cases which allowed for the production of three sets of regression-based scoring algorithms. Scores were produced for a sample of examinees that had completed all four of the cases. These data allowed for a fully crossed person by case by group design. Additionally, the ratings of the individual raters were used to develop rater-specific scoring algorithms for each of the cases. This provided a basis for an analysis within a person by case by rater nested in groups design.

Table 5.5 presents the estimated variance components for the person by case by scoring group design. The scoring group effect impacts four of these variance components. The results indicate that the group effect is substantial, but the interaction terms that include group are relatively small. The reasonably large magnitude for the scoring group effect indicates that the groups differ in severity; the average score across the sample of examinees and cases varies across groups. The relatively small magnitude of the group by case interaction term indicates that there is little difference in the way the three groups rank-order the cases by difficulty. The correspondingly small magnitude of the examinee by group interaction indicates that the three groups rank order examinees similarly. The examinee by case by group term is a residual error term that would be sensitive to the extent to which examinees who perform unexpectedly well (or poorly) on a single case do similarly well or poorly based on scores from the three groups. Again, this term is relatively small which therefore suggests that there is little difference across groups.

The results presented in Table 5.5 are supportive of the generalizability of scores across randomly equivalent groups of expert raters. If the interaction terms were large, group differences could be problematic. The fact that the group effect is relatively large is less of a problem for two reasons. In practice, the scoring algorithm for a single case is developed by a single committee;

different committees develop algorithms for different cases. With this design, the group effects will tend to average out across multiple cases on a test form. The group variance component will be reduced by a factor equal to the number of groups represented on the test form. If a different group develops each case on the form, this factor will be equal to the number of cases on the form. In addition, because the difficulty of the case is confounded with the severity of the group of experts who developed the scoring algorithm, any statistical procedures for equating would be applied to limiting the impact of the combined differences in difficulty. Taken together, these two effects should substantially reduce this source of error.

Table 5.6 presents the variance components from the person by case by raters nested in groups design. The variance components associated with raters are consistently small, suggesting that it is the rating group and not the individual raters within the group that is associated with the larger sources of error. This might suggest that the within-group discussions that take place as the rating algorithms are being developed lead to a near elimination of the between-rater differences. Because there are no between-group discussions, these differences are not eliminated.

TABLE 5.5
Variance Components From a Generalizability Analysis Using a Person by
Person Scoring Group Design (PxCxG).[*]

Source of Variance	Single Observation	Mean Score
Person (P)	0.872	0.872
Case (C)	1.247	0.125
Group (G)	0.323	0.323
PC	3.144	0.314
PG	0.009	0.009
CG	0.076	0.008
PCG	0.157	0.016
Person (P)	0.872	0.872

Note. [*]Copyright © (2000) by the National Council on Measurement in Education; reproduced with permission from the publisher.

TABLE 5.6
Variance Components From a Generalizability Analysis Using a Person by
Case by Rater Nested in Group Design (PxCxR:G).[*]

Source of Variance	Single Observation	Mean Score
Person (P)	0.8710	0.8710
Case (C)	1.2476	0.1248
Group (G)	0.3197	0.3197
Rater:Group (R:G)	0.0137	0.0034
PC	3.1427	0.3143
PG	0.0069	0.0069
PR:G	0.0062	0.0016
CG	0.0604	0.0060
CR:G	0.0626	0.0016
PCG	0.1314	0.0131
PCR:G	0.1042	0.0026

Note. [*]Copyright © (2000) by the National Council on Measurement in Education; reproduced with permission from the publisher.

The results of these various analyses make a strong argument that the scores from the regression-based procedure generalize across cases. Clearly, measuring a proficiency that is entirely tied to the specifics of the individual case would be problematic. However, the scoring algorithms for individual cases being too general would also be problematic. In principle, what is good medical practice in managing one patient or problem would be poor practice in managing a different patient or problem. An algorithm developed for a specific case that produces similar scores when applied to a different unrelated case would raise questions about the extent to which the algorithm adequately captures case-specific content and context. This may imply that the scoring focuses on superficial characteristics of performance. It may also suggest that the test scored with such an algorithm would be coachable in the sense that examinees could be taught strategies that would lead to higher scores but that would not improve their management of the types of patient conditions represented on the test.

To examine this aspect of the performance of the scoring algorithm, six cases were selected from the pool of cases used as part of operational testing in 2002. Performances for a sample of 200 examinees who had completed one of the cases as part of the USMLE Step 3 examination were then scored six times:

once using the algorithm associated with that case and again using the algorithm from each of the five other cases. Ratings were also available for each of the 200 performances on each of the six cases. These ratings were produced for use in developing the operational scoring algorithms for these six cases.

Table 5.7 presents the results for a sample case (Case 3). The results for each of the six cases were similar. The table shows the correlations between the rating of the performances for Case 3 and the scores produced using the six case-specific algorithms. The score produced using the Case 3 algorithm correlated at .88 with the rating of the Case 3 performance. By contrast, the scores produced for the other five algorithms have near-zero correlations with the ratings. The table also shows the correlations between the scores produced using the Case 3 algorithm and those produced using the other five algorithms. Again, each of these values is low. Demonstration of a low correlation is, however, not sufficient evidence in this context. An equally important question is that of how the relative magnitudes of the scores from the different algorithms compare and how these scores compare to the ratings. Figures 5.7 through 5.10 provide scatter plots that illuminate the relationship between the ratings and the scores. The algorithm for Case 3 produces scores that cover most of the range of the ratings (Fig. 5.7). By contrast, the scores produced based on the algorithms for Cases 1, 2, and 4 (Figs. 5.8, 5.9, and 5.10) produce scores with a range well below that of the ratings (these cases are presented as examples, the results for the other algorithms are similar).

TABLE 5.7
Correlation Between the Rating and Score for One CCS Case (Case 3) and the
Scores Produced Using the Six Case-Specific Scoring Algorithms

	Case 1 Score	Case 2 Score	Case 3 Score	Case 4 Score	Case 5 Score	Case 6 Score
Case 3 Rating	.061	.183*	.884*	−.113	.076	−.105
Case 3 Score	.118	.241*	--	−.012	.143	−.050

Note. *Significant at .05 level.

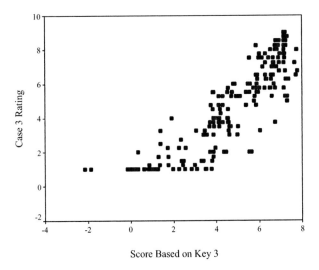

Score Based on Key 3

FIG. 5.7: Scores produced using the scoring key for Case 3 plotted against the ratings for Case 3.

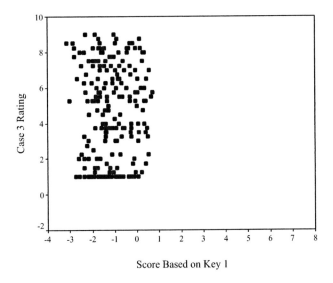

Score Based on Key 1

FIG. 5.8. Scores produced using the scoring key for Case 1 plotted against the ratings for Case 3.

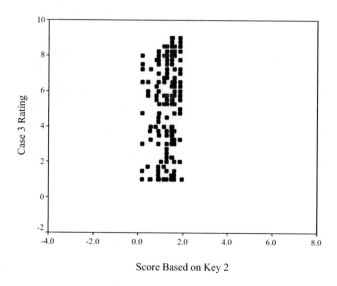

FIG. 5.9. Scores produced using the scoring key for Case 2 plotted against the ratings for Case 3.

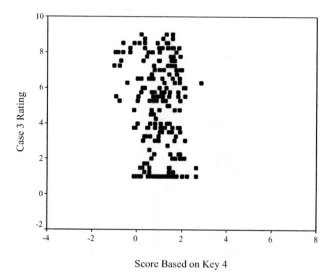

FIG. 5.10. Scores produced using the scoring key for Case 4 plotted against the ratings for Case 3.

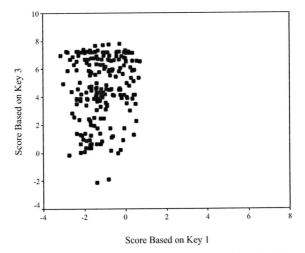

FIG. 5.11. Score on Case 3 using Case 3 scoring key plotted against the score on Case 3 using the Case 1 scoring key.

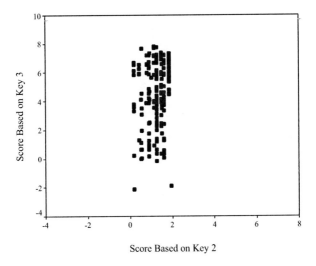

FIG. 5.12. Score on Case 3 using Case 3 scoring key plotted against the score on Case 3 using the Case 2 scoring key.

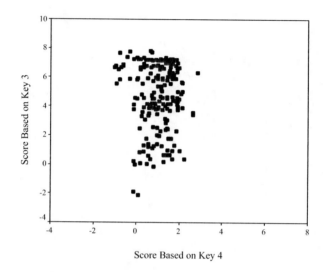

FIG. 5.13. Score on Case 3 using Case 3 scoring key plotted against the score
on Case 3 using the Case 4 scoring key.

Figures 5.11, 5.12, and 5.13 present scatter plots of the scores on Case 3
scored with the algorithm for Case 3 plotted against the scores for Case 3 scored
with the algorithms for Case 1, Case 2, and Case 4 (again, these examples are
similar to those for the other algorithms). As with the plots relating ratings to the
scores, the ranges of scores produced using alternative algorithms are well
below that for the scores produced using the Case 3 algorithm. This suggests
that the scoring algorithms are, in fact, highly case specific and therefore not
sensitive to generic (and potentially coachable) "appropriate" management.

Performance Results

To this point, the empirical results have focused on evaluating the performance
of the scoring algorithm. This section presents results that examine how the
scores relate to other estimates of examinee proficiency and how examinee
performance varies across different examinee groups.

As a reminder, the Step 3 Examination consists of both MCQs and CCSs.
The first study presented in this section examines the relationship between
scores from those two components of the test. The justification for the
considerable effort expended in developing the computer-based case simulation
format rests on the assumption that this format measures an aspect of examinee
proficiency that is distinct from that measured by multiple-choice items. If this
assumption is not justified, the less efficient simulation format may contribute to

the appearance of validity but it would not contribute to improved measurement. This study used an analysis based on multivariate generalizability theory to estimate the generalizability (reliability) of the two formats and to estimate the universe score correlation (true-score correlation) between the formats. Classical test theory assumptions were used to estimate the potential contribution that the simulation format might make to a composite score given assumptions about the proficiency that the composite was intended to measure.

In order to examine this relationship, samples were selected from the full group of examinees who completed the Step 3 examination during the first 2 years of administration (November 1999 to November 2001). Because the test is administered continuously throughout the year, numerous test forms are constructed so that any two examinees completing the test will have a low probability of seeing the same items. In order to estimate the correlation between the proficiency estimates based on these two-item formats, it was necessary to have a sample of examinees that had completed the same test form. Sub-samples of examinees meeting this requirement were selected and sub-samples were identified that represented 10 of the numerous possible test forms. For each of these ten sub-samples, data from 250 examinees were used in a multivariate generalizability analysis that treated the item format as a fixed multivariate facet. Within each level of the fixed facet, a person by item (crossed) design was used. The variance components resulting from each of the ten individual analyses were then averaged; these average components are presented in Table 5.8.

The results in Table 5.8 provide information about generalizability of the separate scoring components as well as information about the relationship between the proficiencies measured by the multiple-choice items and the case simulations. For the person effect, the table includes a variance-covariance matrix. The values on the diagonal for the person effect are the variance estimates that would have been produced if generalizability analyses had been conducted separately for the MCQ items and the case simulations. The value on the lower off-diagonal is the covariance representing the relationship between these two measures. The universe-score correlation between these two variables is shown in the upper off-diagonal and is estimated by dividing the universe score covariance (i.e., the person covariance in Table 5.8) by the square-root of the product of the variances; this correlation is conceptually similar to a true-score correlation. In the present instance, the universe-score correlation is .69 and represents a reasonably strong relationship between the proficiencies measured by the two formats. There is also a substantial difference in the generalizability of the scores produced using the two formats. For example, if the approximately 10 hours of testing time currently allocated to multiple-choice items were used to deliver scored items (as opposed to scored and pre-test items), the resulting 500-item test would have a generalizability of .93. The 4 hours (approximately) of testing time currently allocated to simulations would have a generalizability of .61 based on delivery of nine cases. To provide a more direct comparison, if 10 hours were allocated to the case simulations, the resulting generalizability would be .81 (again, as opposed to .93 for the MCQ items).

Given these results, the more generalizable MCQ items would be preferred if the two formats were presumed to measure the same proficiency. Similarly, if the two formats measured entirely different proficiencies, the discrepancy between levels of generalizability would be irrelevant; the issue then would be one of identifying the proficiency of interest. The actual results fall between these two conceptual extremes. The proficiencies assessed by these two item formats are related but not identical. This is consistent with the expectations of the test developers.

TABLE 5.8
Mean variance and covariance components for CCS case simulations and multiple-choice items from a generalizability analysis using a person by items design (PxI)

Source of Variance/Covariance	Case Simulations	MultipleChoice
Person (P)	0.1917	0.6931
Task (C)	0.0200	0.0045
	0.3160	0.0259
PC	1.0898	0.1712

Wainer and Thissen (1993) argued that, in this circumstance, it can be more effective to allocate all available testing time to the more reliable format, even if the proficiency of interest is associated with the less-reliable format. To assess the extent to which the scores from the simulations contribute to measurement of the proficiency of interest, two alternative assumptions were made: (1) it was assumed that the proficiency of interest was assessed using an equally weighted composite of the proficiencies measured by the multiple-choice items and the case simulations; and (2) it was assumed that the proficiency of interest was that assessed by the simulations. Using either of these assumptions along with the information in Table 5.8, classical test theory makes it possible to estimate the correlation between the proficiency of interest and the observed score on a test of a given length and composition (see Clauser, Margolis, & Swanson, 2002, for additional information regarding the details of how these estimates were produced).

Figure 5.14 presents results for a test that is approximately as long as the current USMLE Step 3 examination (2 days of testing). The four lines represent the correlations between the criteria and the observed scores as the proportion of testing time allocated to the simulations is adjusted from 0% to 100%. Two lines are presented for each of the two criteria (i.e., a score representing the proficiency measured by case simulations and a score representing an equally weighted composite of the proficiencies measured by case simulations and MCQ items). One of these lines represents a condition in which the raw scores from the simulation and MCQ components of the test have been weighted by the proportion of time allocated to each, and the other line represents a condition in which the components have been weighted to maximize the correlation between the resulting composite score and the criterion.

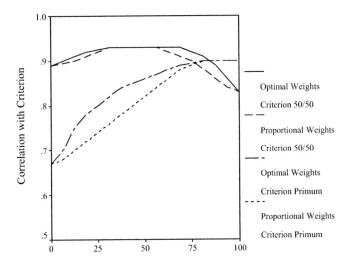

Proportion of Testing Time Used for Primum

FIG. 5.14. Correlations between the assessment criteria (differently weighted case simulation and MCQ item composites) and the observed scores as the proportion of testing time allocated to case simulations increases from 0% to 100%. Test length is approximately equal to current USMLE test length (2 days).

Results suggest that when the criterion of interest is an equally-weighted composite of the proficiencies represented by the two formats, the correlation between the observed scores and the criterion is at a maximum when approximately 50% of the testing time is allocated to case simulations. When the criterion of interest is the proficiency measured by the simulations, the correlation was at a maximum when all available testing time was allocated to the simulations. These results are directly relevant to the context in which the simulations are implemented. It is important to note, however, that these results are a function of test length.

Figure 5.15 shows the same information presented in Fig. 5.14 based on a test that is 8 hours long. In this instance, the overall pattern of results is similar but the correlations are lower. Figure 5.16 presents analogous information for a 2-hour test. In this circumstance, the pattern is significantly different. For this shorter (i.e., less reliable) test, when the criterion is an equally weighted composite, the correlation with that criterion is highest when the entire test is allocated to MCQ items. When the criterion is the proficiency measured by the simulations, the maximum correlation is achieved when 75% of the testing time is allocated to the simulations.

The results presented in Figs. 5.14 through 5.16 indicate that the extent to which the case simulations have the potential to make a contribution to assessment depends both on the criterion of interest and on the length of the test. For the 2-hour test length, the potential contribution of the simulations is modest even when the criterion is the proficiency measured by the simulations. Inclusion of the simulations is counterproductive when the criterion of interest is an equally weighted composite. This result is similar to the results reported by Wainer and Thissen (1993). Their work was similarly based on reasonably short tests. With the longer test lengths, the inclusion of simulations increases the correlation with the criterion. Whether that improvement is substantial or modest depends on the choice of criteria.

The study described in the previous paragraphs examines the relationship between the scores produced using the case simulations and those based on the multiple-choice items. In general, the results suggest that the simulations may contribute evidence about examinee proficiency that is not available in an assessment comprised solely of MCQs. It is reasonable to be concerned about how including this additional information may impact subgroups of examinees. For example, if international graduates have less familiarity with computers than U.S. graduates, unexpected score differences between these groups could be evidence that the simulations are sensitive to computer experience. Similarly, if examinees with English as a second language (ESL) perform unexpectedly poorly, it could suggest that the assessment is sensitive to English proficiency.

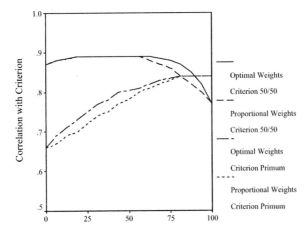

Proportion of Testing Time Used for Primum

FIG. 5.15. Correlations between the assessment criteria (differently weighted case simulation and MCQ item composites) and the observed scores as the proportion of testing time allocated to case simulations increases from 0% to 100%. Test length is 8 hours.

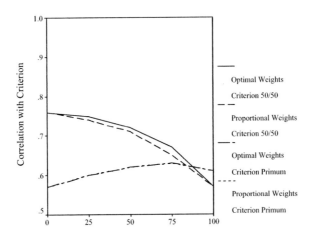

Proportion of Testing Time Used for Primum

FIG. 5.16. Correlations between the assessment criteria (differently-weighted case simulation and MCQ item composites) and the observed scores as the proportion of testing time allocated to case simulations increases from 0% to 100%. Test length is 2 hours.

To the extent that these proficiencies are considered unrelated to the construct that the assessment is intended to measure, their impact on examinee scores could be considered a threat to validity. Analyses comparing the performance of examinee groups which potentially could differ in reading or English language skills or level of familiarity with computers were therefore completed to assess the presence of such construct-irrelevant variance in simulation scores. Using a sample of approximately 20,000 examinees that had completed the USMLE Step 3 examination, comparisons were made between males and females, between examinees who attended U.S. or Canadian medical schools and those trained outside of the U.S. or Canada, and between examinees who reported English as a second language and those who did not. Table 5.9 presents the sample sizes for these groups and the means and standard deviations for group performance on the case simulations. (The scores are on the logit scale used by USMLE for scaling. This allows for the comparison of performance across examinees that completed different test forms.)

Table 5.9 shows the difference in mean scores for the various groups of interest. Because there was no reason to assume that these groups of examinees were similar in proficiency, a direct comparison between groups would provide no direct evidence of the existence of unexpected construct-irrelevant group differences. To provide a more appropriate comparison, an analysis of covariance was implemented. The groups were matched based on proficiency (as measured by the multiple-choice component of the test) and on choice of residency program. This latter variable was included because previous research provided evidence that examinees from different residency training programs may perform differently on specific content areas in ways that cannot be accounted for by overall MCQ performance (Clauser, Nungester, & Swaminathan, 1996).

The analysis of covariance showed no significant differences between groups defined by gender, U.S./Canadian versus foreign training, or ESL status. This initial analysis compared group proficiencies based on all scored case simulations completed by each examinee. As a follow up, similar analyses were conducted using the scores from 18 individual cases included in the larger pool of cases completed by this examinee sample. In general, the results of these follow-up analyses were consistent with the original analysis. A modest but significant difference in performance between males and females was found for two of the 18 cases. Similar significant differences were found for one of the cases in the comparisons based on ESL status and one of the cases in the comparison based on U.S./Canadian versus foreign-trained examinees. Given that this latter analysis included 54 significance tests, the number of significant results is not unexpected.

TABLE 5.9
Sample Sizes and Mean (SD) Case Simulation Candidate Subgroup Performance

Subgroup	N	Mean (SD)
Gender		
Male	13,093	1.09 (.77)
Female	8,874	1.12 (.76)
LCME		
Yes	13,225	1.26 (.73)
No	8,520	.87 (.75)
ESL		
Yes	6,631	.93 (.77)
No	9,580	1.27 (.74)
Residency		
Anesthesiology	1,049	.80 (.71)
Combined Med/Peds	294	1.38 (.79)
Dermatology	44	1.03 (.81)
Emergency Medicine	626	1.37 (.72)
Family Practice	2,578	1.25 (.72)
Internal Medicine	5,749	1.36 (.79)
Neurological Surgery	105	.96 (.58)
Neurology	277	.95 (.73)
Nuclear Medicine	35	.75 (.75)
Ob/Gyn	861	1.10 (.66)
Opthamology	104	.87 (.63)
Orthopedic Surgery	370	1.13 (.67)
Otolaryngology	129	1.23 (.70)
Pathology	618	.79 (.67)
Pediatrics	2,173	.95 (.64)
Physical Medicine/Rehab	233	.99 (.72)
Plastic Surgery	47	1.24 (.95)
Prevent Med/Pub Health	32	.51 (.80)
Psychiatry	1,168	.90 (.72)
Radiation Oncology	50	.90 (.84)
Radiology	324	.90 (.65)
Surgery	1,517	1.08 (.69)
Transitional	944	1.26 (.72)
Urology	130	1.18 (.70)
Total Test	21,980	1.10 (.76)

These results argue against the presence of a pervasive differential impact on examinee subgroups associated with the introduction of case simulations into the examination. Such an effect, if it existed, would not necessarily represent a threat to validity, but it would certainly suggest the need for additional research.

The absence of such an effect is supportive of the view that the scores on the simulations are relatively insensitive to sources of construct-irrelevant variance associated with the characteristics on which these groups differ.

REFINING AND EXTENDING THE PROCEDURE

This chapter provides an overview of the use of regression procedures to approximate expert judgments and summarizes the NBME's application of this approach to scoring computer-based case simulations. Regression procedures have a long history of success in approximating expert judgment (Meehl, 1954; Page, 1966; Page & Petersen, 1995); their use in scoring case simulations extends that history. Page's work demonstrated that regression procedures could be used to score complex constructed-response test items. The research presented in this chapter extends that work by showing how these procedures can be applied to a different type of response format. This research also substantially extends previous research both by comparing the performance of the regression-based procedure to that of other automated scoring approaches and by providing a more sophisticated psychometric evaluation of the resulting scores. In the research presented in this chapter, the regression-based procedure was compared to a rule-based procedure that was conceptually similar to that described in chapter 6 of this volume. The results indicate that the regression procedure produced scores that were both more reliable than those produced by the rule-based procedure and more highly correlated to the ratings that were used as the criterion measure. Analyses indicated that the generalizability of the scores produced using the regression-based procedure compared favorably to that of ratings provided by trained expert raters; the scores produced using the automated system were approximately as generalizable (i.e., reliable) as those produced using two raters to rate each performance. Additional analyses showed that the proficiency assessed by the regression-based system was essentially perfectly correlated with the proficiency assessed by the expert raters. Subsequent analysis also showed that that correlation remained at unity when the criterion was a mean rating produced by a group of expert raters independent of the group that produced the ratings used to model the scoring algorithm.

Using data from the operational USMLE Step 3 examination, it was possible to demonstrate that the simulations, scored with the regression-based procedure, had the potential to make an important contribution to the estimation of examinee proficiency. Analyses based on operational data also indicated that scores provided evidence of examinee proficiency that made a potentially important contribution above and beyond that which was available from the MCQ items and that the scores had at most a trivial differential impact on subgroups of examinees defined by gender, ESL status, and U.S./Canadian versus international medical training.

Taken together, these results provide impressive support for the usefulness of the regression-based scoring procedure in the present application. Fortunately, the general applicability of the model suggests that the potential advantages this approach offers to scoring computer-based case simulations also may apply to a wide variety of other scoring situations. Any time the characteristics of an examinee performance can be quantified and the overall quality of the performance can be judged by raters, regression procedures have potential applicability. In the procedure applied to score CCS cases, the quantified characteristics of the performance (the independent variables in the regression) are primarily counts of actions or other ordered variables; nominal variables, however, are equally as applicable. For example, in scoring a graphics design problem in which the examinee must select from a limited list of fonts or background colors, the choice can be captured and used as a variable in scoring. Similarly, the CCS application uses a rating on a scale from one to nine as the predicted (dependent) variable. Moving from linear to logistic regression would allow for predicting a dichotomous expert judgment (e.g., acceptable/unacceptable).

These types of changes extend the applicability of the procedure. Other modifications may improve the efficiency of the procedure; if the CCS experience is typical, however, fine tuning and experimentation to modify the procedure may be useful but the resulting improvements likely will produce only a modest change in the scores. This conclusion is certainly borne out if the earliest results for CCS scoring (e.g., Clauser, et al., 1993) are compared to those from subsequent research (e.g., Clauser, Ross, et al., 1997). The primary modifications in the procedure during this period include: (1) a change from modeling test-level weights to modeling case-level weights; and (2) changes in how the independent variables were defined. These limited modifications should not be taken as evidence of an assumption that the procedure could not be improved. In fact, several studies focused on assessing the impact of making some basic alterations to the regression procedure (Clauser & Clyman, 1999; Clauser, B. E., Ross, L. P., Fan, V. Y., & Clyman, S. G. 1998; Ross, Clauser, Fan, & Clyman, 1998); two of these will be described briefly.

The first of these efforts, reported by Ross et al. (1998), was motivated by a concern that linear regression may fail to capture the actual relationship between the independent variables and the criterion. For example, it was hypothesized that experts might overlook an examinee's decision to order one or two non-intrusive and non-risky (non-indicated) actions, but that if an otherwise identical examinee performance had included five or six such actions it would have been taken as evidence of an important flaw in the examinee's decision process. This type of relationship would be captured with a nonlinear function (e.g., the square or cube of the count of such actions rather than the count). The Ross et al. (1998) study examined the extent to which the modeling of expert judgments was improved by the addition of nonlinear functions. The simple answer was that nonlinear functions were useful in relatively few of the studied cases and that there was no consistent pattern in terms of which variables could be improved by transformation. The results led to the decision to limit the models used in operational scoring to linear functions.

The study by Clauser and Clyman (1999) examined the impact of making a more basic change in the modeling procedure in an attempt to produce a score that better generalized across cases. It is well documented that a major factor limiting the generalizability of performance assessments is "task specificity" (Brennan, 1996; Clauser & Clyman, 1999; Clauser et al., 2000; Clauser, Margolis, & Swanson, 2002; Margolis, Clauser, Swanson, & Boulet, 2003; Swanson, Norman, & Linn, 1995). From a generalizability perspective, this source of error variance is associated with the examinee by task interaction. Clauser and Clyman (1999) hypothesized that it might be possible to produce a more generalizable score for the computer-based case simulations if the criterion used in modeling the scores (the dependent measure) represented a more general examinee proficiency in patient management rather than the judged performance on the specific case. Following this logic, regressions were implemented to estimate weights for the same set of scoring elements used in the previously described scoring procedure, but with a dependent measure that represented the mean rating received by that examinee across a set of 16 cases. Again, the hypothesis was that weights derived in this way would appropriately represent the relationship between the independent measure on the specific case and examinee case management across cases. The result was, in fact, a more generalizable score. Unfortunately, the correlation between the resulting test scores and the criterion (the test score based on expert ratings) did not increase. This result suggests that the true correlation between the scores and the ratings decreased; such a decrease is a threat to score validity because it indicates that the procedure was capturing systematic construct-irrelevant variance. As with the previous research, the results led to a decision not to pursue this methodology for use in operational testing.

The fact that the two studies described in the previous paragraphs represented Research and Development projects that were not subsequently included in the operational procedure might be considered both good news and bad. Both studies were motivated by the desire to improve the procedure; the subsequent realization that these procedures would not improve the operational test was therefore somewhat disappointing. At the same time, an alternative interpretation of the "bad news" suggests that it is actually good news that the simple version of the regression-based procedure is so useful and so difficult to improve. It suggests that test developers wishing to examine the feasibility of a regression-based procedure for automated scoring of a computer-delivered performance assessment can expect conclusive answers based on reasonably simple models.

The flexibility and simplicity of simple regression models has proven to be extremely effective in the application described in this chapter. These positive results have led to efforts to apply similar procedures to the scoring of other types of complex performance assessments. The first of these used a regression procedure to weight items on a checklist used to score examinees on a performance assessment of physicians' clinical skills (Clauser, Margolis, Ross, Nungester, & Klass, 1997). Optimal weights were derived to produce weighted checklist scores that approximated the rating that expert clinicians gave to the same performances. The results suggested that, depending on the clinical context, these weights could improve the relationship between the scores and the ratings substantially. Such an improvement has the potential to enhance the validity of resulting test scores.

More recently, regression-based procedures were used as part of a process for scoring patient notes (Swygert, Margolis, King, Siftar, & Clyman, 2003). As in the previous application, these notes were written by examinees as part of a performance assessment of physicians' clinical skills. After interviewing an individual trained to play the part of a patient and completing a physical examination, the examinees recorded their findings and impressions in a structured patient note. The notes were entered online and the electronic file was then scored using software that assesses the similarity between the content of that note and notes having predefined scores produced by expert raters. The software produced six subscores for each note. These subscores were then combined using a regression procedure that maximized the relationship between the weighted composite score and the expert rating of the same performance. The resulting cross-validated score was shown to correlate with the ratings of a group of expert judges more highly than an individual expert's ratings would correlate with the ratings of that same group of experts. Examination of the potential to use this technology in large-scale, high-stakes testing is ongoing.

These examples of applications of regression-based procedures are all within the realm of medical education. By extension, it is clear that applications of this approach would be beneficial in any situation where a large number of expert ratings would be needed to assess the quality of complex performance assessment tasks.

CONCLUSIONS

Although the potential broad application of these models makes them attractive, their use for scoring complex examination formats is not necessarily simple and is certainly not likely to be inexpensive. The development of the keyed information to which the regression models are applied is time consuming and the iterative quality assurance procedures required to insure that the algorithm is functioning properly are labor intensive. It should be remembered that although the computer can apply these algorithms with great efficiency, if errors exist in the algorithm, the computer will make errors with equal efficiency. In small-scale testing applications, these steps are likely to make automated scoring procedures more expensive than the use of expert raters. It is also important to note that much of the research reported in this chapter is also basic validity evidence for the specific application; much of this research would need to be repeated in a new application.

As the use of computers in test delivery becomes more commonplace, it is likely that test developers will make increasing use of the potential to deliver complex constructed-response item formats. For these formats to be efficient, it will be necessary for the computer to be responsible not only for item administration but also for item scoring. This chapter has described a regression-based procedure for scoring such complex constructed-response items. Continued application of this procedure has considerable potential to provide practitioners in a variety of fields with an efficient means of producing scores for complex, large-scale assessments.

REFERENCES

Brennan, R. L. (1996). Generalizability of performance assessments. In G. W. Phillips (Ed.), *Technical issues in large-scale performance assessments* (pp. 19–58). Washington, DC: National Center for Educational Statistics.

Brennan, R. L. (2001). *Generalizability theory*. New York: Springer-Verlag.

Camerer, C. F., & Johnson, E. J. (1991). The process performance paradox in expert judgment: How can experts know so much and predict so badly? In K. A. Ericsson & J. Smith (Eds.), *Toward a general theory of expertise: Prospects and limits* (pp. 195–217). New York: Cambridge University Press.

Clauser, B. E., & Clyman, S. G. (1999, April). *A strategy for increasing the generalizability of scores for performance assessments scored with automated scoring algorithms.* Paper presented at the Annual Meeting of The American Educational Research Association, Montreal.

Clauser, B. E., Harik, P., & Clyman, S. G. (2000). The generalizability of scores for a performance assessment scored with a computer-automated scoring system. *Journal of Educational Measurement, 37,* 245–262.

Clauser, B. E., Kane, M. T., & Swanson, D. B. (2002). Validity issues for performance based tests scored with computer-automated scoring systems. *Applied Measurement in Education, 15,* 413–432.

Clauser, B. E., Margolis, M. J., Clyman, S. G., & Ross, L. P. (1997). Development of automated scoring algorithms for complex performance assessments: A comparison of two approaches. *Journal of Educational Measurement, 34,* 141–161.

Clauser, B. E., Margolis, M. J., Ross, L. P., Nungester, R. J., & Klass, D. K. (1997). Regression-based weighting of items on standardized patient checklists. In A. J. J. A. Scherpbier, C. M. P. Van der Vleuten, J. J. Rethans, & A. F. W. Steeg (Eds.) *Advances in medical education* (pp. 420–423). Dordrecht: Kluwer.

Clauser, B. E., Margolis, M. J., & Swanson, D. B. (2002). An examination of the contribution of the computer-based case simulations to the USMLE Step 3 examination. *Academic Medicine, 77* (RIME Supplement), S80–S82.

Clauser, B. E., Nungester, R. J., & Swaminathan, H. (1996). Improving the matching for DIF analysis by conditioning on both test score and an educational background variable. *Journal of Educational Measurement, 33,* 453–464.

Clauser, B. E., Ross, L. P., Fan, V. Y., & Clyman, S. G. (1998). A comparison of two approaches for modeling expert judgment in scoring a performance assessment of physicians' patient-management skills. *Academic Medicine, 73* (RIME Supplement), S117–S119.

Clauser, B. E., Subhiyah, R., Piemme, T. E., Greenberg, L., Clyman, S. G., Ripkey, D. R., & Nungester, R. J. (1993). Using clinician ratings to model score weights for a computer simulation performance assessment. *Academic Medicine, 68* (RIME Supplement), S64–S67.

Clauser, B. E., Subhiyah R., Nungester R. J., Ripkey D. R., Clyman S. G., & McKinley D. (1995). Scoring a performance-based assessment by modeling the judgments of experts. *Journal of Educational Measurement, 32,* 397–415.

Clauser, B. E., Ross, L. P., Clyman, S. G., Rose, K. M., Margolis, M. J., Nungester, R. J., Piemme, T. E., Pinceti, P. S., Chang, L., El-Bayoumi, G., & Malakoff, G. L. (1997). Developing a scoring algorithm to replace expert rating for scoring a complex performance based assessment. *Applied Measurement in Education, 10,* 345–358.

Clauser, B. E., Swanson, D. B., & Clyman, S. G. (1999). A comparison of the generalizability of scores produced by expert raters and automated scoring systems. *Applied Measurement in Education, 12,* 281–299.

Cronbach, L. J. (1955). Processes affecting scores on "understanding of others" and "assumed similarity." *Psychological Bulletin, 52,* 177–194.

Cronbach, L. J. (1980). Validity on parole: How can we go straight? *New directions for testing and measurement: Measuring achievement over a decade, 5* (pp. 99–108). San Francisco: Jossey-Bass.

Cronbach, L. J., & Gleser, G. C. (1953). Assessing similarity between profiles. *Psychological Bulletin, 50,* 456–473.

Dawes, R. M., & Corrigan, B. (1979). Linear models in decision making. *Psychological Bulletin, 81,* 95–106.

Dawes, R. M., Faust, D., & Meehl, P. E. (1989). Clinical versus actuarial judgment. *Science, 243,* 1668–1674.

Hubbard, J. P., & Levit, E. J. (1985). *The National Board of Medical Examiners: The first seventy years.* Philadelphia: National Board of Medical Examiners.

Kelley, T. L. (1924). *Statistical method.* New York: The Macmillan Company.

Kelley, T. L. (1947). *Fundamentals of statistics.* Cambridge, MA: Harvard University Press.

Margolis, M. J., Clauser, B. E., Swanson, D. B., & Boulet, J. (2003). Analysis of the relationship between score components on a standardized patient clinical skills examination. *Academic Medicine, 78*(Supplement), S68–S71.

Meehl, P. E. (1954). *Clinical versus statistical prediction.* Minneapolis, MN: University of Minnesota Press.

Meehl, P. E. (1986). Causes and effects of my disturbing little book. *Journal of Personality Assessment, 50,* 370–375.

Melnick, D. (1990). Computer-based clinical simulation: State of the art. *Evaluation in the Health Professions, 13,* 104–120.

Melnick, D., & Clyman, S.G. (1988). Computer-based simulations in the evaluation of physicians' clinical competence. *Machine-Mediated Learning, 2,* 257–269.

Miller, G.E. (1990). The assessment of clinical skills/competence/performance. *Academic Medicine,* S63–67.

National Board of Medical Examiners (1987). *Bulletin of information and description of national board examinations.* Philadelphia, PA: National Board of Medical Examiners.

National Board of Medical Examiners (1988). *Bulletin of information and description of national board examinations.* Philadelphia, PA: National Board of Medical Examiners.

Naylor, J. C., & Wherry, R. J., Sr. (1965). The use of simulated stimuli and the "JAN" technique to capture and cluster the policies of raters. *Educational and Psychological Measurement, 25*(4), 969–986.

Page, E. B. (1966). Grading essays by computer: Progress report. *Proceedings of the 1966 Invitational Conference on Testing.* Princeton NJ: Educational Testing Service.

Page, E. B., & Petersen, N. S. (1995). The computer moves into essay grading. *Phi Delta Kappan, 76,* 561–565.

Pearson, K. (1915). On the problem of sexing osteometric material. *Biometrika, 10,* 479–487.

Ross, L. P., Clauser, B. E., Fan, V. Y., & Clyman, S. G. (1998, April). *An examination of alternative models for automated scoring of a computer-delivered performance assessment.* Paper presented at the Annual Meeting of the American Educational Research Association, San Diego.

Sebrechts, M. M., Bennett, R. E., & Rock, D. A. (1991). Agreement between expert-system and human raters on complex constructed-response quantitative items. *Journal of Applied Psychology, 76,* 856–862.

Swanson, D. B., Norman, G. R., & Linn, R. (1995). Performance-based assessment: Lessons from the health professions. *Educational Researcher, 24*(5), 5–11, 35.

Swygert, K., Margolis, M. J., King, A. M., Siftar, T, Clyman, S. G., Hawkins, R., & Clauser, B. E. (2003). Evaluation of an automated procedure for scoring patient notes as part of a clinical skills examination. *Academic Medicine, 78*(Supplement), S75–S77.

Tabachnick, B.G., & Fidell, L. S. (1996). *Using multivariate statistics.* New York: Harper Collins College Publishers.

Thorndike, E. L. (1918). Fundamental theorems in judging men. *Journal of Applied Psychology, 2,* 67–76.

Wainer, H. (1976). Estimating coefficients in linear models: It don't make no nevermind. *Psychological Bulletin, 83,* 213–217.

Wainer, H., & Thissen, D. (1993). Combining multiple-choice and constructed-response test scores: Toward a Marxist theory of test construction. *Applied Measurement in Education, 6,* 103–118.

Webster, G. D., Shea, J. A., Norcini, J. J., Grosso, L. J., & Swanson, D. B. (1988). Strategies in comparison of methods for scoring patient management problems. *Evaluation in the Health Professions, 11*, 231–248.

Wherry, R. J. Sr., Naylor, J. C., Wherry, R. J. Jr., & Fallis, R. F. (1965). Generating multiple samples of multivariate data with arbitrary population parameters. *Psychometrica, 30*, 303–313.

6

An Application of Testlet Response Theory in the Scoring of a Complex Certification Exam

Howard Wainer
National Board of Medical Examiners

Lisa M. Brown
American Board of Internal Medicine

Eric T. Bradlow
The Wharton School of the University of Pennsylvania

Xiaohui Wang
University of North Carolina

William P. Skorupski
University of Massachusetts

John Boulet
Educational Commission for Foreign Medical Graduates

Robert J. Mislevy
University of Maryland

> *The sciences do not try to explain, they hardly even try to interpret, they mainly make models. By a model is meant a mathematical construct which, with the addition of certain verbal interpretations, describes observed phenomena .The justification of such a mathematical construct is solely and precisely that it is expected to work.*—Johann Von Neumann; retrieved January, 2006, from www.quotationspage.com.

I: INTRODUCTION

What Is a Testlet?

In 1987 Howard Wainer and Gerald Kiely coined the term *testlet* to represent a unit, generally smaller than the entire test, out of which the test is constructed. A testlet might be a reading passage and a set of items associated with it; it might be a graph followed by a set of items; or it might be a data set and associated items that perhaps ask about the validity of certain inferences from those data.

At an extreme, a testlet could be a single item, or it could be the entire test, although both of these are degenerate cases of the concept. Thus, in a very general sense, virtually all tests are constructed of testlets.

The idea of a testlet can be extended to the context of more complex performance tasks than those listed previously, when multiple aspects or components of the same performance are evaluated; that is, in terms of evidence-centered design (ECD) models (Mislevy, Steinberg, & Almond, 2003), the work product(s) from a given task provide values for a set of observable variables. The issue of conditional dependence within such a set arises regardless of whether the values have been determined by score-key matching, human judgment, or automated scoring procedures. Testlet response theory therefore addresses a problem of test scoring, or evidence accumulation, as opposed to a problem of item scoring, or evidence identification.

How Are Tests Made Up of Testlets Scored?

What makes a multi-item testlet special is the mutual dependence among the items within the testlet caused by some common element (e.g., all based on a common passage, a common figure). If all items relate to the same passage, for example, and the examinee has a poor understanding of the passage, he or she will probably not do as well on all the items relating to that passage.

It is useful at this point to distinguish between item-level scoring (evidence identification) and test-level scoring (evidence accumulation). Item-level scoring concerns the evaluation of students' work in order to produce values of the variables that will be addressed with a test-level statistical model. The determination of a whether each multiple-choice item response is right or wrong, for example, is a phase of evidence identification. The analysis of the resulting vector of responses with an item response theory (IRT) model is evidence accumulation.

Traditionally, analyses of item-based tests with common stimulus materials have ignored any local dependence caused by the testlet structure of the test. That is, a vector of right/wrong scores was determined, and analyzed with an IRT model that assumed the responses were conditionally independent given the ability parameter in the model. Prior research has shown that this practice, while not being formally correct, has not led to serious difficulties because the length of testlets in professionally produced tests were typically modest (e.g., 4 to 5 items per reading passage) and because test developers aimed the questions at different features of the materials or different aspects of knowledge. In addition, ignoring the local dependence has no practical effect on the estimate of the examinee's ability, although it does induce an overestimate, sometimes substantial, of the precision of measurement (Sireci, Wainer, & Thissen, 1991). These conservative characteristics of traditional testlets limit the impact of local dependence. As they are exceeded, which can occur with more complex computerized simulations, the increasing impact of local dependence on estimation jeopardizes conditionally-independence IRT evidence accumulation processes.

Initial attempts to deal with the local dependence caused by testlets scored a test that was comprised of binary items with a polytomous IRT model and treated each testlet as a single polytomous item score (e.g., Sireci, Wainer, & Thissen, 1991; Wainer & Lewis, 1990). This process collapsed the information across the individual items that comprise a testlet into a single, aggregated, observable variable (effectively a second phase of evidence identification). These testlet-level aggregates were then treated, appropriately, as conditionally independent for test scoring, using an IRT model designed for polytomous responses. This approach was generally successful and was used in operational programs (e.g., Wainer, 1995), but had some important drawbacks. One drawback was that scoring a testlet only using the number of binary items within it that were responded to correctly was inefficient because it ignored the pattern of correct responses. Another drawback was that the parameters of polytomous IRT models are harder to interpret than the better know parameterizations for binary items. Thus in those circumstances where a polytomous representation can be avoided interpretation can be facilitated. As we show, this is not always possible.

These problems were overcome with the development and refinement of Testlet Response Theory—TRT (Bradlow, Wainer, & Wang, 1999; Glas, Wainer, & Bradlow, 2000; Wainer, Bradlow, & Du, 2000; Wang, Bradlow, & Wainer, 2002). Although the observable variables from the original item scoring are again obtained from item-level scoring, the test-level scoring is carried out using a model that accounts for the conditional dependence among items within testlets. The model proposed for this adds an additional parameter to the usual IRT model that represents an interaction between the examinee and the testlet. This parameter, $\gamma_{id(j)}$, the effect of administering testlet d(j) to examinee i, allows the model to represent within testlet dependence while maintaining all of the advantages of standard IRT test scoring models.

How Can This New Model Be Used?

Although this new model is sufficiently general to be used on almost any sort of test, its benefits manifest themselves most when it is applied to a test made up of testlets that are of a nontrivial size. We demonstrate its use in the scoring of a clinical skills assessment taken by graduates of international medical schools seeking certification. This is a high-stakes exam where physician candidates must demonstrate their ability to effectively interview and examine a series of patients in a variety of clinical encounters. In this chapter, we analyze the performance of the approximately 6,000 doctors on a set of 60,000 encounters treating each clinical encounter as a testlet. Although these particular data have not been produced by an automated scoring method, the same problem of conditional dependence and the same solution of testlet response theory applies to automated scoring when multiple observable variables are evaluated from the same complex performance.

Outline of This Chapter

In Part II, we describe the test to which we apply our model and some of the inferences we want to draw from the scores. In Part III, we describe the testlet model and the estimation method. Part IV contains the results obtained from fitting the model to these data; and, finally, in Part V we describe the inferences that can be made and compare these results with what we would have inferred using an alternative method.[1]

II: CLINICAL SKILLS ASSESSMENT—BACKGROUND AND SCORING

The use of performance assessments for high-stakes certification and licensure decisions is becoming more prevalent (Ben David, Klass, Boulet, DeChamplain, King, et al., 1999; Educational Commission for Foreign Medical Graduates (ECFMG), 1999; Reznick, Blackmore, Dauphinee, Rothman, & Smee, 1996; Whelan, 2000). In medicine, standardized, structured, clinical evaluations have been used for a number of years to assess the clinical skills of medical students. These types of assessments commonly employ standardized patients (SPs), laypeople who are trained to model the actions, mannerisms, and conditions of real patients. The use of such "high-fidelity" performance tasks in the evaluation process ensures that important skills, not easily measured via traditional paper-and-pencil assessment methods, are evaluated.

The utility, reliability, and validity of performance assessments in the field of medicine, have been reported by various authors (Boulet, McKinley, Norcini,

---

[1]The alternative method we are referring to here is the scoring procedure that is currently in use by the Educational Commission for Foreign Medical Graduates, the organization that administers the test we analyze here.

& Whelan, 2002; Brailovsky & Grand'Maison, 2000; Swanson, Norman, & Linn, 1995; Vu & Barrows, 1994). Unfortunately, these types of evaluations can vary widely in terms of scope, content, length, stakes, and intended purpose, making direct comparisons of the psychometric qualities of the scores difficult. Overall, although the use of SP-based assessments can generally be supported from a score validity perspective, measurement errors associated with checklists and rating scales can be quite large, especially when few encounters are employed for each examinee. In addition, the dependencies inherent in the case-specific rating tools, used for item-level scoring, are ignored. This potentially compromises the utility of the resultant scores. Therefore, research aimed at developing alternate scoring strategies at the item- and/or test-level, especially ones that acknowledge the structure of the data and minimize measurement error, has been encouraged.

The Educational Commission for Foreign Medical Graduates (ECFMG®) is responsible for the certification of graduates of international medical schools who wish to enter graduate medical education training programs in the United States. Internationally trained physicians who obtain a certificate are eligible to apply to such programs in the United States. The issuance of this certificate is dependent on a number of criteria, including a passing score on the performance-based Clinical Skills Assessment (CSA®).

Clinical Skills Assessment (CSA)

The CSA®, instituted in July 1998, is one requirement for ECFMG certification. The assessment takes approximately 8 hours and involves 10 scored simulated encounters with SPs. These encounters represent a cross-section of common reasons for patient visits to a physician. The candidates are given 15 minutes to interview the SP and perform a focused physical examination. Following the encounter, the candidates are required to summarize their findings in the form of a patient note. They are given 10 minutes, plus any surplus time accumulated from leaving the examination room early, to complete this written post-encounter exercise.

The specific purpose of CSA is to ensure that international medical school graduates can demonstrate the ability to gather and interpret clinical patient data and communicate effectively in the English language at a level comparable to students graduating from United States medical schools (Educational Commission for Foreign Medical Graduates, 2002). Extensive research on CSA indicates that valid and reliable scores can be obtained provided that test administration is standardized, the candidates are measured over a sufficient number and breadth of clinical encounters, the SPs are properly trained, and detailed scoring rubrics are followed (Boulet, Ben David, Ziv, Burdick, et al., 1998; Boulet, van Zanten, McKinley, & Gary, 2001; Boulet et al., 2002; Boulet, McKinley, Whelan, & Hambleton, 2003; Whelan, McKinley, Boulet, Macrae, & Kamholz, 2001). Currently, approximately 9,000 candidates per year register for and take the CSA, resulting in approximately 100,000 encounter-level scores.

The generation of forms (sets of cases) for CSA is based on detailed test specifications, including constraints related to medical content, patient age, gender, acuity, etc. For a given test session, which normally includes 10 or 11 candidates (examinees), all individuals see the same cases and SPs, albeit each starting the assessment with a different encounter. Candidates rotate from one examination room to the next in a fixed order. Between any two test sessions, the cases may vary in overall difficulty and the SPs may differ in average stringency. Therefore, adjustments to candidate scores are necessary to ensure the comparability of assessments.

The CSA has two constituent scores, each of which has two components:

1. An Integrated Clinical Encounter score, made up of a data gathering checklist score and a patient note score, and

2. A Doctor–Patient Communication score, made up of a score on interpersonal skills and one on spoken English proficiency.

Description of CSA Components

The descriptions of CSA components are summarized in Table 6.1: The Structure of the Clinical Skills Assessment (CSA).

TABLE 6.1
The Structure of the Clinical Skills Assessment (CSA)

CSA Component	What is evaluated?	How is it measured	Who provides the scores?	Summary Measure
Data Gathering	History taking, questions, and relevant physical examination maneuvers	Case-specific checklists scored (0, 1) for each checklist item	Documented by the standardized patient (following the clinical encounter)	% of items credited
Patient Note	Written summary of clerical findings	Holistic rating (1–9)	Physician raters	Individual rating
Interpersonal Skills	Interviewing, counseling, personal manner, rapport	Holistic rating (1–4) for each of 4 dimensions	Evaluated by the standardized patient (following the clinical encounter)	Sum of 4 dimension ratings
Spoken English Proficiency	English comprehensibility	Holistic rating (1–4)	Evaluated by the standardized patient (following the clinical encounter)	Individual rating

Data Gathering Checklist. In addition to performing the case role, SPs record whether candidates asked specific medical history questions during the encounter. Checklists comprised of dichotomously scored items are used to document the specific case-related inquiries that candidates make. The history-taking checklist includes the key inquiries candidates are expected to make in the course of taking the patient's history. SPs also document the physical examination maneuvers that are performed. The physical exam checklist includes all of the key maneuvers candidates should perform during the course of doing a physical exam on a patient with a specific medical complaint. The vector of indicators of whether the checklist items have been checked constitutes a set of observable variables from a first phase of evidence identification, carried out by the SPs. The data gathering score for a particular case, which is based on a total of 12 to 24 checklist items, is the percentage of medical history questions asked and physical examination maneuvers performed correctly. Individual checklist items all count equally in the derivation of a case score. Likewise, candidates are not penalized for asking superfluous questions or performing physical examination maneuvers that are not indicated. The overall data-gathering score obtained in this way is tantamount to an evidence accumulation process, with the score implicitly a statistic for a one-dimensional unobservable student-model variable.

Cases can vary in difficulty, hence equating candidate data-gathering scores across cases is necessary and is accomplished through the use of common cases in standardized conditions. As a result, any candidate's score can be adjusted based on the difficulty of the set of cases, and stringency of SPs, used in the particular test form that he or she received.

Patient Note. After leaving the examination room, candidates complete a patient note. In an actual medical practice setting, the patient note would be used to communicate findings with other health professionals who may see the patient at a later date. The candidates document the pertinent positive and negative findings, including a differential diagnosis and diagnostic management plan. Specially trained physician–patient-note-raters score the notes at a later date on a scale from 1 to 9. This Process represents item-level scoring carried out by human judgment.

There are three performance levels (unacceptable, acceptable, and superior) defined on the scoring rubric and three defined gradations within each level. Only a single rating of each note is used to generate final candidate scores, although some patient notes are double-rated for quality assurance purposes.

Similar to the strategy employed for the data-gathering component, candidate patient-note scores are adjusted based on the difficulty of the cases encountered but not on the choice of raters (specially trained physicians) who score a given candidate's notes.

Interpersonal Skills. In each encounter, the SP portraying the scenario provides ratings of the candidate's interpersonal skills. These ratings, which can range from 1 (*unsatisfactory*) to 4 (*excellent*), are provided in four dimensions: interviewing and collecting information; counseling and delivering information; rapport (connection between doctor and patient); personal manner. The SPs use detailed, behaviorally anchored, scoring rubrics to determine ratings for each dimension, again values of observable variables determined by human judgment. The final interpersonal skills score is simply the sum of the four dimension ratings, and ranges from 4 to 16.

Spoken English Proficiency. The SPs also evaluate the spoken English proficiency of each candidate in every encounter. Criteria such as pronunciation, grammar, and the amount of effort required by the SPs to understand the candidate are used in this assessment. The comprehensibility of each candidate's spoken English can range from 1 (*low*) to 4 (*very high*).

Composite Scores

Current ECFMG practice is to combine the fundamental scores described previously into a set of composite scores that, in turn are used to make certification decisions.

Integrated Clinical Encounter. The integrated clinical encounter composite is the weighted sum of the data gathering and patient note scores, averaged over the 10 scored CSA encounters. The effective weighting of the data gathering and patient note components within the composite is 60%:40%, respectively. A candidate must achieve a passing score on the integrated clinical encounter to pass CSA.

Doctor–Patient Communication. The doctor–patient communication composite is simply the sum of spoken English and four Interpersonal Skills ratings. Averaging the doctor–patient communication ratings over the 10 encounters derives a total assessment score. A candidate must achieve a passing score on the communication composite to pass the CSA.

Reliability of CSA Scores

Unlike typical multiple-choice examinations, reliability of scores from SP examinations tends to be relatively low, and is dependent on a number of factors including: the number and selection of encounters and the choice of raters (Swanson, Clauser, & Case, 1999). Similar to other performance-based assessments, task (case) specificity has been shown to be a major factor limiting the reproducibility of scores. For the CSA data-gathering component, a reliability of 0.64 for a 10-encounter assessment has been reported (Boulet et al., 2003). Based on a generalizability study, there was significant variance attributable to the choice of case and the choice of SP performing the case. This indicates that the cases are not of equal difficulty and that a candidate's score may vary as a function of which SP is performing. The reliability of the patient note component has been reported to be 0.71 (Boulet, Rebbecchi, Denton, McKinley, & Whelan, in press). In our data, the percent of variance attributable to the case was relatively low (3.4%). However, a significant proportion of the total variance could be ascribed to the choice of physician rater for a given case.

The reliability of the spoken English language ratings, over 10 encounters, is 0.95 (Boulet et al., 2001). The reliability of the mean interpersonal skills score is 0.85 (Boulet et al., 1998). The variance components for the doctor–patient communication composite have also been reported (Boulet et al., 2003). The reliability of the total communication composite score, on a scale from 5-20, was 0.87. While relatively little variance was attributable to the choice of case, mean candidate scores can vary as a function of which SP was performing the case.[2]

III: MODEL AND ESTIMATION

Our approach to assessing the degree of testlet dependence, in the CSA, is parametric in nature and extends the approaches described in Bradlow, Wainer, and Wang (1999) and Wang, Bradlow, and Wainer (2002). Specifically, at the kernel of our approach are the three-parameter IRT model laid out by Birnbaum (1968) and the ordinal response IRT model laid out by Samejima (1969), but extended to allow for TRT dependence and covariates that describe the variation in parameters.

---

[2]The variance attributable to the choice of SP for a given case is significant, indicating that the various SPs differed in average stringency.

Model for Binary Response Items

For binary responses, we model the probability subject i correctly responds to diagnostic item j, $\text{Prob}(Y_{ij} = 1|\Omega_{ij})$, as

$$\text{Prob}(Y_{ij} = 1|\Omega_{ij}) = c_j + (1 - c_j) * \text{logit}^{-1}(a_j(\theta_i - b_j - \gamma_{id(j)})) \tag{1}$$

where a_j, b_j and c_j are the commonly utilized item discrimination (slope), difficulty, and guessing parameters, $\text{logit}^{-1}(x) = \exp(x)/(1+\exp(x))$, θ_i is the person ability, $\gamma_{id(j)}$ is the testlet effect (interaction) for when person i takes any of the items j nested within testlet $d(j)$, and Ω_{ij} is the vector of parameters (a_j, b_j, c_j, θ_i, $\gamma_{id(j)}$) for when person i takes item j. The term $\gamma_{id(j)}$ represents, in a parametric way, the dependence between items that are nested within the same testlet, as they "share" the additional common linear predictor, $\gamma_{id(j)}$, of test item score. Hence, items within the same testlet have a greater marginal covariance, even conditional on θ_i, than items across different testlets (hence a TRT-IRT model). Of course, if item j is an independent item (i.e., in a testlet of size 1) then by definition $\gamma_{id(j)} = \gamma_{ij} = 0$.

From the perspective of the ECD models, the testlet effect parameters, $\gamma id(j)$ effectively play the role of student model variables in the response model, as they can be thought of as student abilities that apply to a given testlet only, above and beyond the overall proficiency that all of the testlets are intended to measure. From the statistician's perspective, however, they are nuisance variables that are included in the model not because we are interested in them for their own sake, but because we wish to partial out their effect from the evidence, we obtain to draw inferences. In technical terms, the inferences we make about θ integrate over the uncertainty about the γs.

To put this parametric approach into perspective, we note that there are three relevant extant research streams that address TRT dependence, albeit in a different way. Much work in the early to mid 1980s, under the rubric of 'appropriateness' measurement' (Drasgow & Levine, 1986; Levine & Drasgow, 1982; 1988) looked at statistics that could be computed based on the examinee's test responses, that would be indicative of increased local item dependence. An additional research stream, also roughly at the same time, described a parametric approach to item dependence called the K-factor model (Gibbons & Hedeker, 1992) that, identical to our approach, posits a marginal covariance structure with K (in our case K is the number of testlets) discrete blocks. What separates our work from theirs (although their approach is in some ways more general) is that our testlet structure is defined *a priori* by the test design (i.e., is not latent), whereas the K factor structure allows for estimation of the unknown latent structure. Finally, more recent work by Zhang and Stout (1999) using a procedure called DETECT, allows one to detect local item dependence using a nonparametric set of procedures. Gessaroli and Folske (2002) accomplish much the same end using a factor analytic approach.

As is common in current testing procedure and practice, we nest the model given in equation (1) in a Bayesian framework (Gelfand & Smith, 1990) to allow for sharing of information across respondents and across items that is likely to exist. This is accomplished by specifying the following prior distributions for the parameter components of Ω_{ij}.

$\theta_1 \sim N(\beta_\theta X_i, ')$

$(\log(a_j), b_j, \text{logit}(c_j)) \sim MVN_3(\beta'Z_j, \Sigma_d)$

$\gamma_{id(j)} \sim N(0, \sigma^2_{d(j)})$

$\log(\sigma^2_{d(j)}) \sim N(\omega'W_{d(j)}, \sigma^2)^3$

where $N(a, b)$ denotes a normal distribution with mean a and variance b, and $MVN_g(a, b)$ denotes a g-variate multivariate normal distribution with mean vector a and covariance matrix b. We note the following about the formulation proposed here.

1. This is an extension of the most recent application of Bayesian parametric TRT in Wang, Bradlow, and Wainer (2002), in that we allow for covariates at the individual level, X_i, to explain variation in abilities, θ_i, covariates, Z_j at the item level to explain item parameter vector $(\log(a_j), b_j, \text{logit}(c_j))$, and covariates at the testlet-variance level, $W_{d(j)}$, to explain why some testlets show greater local dependence than others.

2. To identify the model, we fix the variance of the ability distribution at 1, and note that the covariates for θ_i do not include an intercept and are mean centered.

3. We utilize the item parameters on the transformed scales, $\log(a)$, b, $\text{logit}(c)$, as is common practice, to make the assumption of multivariate normality more plausible.

4. We specify that the covariance matrix of the multivariate normal for the binary response items is Σ_d, as opposed to Σ_p, that we will posit in the

---

[3] Note that if there are no covariates for the testlet variances, then $\sigma^2_{d(j)}$ is drawn from an inverse gamma with small number of degrees of freedom.

following section for the polytomous items, reflecting the fact that item parameter dependence is likely to vary across different formats.

Slightly informative and proper hyperpriors are put on the parameters governing the prior distributions to insure proper posteriors. Sensitivity analyses to these choices suggested little effect.

Model for Polytomous Items

The model we utilize for polytomous CSA (e.g., English proficiency score) items is an extension of the Samejima ordinal response model allowing for testlet dependence. Specifically, we utilize a probit response model for response category $r = 1,..,R$, given by

$$P(Y_{ij} = r | \Omega_{ij}') = \Phi(g_r - t_{ij}) - \Phi(g_{r-1} - t_{ij}) \tag{2}$$

where g_r represents the latent "cutoff" for observed score r, t_{ij} is the latent linear predictor of response score r modified to include a parameter, $\gamma_{id(j)}$, reflecting increased local dependence of items within the same testlet, and $\Phi(a)$ is the normal cumulative distribution function evaluated at a. Note, that as above, $t_{ij} = a_j(\theta_1 - b_j - \gamma_{id(j)})$. In essence, the Samejima model posits that the probability of falling in the r-th category is the probability that a normally distributed latent variable with mean t_{ij} and variance 1, falls between cutoffs g_r and g_{r-1}. We note that $g_0 = -\infty$, $g_R = \infty$, and $g_1 = 0$ to identify the model.

For the parameters describing the model in (2), we utilize the following priors to nest this piece within a Bayesian framework as shown earlier.

$\theta_1 \sim N(\beta'_\theta X_i')$

$(\log(a_j), b_j) \sim MVN_2(\beta' Z_j, \Sigma_p)$

$\gamma_{id(j)} \sim N(0, \sigma^2_{d(j)})$

$\log(\sigma^2_{d(j)}) \sim N(\omega' W_{d(j)}, \sigma^2)$

$g_r \sim Unif(g_{r-1}, g_{r+1})$

Again, slightly informative priors were utilized for all parameters to ensure proper posteriors but also to let the data "speak."

Inference Under the Model

To derive inferences under the model described above, we obtained samples from the marginal posterior distributions of the parameters, given the CSA test scores, using Markov Chain Monte Carlo, MCMC, techniques (Bradlow,

Wainer, & Wang, 1999; Gelfand & Smith, 1990; Patz & Junker, 1999a, 1999b) implemented in the Bayesian TRT software program SCORIGHT version 3.0 (Wang, Bradlow, & Wainer 2004). We provide a very brief description of the MCMC approach; details are available from the authors on request, including access to the software and a user's manual.

The Markov chain approach employed by SCORIGHT is as follows.

- [Step 1] Start the program at an initial guess of all model parameters, for multiple Markov chains. We note that these starting values can typically be obtained from nontestlet-based software such as MULTILOG (Thissen, 1991) or BILOG (Mislevy & Bock, 1983), or generated by SCORIGHT.

- [Step 2] Run each Markov chain for a large number of iterations M, called a burn-in period, for which the effects of the starting values are mitigated, and the posterior draws are traversing to the high-density region of the parameter space. We note that SCORIGHT contains the F-test diagnostic of Gelman and Rubin (1992) to assess convergence of the MCMC sampler.

- [Step 3] After convergence, run the MCMC sampler for an additional N iterations to obtains samples from the marginal posterior distributions that will be utilized to estimate facets of the posterior distributions of interest (e.g., mean, median, any quantile, etc...).

As standard output from the Markov chain, SCORIGHT produces posterior means and standard deviations for all parameters of the models described in the previous section, as well as the posterior draws themselves that can be utilized for further analysis.

For the CSA data analyzed here, SCORIGHT was run using two independent chains for an initial burn-in period of 9,000 draws and 1,000 iterations thereafter. We kept only every 20th draw after the initial 9,000 to leave the draws relatively uncorrelated so that standard variance estimates on the estimated parameters themselves could be applied. We next present the detailed findings from SCORIGHT as applied to the CSA data.

IV: CSA ANALYSIS

This example involves fitting our TRT model to the data from all of the examinees who took the CSA over an entire year beginning on June 29, 2001 until June 28, 2002. The analyses performed to fit this test were different in an important way from those done previously (Wang, Bradlow, & Wainer, 2002). In our earlier use of the testlet-scoring model, we fit tests that had a relatively large number of examinees and a relatively small number of testlets. In this application we have a large number of testlets and a great deal of missing data. There are more than 100 testlets (cases), but most examinees were only presented with 10 of them. The overlapping design allowed us to place all testlets on the same scale, but this application provided a serious test to the fitting software SCORIGHT v. 2.0 (Wang, Bradlow, & Wainer, 2003). In this description, we present only a small, but representative, sample of our results.

Doctor–Patient Communication

When we fit the 101 testlets that represent all the different cases administered during this 1-year time period, we obtained a value of proficiency representing each examinee's performance on the four IPS items and the one English proficiency item. Almost all examinees responded to 10 testlets (cases) comprised of five polytomous items. SCORIGHT yielded the posterior distribution of each examinee's proficiency. We used the posterior mean of each examinee's distribution as the point estimate of proficiency ($\hat{\theta}$) and the posterior standard deviation is used to calculate an estimate of its standard error. In Fig. 6.1 is a plot of these estimates for 1,000 randomly selected examinees as well as their scores obtained through the current ECFMG scoring methodology (sum of IPS and English ratings).

The correlation between these two estimates of performance is 0.98 and demonstrates that both scoring procedures are utilizing the information in essentially the same way. But the details contained in the differences are important. We see that a range of communication scores represents the same IRT score. As we shall see shortly, this has important consequences.

Following the recommendation of Green, Bock, Humphreys, Linn, and Reckase (1984), we calculated the marginal reliability of the communication scale using:

Marginal Reliability = var[true score)] / [Var(true score) + var(error)]   (3)

To get var(true score), we need both components of a conditional variance decomposition: the variance of the posterior means across examinees plus the mean of each examinee's posterior variance.

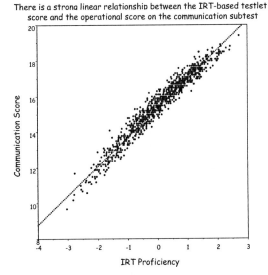

There is a strong linear relationship between the IRT-based testlet score and the operational score on the communication subtest

FIG. 6.1. It is hard to know how much better one scoring model is than another, but we do know that if a scoring model does not yield scores that have a serious similarity to those obtained from a simple score it is likely to be problematic. In this display, we show that the scores yielded by the Bayesian testlet model are very close to those obtained from the current scoring system for the communication subscore.

We estimate error variance using an approximation based on decomposing posterior precision (the reciprocal of each examinee's posterior variance). For a given examinee, the posterior precision is, under a normal approximation, the prior precision plus precision from their responses. The prior precision is the reciprocal of the true score variance. Thus subtracting prior precision off the posterior precision for any given examinee gives the precision from the data for that person. Its reciprocal approximates measurement error variance for that person. The average of these across examinees yields the average measurement error variance.

For the communication score the true score variance was estimated to be .986 and the error variance .15. Combining these in equation (3) yields a reliability estimate of .87. This estimate of reliability matches quite closely what was expected from prior analyses.

The examinee cohort we fit was made up of two quite different kinds of individuals: only 1,543 examinees spoke English as their first language, the remaining 4,523 examinees (the ESL group) did not. The native English group performed almost a standard deviation higher on average than the ESL group (0.92 σ), (see Fig. 6.2) and so we expected that this reliability estimate might be inflated because of the group differences (Fig. 6.3). Thus, we felt that we might get a more informative estimate of the test's reliability if we were to look at the performance on the test of these two groups separately.

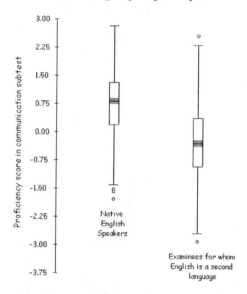

FIG. 6.2. The distributions of TRT scores on the communication subtest show a difference of almost a full standard deviation between native English speakers and those for whom English is a second language.

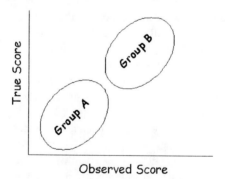

FIG. 6.3. An illustration in which the within group reliabilities could be smaller than the total group reliability due to the difference in the mean performance within each group.

What we found was surprising and instructive. First the test was <u>more</u> reliable within each group than it was when the two groups were combined, with both reliabilities above 0.9. This result seemed remarkable. But if the bivariate distributions of observed score vs. true score looked like those in Fig. 6.4 we would obtain the result we did. In retrospect, this seems plausible given the character of the two examinee groups. When we examined the error variance obtained from the separate analyses we found that it was considerably smaller in each group (0.11 and 0.07) than it was when they were fit together (0.15), signifying a better fit for the model within group. Because the true score variance remained about the same, the reliability (from equation 3) had to increase.

Despite the overall group differences, in a testlet-based analysis of their differential function—Differential Testlet Functioning or DTF for short, see Wainer, Sireci, & Thissen, 1991—we found that once overall differences in proficiency were accounted for what little differential performance that was observed seemed to *favor* the ESL group. The worst DTF seen was on testlet 98 (Fig. 6.5); testlet 67 demonstrated median DTF (Fig. 6.6). Testlet 67 represents the amount of DTF seen in 85 of the 101 testlets administered during the year represented by our data—that is there was less than a single point of differential functioning anywhere in the plausible range of proficiencies. In 11 testlets there was between one and two points advantage for the ESL group, and in 5 testlets there was between 1 and 2 points advantage for the native English group.

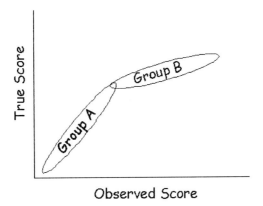

FIG. 6.4. An illustration in which the within group reliabilities could be larger than the total group reliability due to the difference in the relationship between true score and observed score within each group.

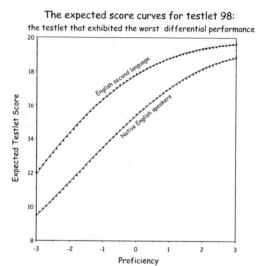

The expected score curves for testlet 98:

the testlet that exhibited the worst differential performance

FIG. 6.5. The expected score curves for testlet 98 showing about a 2 point advantage to examinees for whom English was a second language. This testlet is the one with the largest amount of differential functioning (DTF).

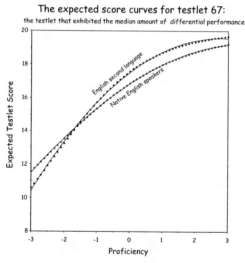

The expected score curves for testlet 67:

the testlet that exhibited the median amount of differential performance

FIG. 6.6. The expected score curves for testlet 67 showing less than a one point advantage to any examinees. This testlet is the one with the median amount of differential functioning (DTF) and is representative of 86% of testlets in the exam.

Measuring the differential functioning of each testlet was not the primary goal of this investigation. If it were, we would have integrated the difference between the two expected score curves with respect to the ESL proficiency distribution to obtain a summary measure of the average differential performance (Wainer, 1993). However our initial look confirmed that differential performance is not a critical issue with this portion of the test. Yet it is interesting to speculate why we see positive DTF for the ESL group. One plausible explanation is suggested by the score distributions for the two components of the communications score (Fig. 6.7). It is not surprising to see a vast difference between the two groups in English, but this difference is ameliorated considerably when this result is mixed with the interpersonal skills score (Fig. 6.2). This suggests that ESL candidates may be stronger students in general than the native English speakers, and this strength manifests itself most among highest levels of proficiency.

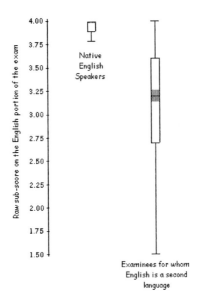

FIG. 6.7. Box plot showing the distributions of the raw scores on the English subscore of the communication test.

The analyses shown thus far parallels analyses that could easily be done using traditional true score theory, except that we have properly accounted for the local dependence and so obtained more accurate estimates of uncertainty. Little of this illustrates the most profound advantages of the testlet model. Of course some results were obtained more gracefully with this model than the traditional one; prominent among these is the outputting of proficiency scores on the same scale without having to do the often tedious equating of the many, many forms that this dataset represents. Instead, simply inputting the data with their overlapping structure provides all the information necessary for the model to place all examinees' scores on a common scale. Next we explore the kinds of questions that the Bayesian-based testlet model can answer easily that are difficult or impossible to approach with traditional scoring methods.

One class of questions for which the Bayesian approach is especially well suited are stochastic; that is those that ask for the probability of a particular outcome. So, for example, suppose we wish to know what is the probability of an examinee passing the test whose proficiency is at some prespecified level. Using standard methods, we might assume normality and use the estimated standard error to calculate the tail probability of interest. Such an approach rests heavily on the viability of the normality assumption; indeed it rests heavily on it holding in the tails of the distribution. Experience has shown repeatedly (Andrews, Bickel, Hampel, Huber, Rogers, & Tukey, 1972) that this is precisely where such assumptions are most likely to be false; often catastrophically so.

The Bayesian approach we utilize here provides the posterior distribution of each parameter and so estimating a probability requires merely counting, not asymptotic inference. For each person, we can sample say 1,000 draws from the posterior distribution of proficiency and count the number that are below the cut-off point. When we do this we find (Fig. 6.8) that there is a substantial chance of someone passing the test even if their true ability is well below the passing score, there is also a non-negligible chance of failing for someone whose true ability is well above the passing score. The slope of this curve provides a strong intuitive meaning to the reliability of the test score. Indeed, it is much better than the reliability, for it measures the reliability of the inference being made. The question of the stability of scores far from the decision point is of much less import than what is happening around the passing score. One might profitably use the slope of this curve at the passing score as a measure of the test's reliability in this application (in this case 0.83). These curves represent the posterior probability of passing (PPoP). The construction of PPoP curves is described in further detail in Wainer, Wang, Skorupski, and Bradlow (2005).

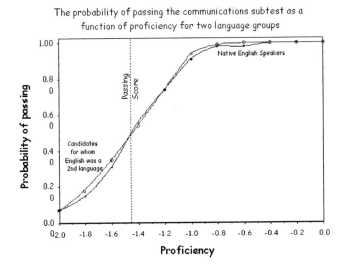

FIG. 6.8. Using the posterior distributions of ability, we can easily calculate the probability of any person passing the communications portion of the exam. In this figure, we show this probability for both native and non native English speakers.

We note in passing that the two curves calculated for native and non native English speakers are almost coincidental, indicating that, at least for these two groups, there is no bias.

Integrated Clinical Encounter

We did many of the same sorts of analyses for the two portions of the integrated clinical encounter (checklist and patient note), as we did for the Doctor–Patient Communication and will not repeat their outcomes here. Instead we briefly mention a few of the findings we found surprising.

1.   Patient Note—The reliability of this section was .66. This is about what was expected from alternative analyses done in the past, which typically found reliabilities in the 0.70 range.

2.   Checklist—The checklist section's reliability was found to be 0.51, which is also in line with expectations.

The combined score for the integrated clinical encounter had a reliability of 0.72, which is modestly higher than prior reports (0.66). This may be due to

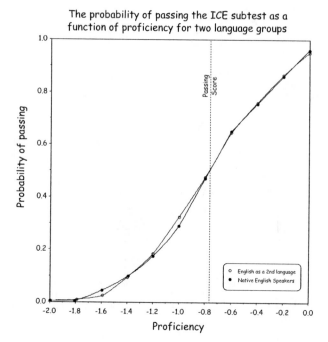

The probability of passing the ICE subtest as a function of proficiency for two language groups

FIG. 6.9. Using the posterior distributions of ability, we calculate the probability of any person passing the ICE portion of the exam. In this figure, we show this probability for both native and non native English speakers.

minor sample fluctuations or to the different methods used in estimating reliability. In either case, our results matched those obtained from prior analyses close enough to assure us that we were on the right track. When we calculate the passing probability curves of the ICE (Fig. 6.9), we discover that once again the difference between the two language groups is negligible.

V: SUMMARY AND CONCLUSIONS

Observations Based on the Clinical Skill Assessment Example

The analyses we have presented here represent a sample of what is possible from the new model described in Part III. Much of what we did might seem like it could be accomplished in a straightforward way using methods more than a half-century old (e.g., Gulliksen, 1950). While it is true that the latent scoring system at the center of all item response models yields results that are very close

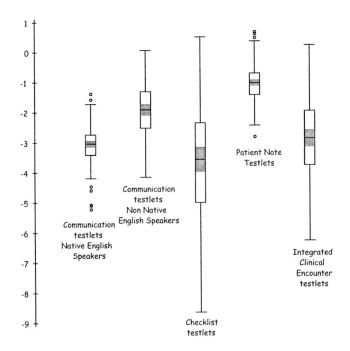

FIG. 6.10. Box plots of the testlet difficulties obtained in five subanalyses showing typical variation. The checklist is unique in its huge range of difficulty.

to scores obtained with much less effort by calculating percent correct, it would be a mistake to underestimate the value of the additional power. The Clinical Skill Assessment is a challenge to score fairly. Figure 6.10 shows the variation in difficulty of the 101 cases used during the course of 1 year of testing in various aspects of the CSA.

Keep in mind that an examinee would receive a sample of only 10 of these testlets and the range of more than 8 logits in the difficulty means that it is possible for the various test forms to vary substantially in their difficulty. In fact, for the communications score the difficulty across forms ranged from −0.30 to − 1.6; this is substantial. Happily, the difficulty of most test forms lay in a much narrower range (Fig. 6.11), but there were certainly some unlucky individuals

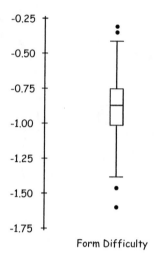

FIG. 6.11. Distribution of form difficulty for communication subscore.

whose tests were far from this middle range.[4] This emphasizes the need to equate forms. But equating this number of different forms is not a task for small children. It involves stringing together many small groups with overlapping testlets and hoping that the strong assumptions underlying the equating model are true enough. The analysis performed here places all test scores on a common scale. It too has assumptions, but it is done in one step and there are many kinds of diagnostics that can be examined to support the validity of the scoring model. Some of these diagnostics grow from the availability of the posterior distributions, whose utility we only briefly touched upon in Part IV. More details on how to use the posterior distributions for model checking are found in Gelman, Carlin, Stern, and Rubin (1995).

---

[4] The variation in unequated difficulty observed here is considerably larger than that commonly seen in other professionally constructed tests. In practice equating can make the quality of decisions unrelated to which particular form was administered, but such large adjustments may be problematic. Frederic Lord emphasized the difficulties in making such large adjustments in his well-known aphorism "Equating is either impossible or unnecessary." Finding a written source of that comment has proved challenging. The closest version is in Lord (1950, "Theorem 13.3.1. Under realistic regularity conditions, scores x and y on two tests cannot be equated unless either (1) both tests are perfectly reliable or (2) the two tests are strictly parallel [in which case x(y) = y]" p. 198). In the specific instance that concerns us in this chapter, none of the test forms we examined had reliability anywhere near perfection, and most forms were not parallel.

But the ease and grace of equating is not the only reason to use this test-scoring model. It also provides a more accurate estimate of the precision of measurement. This information can be used by test developers to measure the efficacy of modifications. Previous approaches to the scoring of testlet-based tests either overestimated precision by not taking into account the within testlet dependence or underestimated precision by collapsing all item response patterns within a testlet into a single polytomous score. The model we propose here more closely mirrors the structure of the test and so estimates test precision more accurately.

The probability of passing curves shown previously in Figs. 6.8 and 6.9 can profitably be placed on the same axes. Even though the two test scores, communication and ICE, are measuring different traits, they are both scaled so that the variability of proficiency of those traits has the same standard deviation. Thus, one can draw sensible inferences when they are plotted together. When this is done (see Fig. 6.12), we can see immediately how much easier it is to pass the communications section (from the amount of displacement to the left). But more importantly, we can see how much more accurately the communications test allows us to make decisions than the ICE (from the differences in the slope; .98 for communications, .74 for ICE). Test developers can do simple analytic experiments by varying the passing score and seeing where the slope is steepest. We can also measure the efficacy of any changes in test content on this very important test characteristic.

There is no free lunch. You cannot eat the Bayesian omelet without breaking the Bayesian egg. The estimation algorithm sketched in Part III takes a while. The analyses reported here typically ran 5 to 6 days. For longer subtests (checklist), it took even longer. Thus this scoring method is not suitable for providing immediate feedback to examinees, unless they are willing to wait at their computer for a week or so. But this practical drawback is temporary. Computers will get faster and storage will get cheaper. The algorithm is well-suited for parallel processing by allowing each processor to calculate a separate chain. In addition, using maximum marginal likelihood estimates of item parameters (assuming local independence) as starting values will speed convergence considerably. Initial experience suggests that this could easily cut the number of iterations required for convergence by a factor of four.

For the Clinical Skills Assessment, this model can be operationally used by fitting the model periodically and including overlapping testlets in the sequential fits and holding constant the parameters from the previous fit. For example, one might fit exams administered January through June, then fit April through

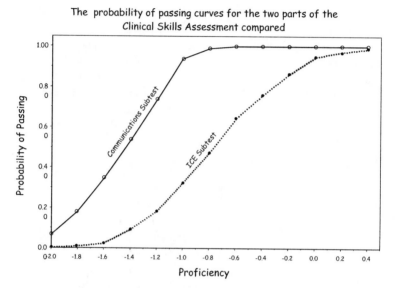

FIG. 6.12. When the P(Passing) curves for both portions of the CSA are plotted on the same axes, we can visually compare their difficulty and precision.

September while holding constant the parameters of the testlets administered in April through June. This would mean that the testlets administered July through September would be on the same scale as the prior scoring.

Extensions

The analyses of the Clinical Skills Assessment used in this chapter to illustrate Testlet Response Theory share two features with traditional test analyses. First, the object of inference in any given subarea we analyzed was an overall proficiency score for each examinee in that area; that is, we used a unidimensional model for each of the analyses we carried out. Second, the testlet structure had a single layer: conditional dependence among item was presumed to be exhausted by their associations within testlets. As tasks increase in complexity, both of these conditions may fail. Both can be accommodated by extensions to the basic TRT model in the following manner.

A multidimensional test-scoring model is one in which more than one student model variable is used to model performance on a task. It may be that different student-model variables are involved for different observable variables, or all are involved but perhaps with different weights. A number of multivariate

IRT models have been proposed for the case in which observable variables are conditionally independent given the now vector-valued student model variable (e.g., Reckase, 1997). In most of these models, the probability of observing a response in category k to task j from examinee i is constructed from logit or probit function of a linear combination of vectors of parameters for the examinee (θ_i) and the task (β_j). For example, one logistic multivariate model for 0/1 items takes the form

$$\text{Prob } (X_{ij} = k | \theta_i, \beta_j) = \text{logit}^{-1} [a_{j1}\theta_{i1} + a_{j2}\theta_{i2} + b_j],$$

and has a two-dimensional examinee ability $\theta_i = (\theta_{i1}, \theta_{i2})$ and an item parameter vector $\beta_j = (a_{j1}, a_{j2}, b_j)$ that consists of two discrimination parameters and a difficulty parameter.

The extension (if not the implementation) to TRT is straightforward: With the same definition for the testlet effect as in Equation 1, the response probability in the multivariate testlet model is $F_{jk} [1 (\theta_i, \beta_j) - \gamma_{id (j)}]$. That is,

$$\text{Prob } (X_{ijk} = k | \theta_i, \beta_j) = \text{logit}^{-1} (a_{j1}\theta_{i1} + a_{j2}\theta_{i2} + b_j - \gamma_{id (j)}).$$

An example of a more complex dependence structure is one in which an examinee takes multiple cases, each case consists of multiple scenarios, and each scenario yields values for multiple items (i.e., observable variables). The response probability for case k could then be modeled as

$$\text{logit}^{-1} (a_{j1}\theta_{i1} + a_{j2}\theta_{i2} + b_j - \gamma_{id (j)} - \eta_{ic (j)}),$$

where $\gamma_{id} (j)$ is the effect for examinee i for the case to which item j belongs and $\eta_{ic (j)}$ is the effect for examinee i for the scenario within that case to which item j belongs. These nested effects are analogous to those encountered in multistage survey sampling, as for example when students are nested within classes within schools within districts within states.

We do not propose these extensions lightly. We have experienced firsthand the challenges of fitting TRT models to essentially unidimensional tests with a single hierarchy of dependence; nevertheless, if it is possible to create more complex tasks, somebody will build them, and will want to score them. We would emphasize the importance of integrating test design and scoring procedures in such cases, ideally iterating between designing prototype tasks and trying scoring methods from the beginning of the project. Only with clean data designs and well-informed expert opinion to suggest model structures and prior distributions for parameters can we expect to make progress with complex scoring models. The worst time to ask, "How do you score it" with respect to complex tasks is after the tasks have already been created, simulation systems and procedures developed, and data gathered (Mislevy, Steinberg, Breyer, Almond, & Johnson, 2002).

A FINAL COMMENT

Much work remains before this methodology is fully ready for prime time, but we believe that it holds great promise for the automatic scoring of tests that are built to match the test developer's vision of what suits the traits of interest, rather than forcing the construction of tests to suit an outdated scoring model.

ACKNOWLEDGMENTS

The National Board of Medical Examiners and the Educational Commission for Foreign Medical Graduates supported this work; we are delighted to have the opportunity here to express our gratitude, although nothing we say here necessarily reflects their corporate views. In addition, the careful reading and helpful suggestions of Ronald Nungester have aided the clarity and correctness of what we say. We would like to thank him for helping us more nearly say what we meant.

REFERENCES

Andrews, D. F., Bickel, P. J., Hampel, F. R., Huber, P. J., Rogers, W. H., & Tukey, J. W. (1972), *Robust Estimates of Location*. Princeton, NJ: Princeton University Press.

Ben David, M. F., Klass, D. J., Boulet, J., De Champlain, A., King, A. M., Pohl, H. S. et al. (1999). The performance of foreign medical graduates on the National Board of Medical Examiners (NBME) standardized patient examination prototype: A collaborative study of the NBME and the Educational Commission for Foreign Medical Graduates (ECFMG). *Medical Education, 33*, 439–446.

Birnbaum, A. (1968) Some latent trait models and their use in inferring an examinee's ability. In F. M. Lord & M. R. Novick, *Statistical theories of mental test scores* (Chap. 17–20). Reading, MA: Addison-Wesley.

Boulet, J. R., Ben David, M. F., Ziv, A., Burdick, W. P., Curtis, M., Peitzman, S. et al. (1998). Using standardized patients to assess the interpersonal skills of physicians. *Academic Medicine, 73*, S94–S96.

Boulet, J. R., McKinley, D. W., Norcini, J. J., & Whelan, G. P. (2002). Assessing the comparability of standardized patient and physician evaluations of clinical skills. *Advances in Health Science Education., 7*, 85–97.

Boulet, J. R., McKinley, D. W., Whelan, G. P., & Hambleton, R. K. (2003). Quality assurance methods for performance-based assessments. *Advances in Health Science Educatio., 8*, 27–47.

Boulet, J. R., van Zanten, M., McKinley, D. W., & Gary, N. E. (2001). Evaluating the spoken English proficiency of graduates of foreign medical schools. *Medical Education, 35*, 767–773.

Boulet, J., Rebbecchi, T., Denton, E., McKinley, D., & Whelan, G. P. (in press). Assessing the written communication skills of medical school graduates. *Advances in Health Science Education.*

Bradlow, E. T., Wainer, H., & Wang, X. (1999). A Bayesian random effects model for testlets. *Psychometrika, 64*, 153–168.

Brailovsky, C. A., & Grand'Maison, P. (2000). Using evidence to improve evaluation: A comprehensive psychometric assessment of a SP-based OSCE licensing examination. *Advances in Health Science Education, 5*, 207–219.

Drasgow, F., & Levine, M. V. (1986). Optimal detection of certain forms of inappropriate test scores. *Applied Psychological Measurement, 10*, 59–67.

ECFMG. (1999, 2002). *Clinical Skills Assessment (CSA) Candidate Orientation Manual.* Philadelphia: Educational Commission for Foreign Medical Graduates (ECFMG).

Gelfand, A. E., & Smith, A. F. M. (1990), Sampling-based approaches to calculating marginal densities, *Journal of the American Statistical Association, 85*, 398–409.

Gelman, A., Carlin, J. B., Stern, H. S., & Rubin, D. B. (1995). *Bayesian Data Analysis.* London: Chapman & Hall.

Gelman, A., & Rubin, D. B. (1992), Inference from iterative simulation using multiple sequences. *Statistical Science, 7*, 457–511.

Gessaroli, M. E., & Folske, J. C. (2002). Generalizing the reliability of tests comprised of testlets. *International Journal of Testing, 2*, 277–295.

Gibbons, R. D., & Hedeker, D. R. (1992). Full Information item bi-factor analysis. *Psychometrika, 57*, 423–436.

Glas, C. A. W., Wainer, H., & Bradlow, E. T. (2000). Maximum Marginal Likelihood and Expected A Posteriori estimates for the testlet response model. In W. J. van der Linden & C.A.W. Glas, (Eds.), *Computerized adaptive testing: Theory and practice* (pp. 271–288). Boston, MA: Kluwer-Nijhoff.

Green, B. F., Bock, R. D., Humphreys, L. G., Linn, R. B., & Reckase, M. D. (1984). Technical guidelines for assessing computerized adaptive tests. *Journal of Educational Measurement, 21*, 347–360.

Gulliksen, H. (1950). *Theory of mental tests,* New York: Wiley. (Reprinted in 1987 by Lawrence Erlbaum Associates, Hillsdale, NJ)

Levine, M. V., & Drasgow, F. (1982). Appropriateness measurement: review, critique and validating studies. *British Journal of Mathematical and Statistical Psychology, 35*, 42–56.

Levine, M. V., & Drasgow, F. (1988). Optimal appropriateness measurement. Psychometrika, 53, 161–176.

Lord, F. M. (1950). *Notes on Comparable Scales for Test Scores* (RB-50-48). Princeton, NJ: Educational Testing Service.

Mislevy, R. J., & Bock, R. D. (1983). *BILOG: Item analysis and test scoring with binary logistic models* [computer program]. Mooresville, IN: Scientific Software.

Mislevy, R. J., Steinberg, L. S., & Almond, R. G. (2003). On the structure of educational assessments. *Measurement: Interdisciplinary Research and Perspectives, 1*, 3–67.

Mislevy, R. J., Steinberg, L. S., Breyer, F. J., Almond, R. G., & Johnson, L. (2002). Making sense of data from complex assessments. *Applied Measurement in Education, 15*, 363–378.

Patz, R. J. & Junker, B. (1999a). A straightforward approach to Markov Chain Monte Carlo methods for item response models. *Journal of Educational and Behavioral Statistics, 24*, 146–178.

Patz, R. J. & Junker, B. (1999b). Applications and Extensions of MCMC in IRT: Multiple item types, missing data, and rated responses. *Journal of Educational and Behavioral Statistics, 24,* 342–366.

Reckase, M. (1997). A linear logistic multidimensional model for dichotomous item response data. In W. J. van der Linden & R. K. Hambleton (Eds.), *Handbook of modern item response theory* (pp. 271–286). New York: Springer-Verlag.

Reznick, R. K., Blackmore, D., Dauphinee, W. D., Rothman, A. I., & Smee, S. (1996). Large-scale high-stakes testing with an OSCE: Report from the Medical Council of Canada. *Academic Medicine, 71,* S19–S21.

Samejima, F. (1969). Estimation of latent ability using a response pattern of graded scores. *Psychometrika Monographs,* (Whole No. 17).

Sireci, S. G., Wainer, H., & Thissen, D., (1991). On the reliability of testlet-based tests. *Journal of Educational Measurement, 28,* 237–247.

Swanson, D. B., Clauser, B. E., & Case, S. M. (1999). Clinical skills assessment with standardized patients in high-stakes tests: A framework for thinking about score precision, equating, and security. *Advances in Health Science Education, 4,* 67–106.

Swanson, D. B., Norman, G. R., & Linn, R. L. (1995). Performance-based assessment: Lessons from the health professions. *Educational Researcher, 24,* 5–11.

Thissen, D. (1991). *MULTILOG user's guide* (Version 6). Mooresville, IN: Scientific Software.

Vu, N. V., & Barrows, H. S. (1994). Use of standardized patients in clinical assessments: Recent developments and measurement findings. *Educational Researcher, 23,* 23–30.

Wainer, H. (1993). Model-based standardized measurement of an item's differential impact. In P. W. Holland & H. Wainer (Eds.), *Differential Item Functioning (pp.123–135).* Hillsdale, NJ: Lawrence Erlbaum Associates.

Wainer, H. (1995). Precision & Differential Item Functioning on a testlet-based test: The 1991 Law School Admissions Test as an example. *Applied Measurement in Education, 8*(2), 157–187.

Wainer, H., Bradlow, E. T., & Du, Z. (2000). Testlet response theory: An analog for the 3-PL. In W. J. van der Linden & C. A. W. Glas (Eds.),*Computerized adaptive testing: Theory and practice* (pp. 245–270). Boston, MA: Kluwer-Nijhoff.

Wainer, H., & Kiely, G. (1987). Item clusters and computerized adaptive testing: A case for testlets. *Journal of Educational Measurement, 24,* 185–202.

Wainer, H., & Lewis, C. (1990). Toward a psychometrics for testlets. *Journal of Educational Measurement, 27,* 1–14.

Wainer, H., Sireci, S. G., & Thissen, D. (1991). Differential testlet functioning: Definitions and detection. *Journal of Educational Measurement, 28,* 197–219.

Wainer, H., Wang, X., Skorupski, W.P., & Bradow, E.T. (2005). A Bayesian method for evaluating passing scores. *Journal of Educational Measurement,* 271–281.

Wang, X., Bradlow, E. T., & Wainer, H. (2004). *User's Guide for SCORIGHT (version 3.0): A computer program for scoring tests built of testlets including a module for covariate analysis.* Research Report 04–49. Princeton, NJ: Educational Testing Service.

Wang, X., Bradlow, E. T., & Wainer, H. (2002). A general Bayesian model for testlets: Theory and applications. *Applied Psychological Measurement, 26*(1), 109–128.

Whelan, G. (2000). High-stakes medical performance testing: The Clinical Skills Assessment program. *Journal of the American Medical Association, 283,* 17–48.

Whelan, G. P. (1999). Educational commission for foreign medical graduates: clinical skills assessment prototype. *Medical Teacher, 21,* 156–160.

Whelan, G. P., McKinley, D. W., Boulet, J. R., Macrae, J., & Kamholz, S. (2001). Validation of the doctor-patient communication component of the Educational Commission for Foreign Medical Graduates Clinical Skills Assessment. *Medical Education, 35,* 757–761.

Zhang, J., & Stout, W. F. (1999). The theoretical DETECT index of dimensionality and its application to approximate simple structure. *Psychometrika, 64,* 213–249.

7

An Application of Bayesian Networks in Automated Scoring of Computerized Simulation Tasks

David M. Williamson
Russell G. Almond
Educational Testing Service

Robert J. Mislevy
Roy Levy
University of Maryland

> *Probability is not really about numbers; it is about the structure of reasoning.*—Glenn Shafer (quoted in Pearl, 1988, p. 77)

There are many ways to address the design of automated scoring systems for complex constructed response tasks. This volume illustrates a variety of such methods, as well as their human scoring alternative, in terms of Evidence-Centered Design (ECD; see Mislevy et al., chap. 2, this volume). Some of these methods are familiar statistical techniques applied in innovative ways, whereas others are relatively new methods to the field of educational measurement. A common theme across all of these chapters is leveraging advances in technology and measurement methods to accomplish assessment goals that were previously impossible. This chapter continues that theme by presenting an application of Bayesian networks (BNs, also called belief networks, Bayesian belief networks, influence diagrams, relevance diagrams, causal probabilistic networks, and Bayes nets) for the evidence accumulation process of automated scoring[1] of a web-based assessment prototype of computer networking ability that uses computerized simulation tasks.

---

[1] See Chapter 2, this volume, for discussion of the distinction between *evidence identification*; the process of extracting and summarizing construct relevant observations, and *evidence accumulation*; the process of using these observations to draw inferences about ability.

A BAYESIAN VIEW OF EVIDENCE ACCUMULATION

Consider for the moment the role of the Evidence Accumulation Process in an Intelligent Tutoring System (because of the real-time and adaptive nature of the tutoring system, this is a harder case than the summary scoring for an end of course assessment). The tutoring system usually maintains some kind of student model, which contains several proficiency variables related to the knowledge, skills and abilities that are the target of assessment claims. At any given point in time, the student model describes beliefs about those variables for a particular student based on the evidence collected so far. Initially, when the student first sits down in front of the computer terminal, one's beliefs about the proficiency variables are diffuse, usually based on the range observed in the target population for the assessment, for example, what is expected from a randomly chosen student of that age, grade level, and previous course experience. Next evidence starts arriving from the tasks that the student performs. This could come as single or multiple observed outcome variables. The latter is the usual case when the tasks involve a complex simulation (as in the example that follows). The Evidence Accumulation process must update the student model to reflect the change in belief based on the new evidence. As information builds up, belief about the student's proficiency variables becomes sharper, and increasingly based on that particular student's performance. At any point in time, the student model could be queried to provide information for score reporting or selecting the next task.

This is essentially the framework laid out in Almond and Mislevy (1999) and it is not specific to Bayesian networks or even Bayesian models. However, it works particularly well with the Bayesian view of using probabilities to represent uncertain states of knowledge. For a Bayesian evidence accumulation process, the student model represents beliefs about the student's proficiencies as a joint probability distribution over the proficiency variables. The updating of these distributions from the observed evidence from tasks can be done via Bayes theorem. At any point in time, any statistic of the current proficiency distribution can be used to produce scores to make inferences about the desired *claims* to make about the student. This use of probability to represent states of knowledge can be criticized as being subjective. However, if such knowledge is established on the basis of empirical observation it is an objective subjectivism (Dempster, 1990) in that the assessment of uncertainty in the probabilistic estimate is based on a shared understanding of prior observations similar to a frequentist perspective. As such, the calculations only encompass a well-defined set of evidence; the evidence from the particular set of tasks seen by the student and the evidence about expected behavior of the intended target population based on prior experience. One advantage of the Bayesian methodology is that it forces the practitioner to be explicit about all of the assumptions that go into the model, whether from expert judgment, prior experience, or observed evidence. As illustrated in subsequent sections, another advantage of Bayesian methodology for modeling is the direct correspondence between the statistical model and cognitive reasoning patterns and structures.

BAYES NETS BRIEFLY DEFINED

As a result of their representational form, Bayesian networks are a convenient class of Bayesian models to work with for building an evidence accumulation scoring process. Formally, Bayesian networks are defined with a graph (see, e.g., Fig. 7.1), the *nodes*, represented as circles in the graph, represent variables in the problem (this includes both the proficiency variables and the observable outcome variables described earlier), and the *edges*, represented as arrows in the graph, represent patterns of conditional independence among the variables in the model in that any two nodes not directly connected by a single arrow are conditionally independent. The edges in the graph are *directed*, indicated by the direction of the arrow and signifying that the value of the variable at the termination of the edge is dependent on the value of the variable at the origin. The variable from which the edge comes is called the *parent* and the variable to which the edge flows is called the *child*. (As discussed later, evidence often flows from child variable to parent variable despite the fact that the relationships are represented directionally from parent to child variable). More importantly, *separation*, in which two variables are not directly connected in the graph, implies conditional independence in the mathematical sense.

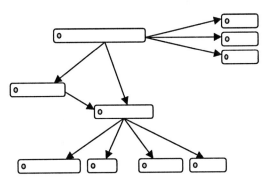

FIG. 7.1. Sample Bayesian network graph.

For example, if an observed outcome variable had Skill 1 and Skill 5 as parents, but no other edges connecting it, then it would be conditionally independent of all other variables in the model given the true states of Skill 1 and Skill 5. Pearl (1988) defined this idea of separation more formally. Finally, all of the variables in the Bayesian network are discrete. This means that there are no integrals required in the algorithms used to update belief about variables in one part of the graph on the basis of values in another part of the graph.

At any time, the probability of any variable in the model can be obtained by querying the corresponding node in the network. The model can be updated with evidence by first *instantiating* a node in the network corresponding to the observed evidence and then transmitting the influence of this observation along the edges of the graph to update values of other variables in the graph. There are several variations on the basic updating algorithm (Almond, 1995; Jensen, 1996; Lauritzen & Speiegelhalter, 1988; Neapolitan, 2004; Pearl, 1988). The algorithm is implemented by readily available software packages including Hugin (http://www.hugin.com/), Netica (http://www.norsys.com/), Ergo (http://www.noeticsystems.com) and Microsoft's MSBNx (http://research.microsoft.com/adapt/MSBNx/). Kevin Murphy maintains a list of Bayes net software packages at http://www.ai.mit.edu/~murphyk/Bayes/bnsoft.html.

Bayesian networks have four advantages that make them particularly useful for diagnostic assessments with complex performance tasks:

1. The graph serves as a common representation for subject matter experts (SMEs) and psychometricians, enabling the experts to more fully share in the model building process. Bayes nets share this property with structural equation models, but the extra restrictions on Bayes nets ensure that the model structure can always be quickly computed.

2. Bayes nets support *Profile Scoring*—providing simultaneous scores on more than one aspect of proficiency. This is particularly useful for diagnostic assessments.

3. Bayes nets support multiple observed outcome variables per task. This is especially important when the tasks involve complex simulations as described later in this chapter.

4. Bayes nets support Bayesian modeling of their parameters. This means that models can be defined with parameters supplied initially by experts, and later refined based on experiential data (Williamson, Almond, & Mislevy, 2000). Contrast this with neural network models that cannot incorporate the expert opinion, and formula score and rule-based systems which do not allow easy refinement on the basis of data.

BAYESIAN NETWORK APPLICATIONS

Bayesian networks have a history of application as the statistical inference engine in expert systems for such fields as agriculture (Jensen, 1996), troubleshooting computer printing problems (Heckerman, Breese, & Rommelse, 1994), computer vision (Jensen, 1996), diagnosis of congenital heart disease (Spiegelhalter, Dawid, Lauitzen, & Cowell, 1993), computing (Jensen, 1996), and weather forecasting (Edwards, 1998). They have also been implemented in fielded intelligent tutoring and assessment systems, including Corbett, Anderson, & O'Brien's (1995) ACT programming tutor; the HYDRIVE tutor for aircraft hydraulics (Mislevy & Gitomer, 1996; Steinberg & Gitomer, 1993), Derry and Hawks' (1993) TAPS tutor for arithmetic story problems, and the OLAE and ANDES physics tutoring systems (VanLehn & Martin, 1998). A number of these systems are designed to improve skills at complex tasks by assessing learner ability and concurrently making interventions to improve abilities the assessment has identified as deficient (Gitomer, Steinberg, & Mislevy, 1995).

This chapter presents basic concepts of Bayesian networks and illustrates their application in NetPASS; a Cisco Learning Institute (CLI) assessment of computer networking skills. NetPASS is performance based and uses web-administered simulation tasks and live interactions with functional hardware to assess student ability in computer network design, implementation, and troubleshooting. The next section discusses the role of Bayesian networks as the evidence accumulation engine for this assessment from an Evidence-Centered Design (ECD) perspective (see chap. 2, this volume). The NetPASS assessment design is used to illustrate concepts of Bayesian networks and the interaction between assessment design and scoring. The subsequent section goes into more technical detail about Bayesian networks and their application to NetPASS. Following this is an illustration of Bayesian networks in operation during assessment administration and the implications for score reporting. The chapter continues with some notes on constructing a Bayesian network and concludes with some notes about special considerations for high stakes assessment.

ASSESSMENT DESIGN AND THE ROLE OF BAYESIAN INFERENCE NETWORKS

An increased emphasis on assessment as a learning tool rather than solely for rank-ordering has resulted in greater emphasis on cognitively-based assessment that leverages research on knowledge acquisition and learning (e.g. Chase & Simon, 1973a; 1973b; de Groot, 1965, on chess; Chi, Feltovich & Glaser, 1981, on physics; Lesgold, Feltovich, Glaser & Wang, 1981, on radiology; Newell, 1990; Newell & Simon, 1988, on general problem solving; Nesher, 1986; Brown & Burton, 1978, on arithmetic). Such assessments shift the target of inference from a singular and continuous trait to a constellation of knowledge structures, strategies and conceptualizations used in problem solving (Masters & Mislevy, 1993). This approach targets a more accurate portrayal of individual abilities for the purpose of more accurate prediction, better selection and placement decisions, more specific and beneficial diagnostic information (e.g. Gitomer & Yamamoto, 1991), more effective educational programs, and to provide a greater understanding of the factors (both internal and external to the individual) that contribute to task performance.

Such interest in cognitively diagnostic assessment suggests de-emphasizing multiple-choice tasks, commonly criticized as requiring a substantially different and less valued set of operations than the criterion of interest to the assessment (Frederiksen & Collins, 1989; Frederiksen 1984), in favor of constructed-response tasks. It is believed that such tasks, particularly computerized simulations, are more capable of providing rich observations required (e.g. Chipman, Nichols, & Brennan, 1995; Collins, 1990; Fiske, 1990) to provide evidence about cognitive processes (Ackerman & Smith, 1988; Ward, Frederiksen, & Carlson, 1980) supporting multivariate cognitive inferences.

The transition from reliance on multiple-choice items for univariate proficiencies to computerized simulations using constructed-response tasks for multivariate cognitive models of proficiency poses new challenges for measurement models and statistical methods of inference. The following sections describe such a challenge posed by an assessment of computer networking ability and some of the successes and challenges in applying Bayesian networks as the statistical inference engine for this assessment.

THE DESIGN OF NETPASS

Context and Purpose

The Cisco Learning Institute collaborates with high schools, community colleges, and vocational schools to provide fundamental computer networking education. The Cisco Networking Academy Program (CNAP) is four-semester curriculum teaching the principles and practice of designing, implementing, and maintaining computer networks capable of supporting local, national, and global organizations. Instruction is provided in classrooms as well as through online curriculum and activities. Assessments are likewise conducted through classroom exercises and online testing. The CNAP uses the World Wide Web for both instruction and assessment administration and data maintenance. World Wide Web usage facilitates global access to educational resources and assessment tools, presenting both opportunities and challenges for educational research. To become accomplished at common networking tasks demands considerable technical knowledge as well as strategic and procedural expertise. As a result, CLI was dissatisfied relying only on multiple-choice assessments of declarative knowledge to determine students' understanding of some of the most important aspects of networking ability.

To prevent over reliance on assessment of declarative knowledge in their educational program, the CNAP, in collaboration with CLI, ETS, and the University of Maryland, redesigned the assessment program to leverage simulation technology and remote connection capabilities to produce an online assessment exercising the *cognitive* (if not physical) aspects of network design, implementation, and troubleshooting. The initial prototype assessment, called NetPASS, uses network simulations with realistic interactive tasks to measure students' abilities and provide targeted educational feedback. This feedback includes reporting on the students' knowledge of networking, their mastery of various networking skills, their ability to carry out procedures and strategies for networking tasks, and their misconceptions about network functionality and operational procedures. An ECD process was employed in this redesign, providing the framework necessary to meet the design needs for such a complex computerized assessment in a technical domain.

The Student Model

The full NetPASS Student Model representing the constellation of proficiencies important for success as a CNAP student is shown as Fig. 7.2 (as are a few associated claims, indicated by stars) and includes the declarative knowledge of the domain (represented as Network Disciplinary Knowledge), which itself is composed of multiple sub-areas of declarative knowledge (IOS, Protocols, etc.). An ability of interest that depends on Network Disciplinary Knowledge is the ability to create mental representations of the structure and function of a computer network, represented as Network Modeling. The strategic and operational proficiency for conducting various computer network activities is represented as Network Proficiency. It is comprised of specific subproficiencies for particular classes of tasks: Implement (for implementing a computer network for a particular design), Design (for designing the structure and function of computer network components), Troubleshoot (for identifying and remediating problems in existing computer networks), Operation (for routine maintenance and use of a computer network), and Planning (for anticipation of computer network characteristics required in anticipation of network function for particular purposes). This full model represents the knowledge, skill and ability necessary for CNAP success as well as the dependencies among them. For example, a student's Network Proficiency (which consists of five interrelated skills) is modeled as dependent on her Network Disciplinary Knowledge (which also consists of multiple components). A subsequent discussion addresses how the dependencies suggested in the graph by the arrows correspond to characteristics of the statistical inference model.

As the NetPASS assessment was developed to address areas of proficiency not easily measured through multiple-choice items, the Student Model implemented in NetPASS, provided as Fig. 7.3, is a restricted version of the model presented in Fig. 7.2. The operational Student Model is restricted to variables of inference from the assessment (those for which scores or other information will be reported). In this model the Design, Implementation, and Troubleshooting components of Network Proficiency are retained but Operation and Planning are removed as a result of being conceptually relevant but bearing no influence on the model or assessment outcomes (and no tasks evoke direct evidence about them). Similarly, the knowledge variables that are components of Network Disciplinary Knowledge are removed as these variables are neither targeted by the assessment nor reported since they are adequately addressed through existing multiple-choice assessments.

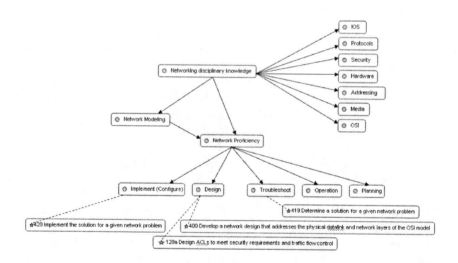

FIG. 7.2. The full Student Model for the NetPASS assessment.

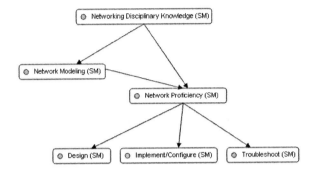

FIG. 7.3. The Operational NetPASS Student Model.

The Student Model provides the starting place for the Bayes net-based evidence accumulation engine. It will provide the initial values for the student model used to track belief about the student proficiencies during the assessment. The Student Model in its initialized state (before the examinee begins testing) is not student specific, but rather population specific, as it refers to what is expected from students who are likely to take the NetPASS assessment. Because the assessment is designed to use a Bayes net-based evidence accumulation engine, the Student Model is likewise expressed as a Bayesian network. This Bayes net provides the core for the scoring algorithm: It updates and maintains the current state of belief about each student's abilities as new evidence is obtained from the Evidence Models.

Task Models

Although it would be possible to construct each task from scratch, Task Models facilitate designing tasks that succeed in posing realistic networking challenges required by the NetPASS assessment. A Task Model is a general framework, or framework hierarchy, for design of tasks that meet certain evidential requirements with respect to the Student Model, as well as meeting other specifications of importance for the test design. That is, a Task Model is a blueprint for task development that allows for some flexibility in creating multiple tasks, each of which is a different instantiation of the Task Model. A task is a particular instantiation of that Task Model, in which the values of model variables are now fixed and the content developed to be consistent with these fixed values. (The distinction between Task Models and tasks is similar to the specification of item model and items in automatic item generation of multiple-choice items (e.g., Irvine & Kyllonen, 2002). Directed development of assessment tasks within flexible but well-defined Task Models facilitates building tasks to be comparable in both difficulty and in targeted discrimination among levels of proficiency, or to vary in controlled ways.

The Task Models specify Task Model variables—task features and possible sets of values—that are important to control in task construction. These task features are used for a variety of purposes, including: (1) defining evidentiary focus (i.e., if these features of a task were changed the nature of the proficiency being measured by the task would also be changed); (2) controlling task difficulty and discrimination; and (3) controlling context (these task features may incidental to both evidentiary focus and difficulty yet are necessary to provide a complete scenario). A portion of a Task Model developed for the Troubleshooting tasks in NetPASS is presented as Fig. 7.4. It shows some of the variables used to define a task in the Troubleshooting family. The possible values for the selected variables are listed in the figure, with the value chosen for a particular task in bold face. The stimulus for the resulting task is shown in Fig. 7.5, which constitutes the upper third of the task screen for the NetPASS assessment. The remaining two-thirds are presented in a subsequent figure. The full Troubleshooting Task Model contains many more variables than are presented here. For greater detail regarding the development of the assessment models and the operational processes for NetPASS see Williamson, Bauer, Steinberg, Mislevy, and Behrens (2004).

Task Model Variable

..... Fault Symptoms → subtle; moderate; **significant**

..... Nature of Claim → Design; Implementation; ***Troubleshooting***

..... Network Complexity → **low**; moderate; high

.... Network Connectivity → **simple**; moderate; rich

.... Number of routers → 0; 1; **2**; 3; 4; 5; 6; 7; 8; 9; 10

..... Network Testing Characteristics → minor; moderate; substantial

.... Number of tests required → 0; **1**; 2; 3; 4; 5; 6; 7; 8; 9; 10

.... Test Types → **ping**; telnet

..... Number of faults → 0; 1; 2; **3**; 4; 5; 6; 7; 8; 9; 10

....

FIG. 7.4. Sample of Task Model instantiation.

Scenario Description:

A small community college campus has two buildings, each housing a router. The college network has been functioning well. Students have been found telnetting to the routers. Suddenly, the East building experiences connectivity problems with receiving e-mail. Users in the Central building are able to receive e-mail from the e-mail server and are not experiencing problems. The e-mail server is located on the LAN in the Central building. Access to the Internet is provided from the East building via S0.

Information about the network:

ISP	East	Central
S0 212.56.25.66 (DCE)	E0 199.100.25.33	E0 199.100.25.97
	S0 199.100.25.65 (DCE)	S1 199.100.25.66
	S1 212.56.25.65	

1. The subnet mask is 255.255.255.224, and IGRP 100 is the routing protocol

2. For testing purposes, the S0 interfaces provide the clocking

3. It is not necessary to represent the LAN in the network diagram

---

FIG. 7.5: Task Stimulus example.

Upon initializing the test with an authorization code, the student is presented with navigation screens that allow the student to self-select the nature of task they would like to attempt (Design, Implement, or Troubleshoot) and the approximate difficulty of the task (Easy, Moderate, or Hard). Once they select a task type and difficulty level, they are presented with the basic scenario providing the context of their work and their work objectives. From that point, they can choose how to begin working, either by completing a network diagram, directly interacting with the network, or by completing a list of identified faults (when applicable for troubleshooting tasks). This process and student options are elaborated further later in the chapter.

As a result of the interactions with the task, a number of work products are recorded and preserved. These work products entail both the work process undertaken and the outcomes of the work itself. In addition, they also include student records of the identified faults, or other self-reports of work conducted when applicable. As an example, the troubleshooting tasks produce four work products (one or more of which could be empty if the student does not complete all parts of the task). They are:

1. A log of all troubleshooting and repair actions taken. This log contains a complete transaction of every command entered.

2. A list of faults which student generates in the process of completing the task. This is a self-report of faults identified and remediated by the student.

3. The final state of the network, after all repairs are completed. This represents the final functioning form of the network once the student has completed all work.

4. A diagram of the network, which the student may construct in analyzing the problem. This diagram allows for the automated analysis of diagrammed objects, their physical and technical relationships to each other, and for comparison to the actual network components and relationships.

Evidence Models

The Evidence Models provide the bridge between the tasks and the Student Models. They are responsible for using the work products that are the output of the student's interaction with the task to update the current set of beliefs about the student's proficiencies. Modeling the evidence separately from a general Task Model rather than a specific task means that the Evidence Model can be used to adapt between a given Student Model and a given Task Model. For example, if the Student Model consists of a single "overall proficiency" variable, then the Evidence Model would implement some kind of univariate scoring. However, if the Student Model addresses multiple aspects of proficiency, then the Evidence model must be much more detailed to reflect the evidence for each of these aspects of proficiency.

Following the ECD framework, the Evidence Models for the NetPASS assessment consist of two components: one for task-level scoring or evidence identification, and the other for drawing inferences about ability, or evidence accumulation. The two parts of the Evidence Model describe (1) how to set the proper values of the observables based on the contents of the work product (evidence identification); and (2) how the observables relate to the proficiency variables (evidence accumulation). The evidence identification engine is custom software that analyzes the work products (e.g., network diagrams and troubleshooting logs) and produces the observed outcome variables. The NetPASS evidence identification engine is itself an example of automated scoring—rule-based scoring, to be specific—and observable variables, which are the output of the evidence identification process, represent summaries of lower level scoring features in a manner similar to Clauser, Subhiyah, Nungester, Ripkey, Clyman et al. (1995).

The evidence accumulation component of an Evidence Model is the mechanism by which student task performance data is used as evidence about student knowledge, skills, and abilities. In particular, this component describes the relationship between the proficiency variables described in the Student Model, and the observable outcome variables. In the case of the Bayes net-based Evidence Accumulation Engine, this part of the Evidence Model is expressed as a Bayes net fragment linking the proficiency variables to the observables. This is only a Bayes net fragment, because it borrows the proficiency variables from the Student Model. It becomes a complete network when it and the other fragments are joined with the Student Model.

If the Evidence Model is a bridge, its keystone is the *observable outcome variables* (*observables* for short). These are the outputs of the Evidence Identification process and the inputs to the Evidence Accumulation process. They are what Thissen and Wainer (2001) called the "scored responses." In a multiple-choice task, the work product is typically what selection the student made and the observable is typically whether or not that selection was correct. In constructed response tasks, there are typically multiple observables from more complex work products. The NetPASS model features the following observables:

- *t2-scr-flst-Correctness of Outcome*—Whether or not the fault list correctly identified all the faults.

- *t2-scr-cfg-Correctness of Outcome*—Whether or not the network was in working order after all troubleshooting and repairs.

- *t2-scr-log-Correctness of Procedure*—Whether or not the correct troubleshooting and repair steps where taken.

- *t2-scr-log-Efficiency of Procedure*—How directly did the student arrive at a solution (or did the student require considerable trial and error or false steps).

- *t2-scr-dgm-Correctness of Outcome*—If the student drew a network diagram, was it a correct representation of the network.

The observables are the key features of the work products, the ones used to draw inferences about the proficiency variables. The five observables above are *final observables*, that is, observables that will be used in evidence accumulation. The NetPASS model also includes some additional *feedback observables* that are used for task level feedback to the student, but not for scoring across the assessment. For example, NetPASS included an observable related to the number of times the student used the help system that was used for task level feedback but not for final scoring.

An example of a summary score Evidence Model fragment for the troubleshooting scenario is provided as Fig. 7.6. This Evidence Model taps three proficiency variables: *Troubleshoot, Network Disciplinary Knowledge,* and *Network Modeling.* The nodes for these variables are annotated with a circle (●) in the graph. The five observable variables (described previously) are marked with a triangle (▼). The edges in the graph show which skills influence performance for which observables. This is referred to as a Bayes net fragment because the proficiency variables are temporarily separated from the rest of the proficiency variables. In this separation they retain their probability distributions they had in the Student Model, and are then updated based on the values of the observables. Then, "docking" the Evidence Model back with the full Student Model will create a complete Bayesian network that can be used to update beliefs about the student (Almond, Herskovits, Mislevy, & Steinberg, 1999).

Scoring using this Evidence Model proceeds as follows: When the Evidence Identification engine receives the work product, it calculates the values for the observables; both the final observables and the ones to be used for task-based feedback. The final observables are sent to the evidence accumulation engine, which "docks" the Bayes net fragment for the appropriate Evidence Model with the current Student Model for the student in question (with any values updated from the previous tasks for this individual). It *instantiates* the observable nodes of this joint network and propagates the information to the Student Model.

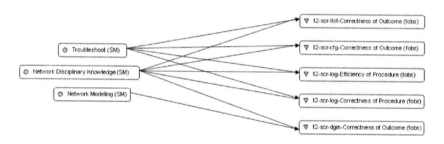

FIG. 7.6.   An Evidence Model for Summary Score reporting from troubleshooting tasks.

The Evidence Model also specifies what will happen if some or all of the work product is missing. For example, completing the fault list is a required step. So if the fault list is empty, that is the same as a wrong answer and the evidence identification engine would pass along the lowest possible value for that observable. The network diagram is an optional step. In this case, if the network diagram part of the task was not attempted, then the value for the corresponding observable would remain uncertain, with the possible values at probabilities conditional on the values of variables that had been observed thus far. In this case, the node would not be instantiated in the network and it would count neither for nor against the student.

Obviously, the NetPASS assessment design poses a number of challenges for measurement. As illustrated in Figure 7.6, which is a fragment of a Bayesian network that becomes a complete network when joined with the Student Model (Figure 7.3), appropriate inference requires that multiple observable variables be computed from multiple work products stemming from a single task. These multiple scorable elements provide evidence about multiple aspects of proficiency. The result is a many-to-many relationship in which multiple, potentially dependent observables from a common task are used as evidence to simultaneously inform multiple proficiency variables. Figure 7.6 already shows the value of the graphical representation of the Bayes net in helping to sort out the many-to-many relationship. The subsequent section shows how Bayesian networks meet the statistical requirements as well.

BAYESIAN NETWORK DEFINITIONS AND THEIR USE

Bayesian networks are a representation of a complex probability distribution using a graph. Efficient computational techniques can exploit this graphical structure to solve problems of inference, such as those posed by the requirements for the Evidence Accumulation Process. This section provides some basic definitions and fundamental properties of Bayesian networks. It describes how to do routine calculations using Bayes nets and how they relate to the Proficiency and Evidence models described above.

Bayesian networks can be used to support probability-based reasoning from a collection of data on examinee performances on complex tasks: evaluation of corroborating and converging evidence as it relates to hypotheses about the strategies, knowledge, and abilities of the examinee; decisions regarding appropriate actions based on that evidence; and decisions about collecting additional data on the basis of current hypotheses and examinee performance.

Through this probability-based reasoning, the Bayes net serves to transmit complex observational evidence throughout a network of interrelated variables. The Bayes net provides the means for *deductive reasoning* (from generals, such as students' knowledge, to particulars, such as their observable behaviors) and *inductive reasoning* (from particulars to generals, such as from students' behaviors to their likely states of knowledge) (Mislevy, 1996; Schum, 1987).

BAYES THEOREM

As the name implies, Bayesian inference networks derive their calculus from Bayes theorem. Bayes theorem is a simple rule for calculating inverse probability, that is, reversing the direction of conditioning in a conditional probability statement. However, Bayes theorem also supports an interpretation of probability as a state of information. A simple example will illustrate this process.

Let A represent the event that a student has a skill of interest, and let B represent the event that the student can correctly perform a given task which requires the skill. (In the ECD language, A is a proficiency variable and B is an observable, in the terminology of item response theory (IRT), it may be helpful for the reader to think of A as θ and B as an item response.) Assume that the prevalence of this skill in the population the student is drawn from is $p(A)$. Next, the operating characteristics of the task are defined. The *sensitivity* of the task is $p(B|A)$, that is, the probability that the student will get the task right given that the student has the required skill. The *specificity* of the task is $p(\neg B|\neg A)$, that is the probability that the student will get the task wrong given that the student lacks the skill. Together, these three probabilities specify the joint probability for A and B. However, the usual situation is that the value B is observed and is used to draw inferences about A. To do this, Bayes theorem is applied:

$$p(A \mid B) = \frac{p(A)p(B \mid A)}{p(B)} \qquad (1)$$

The terms *sensitivity* and *specificity* come from the field of signal processing and are commonly used in medical testing. However, they are desirable properties of educational tests as well and best practice in test design tries to maximize them. In particular, a test with low sensitivity will be very difficult and almost nobody will perform well; therefore, it will provide poor evidence for the skill (assuming the skill is more prevalent in the population). Similarly, a test with low specificity will be too easy and almost everybody will perform well; therefore it will not provide good evidence. Good (1950) formalized this idea calling it the *weight of evidence*. Mislevy (1994) characterized it as follows:

- Prior to observing a datum, relative belief in a space of possible propositions is effected as a probability (density) distribution, namely, the prior distribution *[p(A)]*.

- Posterior to observing the datum, relative belief in the same space is effected as another probability (density) distribution, the posterior distribution *[p(A|B)]*.

- The evidential value of the datum B is conveyed by the multiplicative factor that revises the prior to the posterior for all possible values of A, namely, the likelihood function p(B|A). One examines the direction by which beliefs associated with any given A change in response to observing B (is a particular value of A now considered more probable or less probable than before?) and the extent to which they change (by a little or a lot?)." (p. 453)

Above, *B* was defined as a single observation relevant to Skill *A*. The usual practice in educational testing is to produce a test that includes multiple opportunities to observe the skills in practice. Thus *B* is replaced with $\mathbf{B} = B_1...B_n$. The likelihood $p(\mathbf{B} \mid A)$ is now the probability of seeing a particular response pattern. Usually to make Bayes theorem tractable in such cases, a *conditional independence* assumption can be made in which B_i and B_j are conditionally independent given *A*. In this case,

$$p(\mathbf{B} \mid A) = \prod p(B_i \mid A).$$

Although this may seem like an assumption of convenience, best practice in test design usually tries to engineer the test so that this assumption holds (Almond & Mislevy, 1999). If the binary skill variable, *A*, is replaced with a continuous θ, the result is an equation that is familiar from Item Response Theory. In this case, the likelihood $p(B_i \mid \theta)$ usually takes on a familiar functional form such as the two-parameter logistic function or the Rasch model.

With this in mind, the Bayesian approach can be contrasted with the maximum likelihood approach. The maximum likelihood estimate for theta is the same as the *maximum a posteriori* (or MAP) estimate from the Bayesian model with the additional assumption that the prior distribution is uniform over the allowed range for theta. The Bayesian method, in contrast, can use a more informative prior, such as the population distribution. If the test is sufficiently long and the pattern of responses is consistent, then the likelihood will be strongly peaked and somewhat narrow. In this case, the posterior distribution will look very much like the likelihood, and the difference between the Bayesian and maximum likelihood estimates will be small. When the test responses are inconsistent (e.g., when a student gets hard items right and easy items wrong because of poor time management), the likelihood will be nearly flat and a change in a single item outcome variable could drive the maximum likelihood estimate from one end of the scale to the other. The Bayesian solution, however, will look much like the prior, saying that in presence of contradictor or insufficient evidence, the best estimate of the student's proficiency is based on the population properties. In these cases, the Bayesian estimate would tend to be towards the center of the scale.

The conditional independence assumption above has interesting implications when the data are delivered in multiple batches. Suppose, for simplicity that there are two batches of responses, $\mathbf{B}_1$ and $\mathbf{B}_2$. Then Bayes theorem can be factored as follows:

$$p(A \mid \mathbf{B}_1, \mathbf{B}_2) = \frac{p(A)p(\mathbf{B}_1 \mid A)p(\mathbf{B}_2 \mid A)}{\sum_A p(A)p(\mathbf{B}_1 \mid A)p(\mathbf{B}_2 \mid A)} = \frac{p(A \mid \mathbf{B}_1)p(\mathbf{B}_2 \mid A)}{\sum_A p(A \mid \mathbf{B}_1)p(\mathbf{B}_2 \mid A)} \qquad (2)$$

Note that the posterior distribution after processing the first batch of data, $p(A \mid \mathbf{B}_1)$, becomes the prior distribution for the subsequent batch. Aside from being a computational convenience, this meets the requirements of the Evidence Accumulation Process in an intelligent tutoring system. The "state" of the student model at any point in time is the posterior distribution over the proficiency variables given the evidence observed so far. As new evidence comes in, Bayes theorem is applied to update the student model. The resulting posterior distribution for variables in the student model becomes the prior distribution of the model for new evidence.

As discussed in a subsequent section, a key idea in Bayesian networks is extending this kind of reasoning to many variables, with varying patterns of theoretical and empirical interrelationships.

BASIC PROPERTIES OF BAYESIAN NETWORKS

The Bayesian view of statistics as described above provides a foundation for the construction of an Evidence Accumulation Process (Almond & Mislevy, 1999; Mislevy, 1995). In implementation the NetPASS model presents two challenges: (1) because NetPASS requires *profile scoring* (reporting on multiple proficiency variables for an individual), there are multiple variables representing knowledge, skills, and abilities in the model; and (2) because the tasks require complex performances, there are multiple variables representing observable outcomes for each task. As the dimensionality of the model increases, so does the computational complexity of applying Bayes theorem. For example, the NetPASS Student Model given in Fig. 7.3 contains six variables each of which can take on five possible states. Calculating the denominator for Bayes theorem requires summing over the 5^6 possible combinations of their values! As presented in the following section, the key to more efficient computation involves expressing the interrelationships among variables in terms of interactions among smaller interrelated clusters of variables, as posited by theory, prior research, and experience.

Conditional Independence

The key to solving any large problem is to split it into smaller pieces. With probability distributions, this is accomplished by exploiting independence relationships among the variables. Two random variables A and B are *independent* if their joint probability distribution $p(A,B)$ is simply the product of their individual probability distributions:

$$p(A, B) = p(A)p(B).$$

If two variables are independent, then observing the value of one variable provides no information about the value of the other. Two random variables A and B are *conditionally independent* if they seem to be related, so that

$$p(A, B) \neq p(A)p(B),$$

but the relationship between these variables can be understood as being determined by the values of one or more other variables, so that

$$p(A, B \mid C) = p(A \mid C)p(B \mid C).$$

The value of exploiting conditional independence relationships in the calculation of the likelihood is discussed previously. However, with a model the size of the NetPASS model the conditional independence conditions become complex and there is a need for a mechanism to facilitate tracking the modeled conditions.

A key feature of a Bayesian network model is to represent the conditional independence relationships with a graph. Nodes in the network represent variables in the graph. Edges in the graph represent patterns of dependence and independence. A Bayesian network is always an *acyclic directed graph*. The term *directed* means that the edges are drawn as arrows indicating a direction of influence pointing from a *parent* node to the *child* node it influences. The term *acyclic* indicates that, starting from a variable in the network and following the edges in the direction of the arrows, it is impossible to return to the originating variable. This has important implications for the consistency of the model, as discussed next.

An advantageous property of Bayesian networks is that separation in the graph implies conditional independence in the network. The notion of separation is somewhat complex, as it depends on the direction of the arrows. In particular, the graph structure must account for the *competing explanation* phenomenon. Suppose there is a task with an observable outcome variable that has as parents two proficiency variables. Suppose that the task is designed so that the application of the skills is in a *conjunctive* manner, that is, both skills are necessary to solve the problem well. Even if the two skills are *a priori* independent (independent in the population), the task design is such that the estimates of these skills (for a particular student) on the basis of task performance may not be independent. Suppose, for example, that the student did not do well on the task. It would be appropriate to infer that either the first or the second (or both) proficiencies were lacking. If it was later learned that the student had likely mastered the first skill, then this would result in the inference that the second skill was the skill that is lacking. Thus, the observation of a value for a child variable for which there are two parent variables renders previously independent variables dependent. Pearl (1988) introduced rules for *d-separation* to formalize this idea.

The graph in Fig. 7.3 expresses the conditional independence relationships in the NetPASS Student Model. The theory of the structure of the domain (i.e., expertise in designing and troubleshooting computer networks) is represented through the deductive reasoning structure by a top-down series of dependencies beginning with Network Disciplinary Knowledge. The Student Model variables of Network Modeling and Network Proficiency represent variables directly dependent on Network Disciplinary Knowledge. Network Proficiency also has a direct dependency on Network Modeling skill. The skills of Design, Implementation, and Troubleshooting are in turn dependent on Network Proficiency. This model was built in a collaborative effort between SMEs and psychometricians. In particular, it represents the psychometric view of the SMEs' view of how the domain is structured.

The importance of using substantive theory to suggest conditional independence relationships cannot be overemphasized. They are critical in defining the topology of the Bayesian network of variables. If this topology is favorable, the Bayesian probabilistic calculations can be carried out efficiently for large networks by means of strictly local operations (Lauritzen & Spiegelhalter, 1988; Pearl, 1988).

Pearl (1988) argued that the specification of intervening variables permitting conditional independence is not a mere technical convenience, but reflects the patterns of relationships in a domain—indeed, represents a natural element in human reasoning about a field of study. He writes:

> It is this role which prompts us to posit that conditional independence is not a grace of nature for which we must wait passively, but rather a psychological necessity which we satisfy actively by organizing our

knowledge in a specific way. An important tool in such organization is the identification of intermediate variables that induce conditional independence among observables; if such variables are not in our vocabulary, we create them. In medical diagnosis, for instance, when some symptoms directly influence each other, the medical profession invents a name for that interaction (e.g. "syndrome," "complication," "pathological state") and treats it as a new auxiliary variable that induces conditional independence; dependency between any two interacting systems is fully attributed to the dependencies of each on the auxiliary variable. (p. 44)

Conditional independence constraints not only permit computation in large networks but, perhaps more significantly, they also serve as a tool for mapping Greeno's (1989) "generative principles of the domain" into the framework of mathematical probability. Such a mapping transforms the substantive theory of a field into structures that embody the principles upon which deductive reasoning in the field is based (Mislevy, 1994). Bayes theorem then enables one to reverse the flow of reasoning through these same structures to one of inductive reasoning, from observations to expressions of belief in terms of the more fundamental concepts of the domain (Mislevy, 1994).

So where do the arrows come from and how do the SMEs know which direction to point the arrows? One possibility is that that the SMEs have a causal conjecture about the domain. In this case, directing the arrow from the "cause" to the "effect" almost always leads to a more efficient representation. For example, as a skill is believed to cause good or bad performance on a task, the arrow almost always points from the skill variable to the observable variable. For this reason, Pearl (1988) emphasized causality when building models.

Although causal conjectures are useful, they are not necessary. All that is necessary is that the variables be statistically related. Howard and Matheson (1981) emphasized that all that is necessary is *relevance*, and Schacter (1986) provides formal mechanics for reversing the direction of edges in the graph. The use of causality has been hotly debated in the field of Bayesian networks, with a large body of work investigating methods of learning causal relationships from data (e.g., Cliff, 1983; Glymour, Scheines, Spirtes, & Kelly, 1987). The usual cautions when trying to draw inferences from observational data apply to this activity. For example, almost all of the formal systems for learning causality are limited in scope to the variables that are included in the model. Shafer (1996) discussed the role of causality in more detail. For the purposes of this chapter, it is sufficient to know that when there are causal conjectures about the domain, they can be exploited in model building.

Recursive Representation and Factorization

Building the Student Model for an Evidence Accumulation Process requires the specification of the joint distribution of the set of proficiency variables. Ordering the variables and conditioning on the previous variables in the order produces what is called the recursive representation of the joint distribution:

$$p(x_1,...,x_N) = p(x_n \mid x_{n-1},...,x_1)p(x_{n-1} \mid x_{n-2},...,x_1)...p(x_2 \mid x_1)p(x_1) = \prod_{j=1}^{n} p(x_j \mid x_{j-1},...,x_1), \quad (3)$$

where for $j = 1$ the term is simply defined as $p(X_1)$. Although this expression is valid for any ordering of the variables, ordering the variables according to the direction of arrows in the Bayesian network produces a computational advantage. In particular, let $pa(x_j)$ represent the parents of node x_j in the graph. Then, because of the conditional independence conditions embodied in the Bayes net, we can write:

$$p(x_j \mid x_{j-1},...,x_1) = p(x_j \mid pa(x_j))$$

and Equation 3 becomes

$$p(x_1,...,x_N) = \prod_{j=1}^{N} p(x_j \mid pa(x_j)) \quad (4)$$

where $p(x_j \mid pa(x_j))$ is an unconditional probability when $pa(x_j)$ is empty.

The recursive representation and the model graph together provide an efficient factorization of the probability distribution. There is a fundamental duality between this factorization and the conditional independence conditions expressed by the graph, and it is difficult to tell which is more important (Almond, 1995). Together, they lead to the efficient computational techniques described below.

PROPAGATING EVIDENCE

Pearl (1982) described an efficient scheme for making calculations with Bayes nets by passing messages in the network. When the value of a variable is observed, then the corresponding node in the graph is *instantiated* by multiplying its probability distribution with a new probability containing a one in the spot corresponding to the observed value of the variable and a zero elsewhere. Messages are passed down the graph (in the direction of the arrows) by applying the recursive partitioning formula (Equation 4). Messages are passed up the graph (against the direction of the arrows) by applying Bayes theorem. After propagation, the posterior (given the instantiated evidence) distribution for any node in the graph can be read by looking at the corresponding node in the graph and reading off the values stored there. Pearl (1988) described the intuition behind this algorithm.

The Pearl (1982) algorithm was limited to polytrees, directed graphs that contain no cycles after dropping the direction of the edges. Pearl (1988) noted that clustering several variables together to make super-variables can get around the polytree restriction. This is essentially the method employed by Lauritzen and Spiegelhalter (1988), they identify groups of variables called *cliques* and form these cliques into a tree. All of the computations necessary can be done by passing messages through the tree of cliques. There are numerous variations on this algorithm (Almond, 1995; Jensen, 1996; Neapolitan, 2004; Spiegelhalter, Dawid, Lauritzen, & Cowell 1993). When conditions are favorable (due to simplifications afforded by conditional independence constraints), these computations are tractable even in very large networks.

The process of defining cliques for evidence propagation is typically transparent to the user of Bayes net software packages. However, some knowledge of the implicit clique structure of models is needed in order to understand model performance and efficiency. The size of the largest clique in the transformed model usually dominates the cost of working with a Bayesian networks. In general, variables with large numbers of parents produce large cliques in the network. Furthermore, loops in the network often must be "filled-in" to produce the tree of cliques, again resulting in big cliques. Accessible descriptions of the stepwise approach to construction of clique structure can be found in Almond (1995) and Mislevy (1995); the former contains a survey of the literature on optimal tree construction and the latter some notes on how to design graphical models to have small clique trees.

THE PROFICIENCY AND EVIDENCE MODELS AS BAYESIAN NETWORKS

The IRT model can be represented by a graphical model (a generalization of the Bayes net in which variables are allow to be continuous) with all of the observable outcome variables conditionally independent given the proficiency variable (θ). This can be generalized to the case where the proficiency is represented by multiple variables. In this case, the complete Bayes network an be split into a *Student Model* containing the variables that describe characteristics of people and the *Evidence Models* which link the proficiency variables to the observed outcome variables for each task.

As evidence comes into the system from a particular task, the Evidence Model for that task can be "docked" with the Student Model and the evidence propagated from one to the other (Almond & Mislevy, 1999; Almond et al. 1999). The Evidence Model is then undocked and discarded. The Student Model contains all of the knowledge of the student's state, which must be maintained across tasks. This split between Student Models and Evidence Models is exactly the same as the division used in the Evidence-Centered Design framework (described above and in chap. 2).

A key assumption for this approach is that the observable evidence from different tasks must be independent given the proficiency variables. This is the same assumption underlying an IRT model and, like the IRT model, an assessment can be designed around this assumption following good design principles. Consistent with this approach, the Task Models used in NetPASS were designed to exhibit conditional independence relationships consistent with the needs of the Evidence Models.

The Student Model

The complete Bayesian network for an assessment is divided between the Proficiency and Evidence Models of the Evidence-Centered Design framework. The Student Model is the realm of variables that are explicit descriptions of people, whereas the Evidence Models are variables describing performance exhibited in the collected data and how these connect to the related proficiency variables. In this separation, the observable variables from different Evidence Models must be conditionally independent given the variables in the Student Model.

The most important parts of the Student Model are the variables representing the knowledge, skills, and abilities that will constitute reporting variables (that are directly represented in score reports). These are tied closely to the claims made by the assessment. Note that the values of the proficiency variables are latent and usually it is never possible to know them with certainty. Following Bayesian principles, the state of uncertain knowledge about the proficiency variables is represented by a probability distribution. This probability distribution is expressed in a Bayesian network. This allows the exploitation of the network structure to make efficient queries about the current value of any proficiency variable.

Initially, without observing any evidence for an individual, the prior distributions for Student Model variables will reflect beliefs about the population. When an examinee begins the assessment, the initial Student Model is opened to updating based on observed evidence from the individual (scoring). As the Evidence Models provide evidence from performance, the values of Student Model variables are updated to reflect the current estimates for the individual examinee. As such, the Student Model, with its posterior distribution based on observed evidence, becomes the representation of examinee ability used for score reporting and for adaptive task selection (in instances of adaptive testing).

The Student Model alone is sufficient for modeling and/or representing the interrelationships between various proficiencies. However, to understand the relationship between proficiency and task performance, it is necessary to examine the Student Model and Evidence Models jointly.

The Evidence Models

Although the Student Model provides the prior (and upon observing evidence from testing, posterior) distribution in the Bayes theorem, the analog of the likelihoods is provided by the Evidence Models (one for each task in the assessment design). The Student Model provides the probability distributions for the proficiency variables, and the Evidence Model provides the conditional probability of the observable outcomes for a task given the value of the relevant proficiency variables.

Of course, Evidence Models alone are a set of fragments of the complete Bayesian network and they must be rejoined with the Student Model to complete the network. The combined proficiency and Evidence Models are called a *motif*. The full motif lays out the relationship between behavior on assessment tasks and inferences about proficiency resulting from those behaviors, as represented by the posterior distributions of variables in the full motif.

Three types of variables appear in the Evidence Model Bayes net fragment. They are proficiency variables (borrowed from the Student Model), observable outcome variables, and, perhaps additionally, intermediate variables introduced for modeling convenience. These intermediate variables are Evidence Model variables that are neither proficiency variables nor directly extracted from work products, but which make construction of the Bayes net easier. They do this either by representing important latent variables that influence performance but aren't part of the Student Model (such as modeling context effects or "testlet" effects) or by combining multiple-parent variables to allow SMEs to more easily specify the conditional distributions for the model. However, the influence of intermediate observables is specific to a single Evidence Model (i.e., relevant only to the assessment task at hand). If they apply to multiple Evidence Models, then they should instead be represented as part of the Student Model.

Fig. 7.6 shows the initial Evidence Model for one of the NetPASS troubleshooting tasks. Note that a circle indicates the proficiency variables and observed outcome variables are indicated by a triangle. A revised version of this model is provided as Fig. 7.7 and includes representations of the probability distributions (table-like boxes) and inclusion of some intermediate variables added for computational convenience. The meaning and function of the intermediate variables is discussed in the following section.

The Bayes net is not the complete representation of the Evidence model. The aspects not represented graphically are the collection of *evidence rules* that describe how to compute the values of the observable outcome variables given the work product(s) from the task, that is, the process of evidence identification. The evidence rules provide the operational definition of the outcome variables. Note that not all outcome variables need be used in evidence accumulation. For example, NetPASS defined several kinds of "feedback" observables for task level feedback, which were never included in the Bayes net fragments, but which were used to help provide instructionally relevant performance feedback to students.

The initial version of one of the Evidence Models is provided as in Fig. 7.6, while the final version of this model, including additional intermediate variables, is provided as Fig. 7.7. These intermediate latent variables are added to the Evidence Model to aid in the specification of the probability distributions. They are neither observed nor used for reporting since they are only specific to one task, and appear in the Evidence Model rather than the Student Model. There are two types of intermediate variables represented: a combined skill variable and a context effect.

Of these additional intermediate variables, the context effect is probably the most significant. The initial model (Fig. 7.6) contained the assumption that given the proficiency variables all five observable outcome variables are independent. This assumption is suspect because all of the observations are part of a common task. For example, if the student misread part of the problem statement, that student would likely get low variables for all observables.

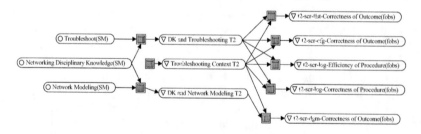

FIG. 7.7.   Refined Evidence Model with intermediate variables and distributions.

Bradlow, Wainer, and Wang (1999) called this a *testlet* effect and introduce a *testlet parameter* to model the dependence of items coming from a common stimulus. The context variable is a similar modeling tool. It is a latent variable that is given two states: *high* and *low*. This variable is not typically reported or interpreted, but instead it is used to account for shared variance between the observable outcome variables that is not the result of the Student Model variables.

The DK and Troubleshooting variable represents a different kind of intermediate variable. This variable represents the direct combination of the Disciplinary Knowledge and Troubleshooting skills. As a result, each of the observables in Fig. 7.7 has two parents (a combined skill variable and the context effect) instead of three (each of the two skills used plus the context effect). This reduces the size of the conditional probability tables that must be specified (from 50 rows to 10 rows as each skill variable has five possible levels) for each observable.

Finally, note that in Fig. 7.7 all variables except the Student Model variables (indicated by circles) have probability distributions associated with them. This is because the Proficiency Variables are actually defined in the Student Model and appear in the Evidence Model to represent the nexus between Student Model and Evidence Model. Therefore, the prior probabilities for Student Model variables in the Evidence Model are uniform distributions until such time as they are "docked" with the Student Model and updated in accordance with realized values of the observable variables.

The Motif: Putting the Pieces Together

The Conceptual Assessment Framework refers to the collection of a Student Model, a set of Task Models, and a corresponding set of Evidence Models. Combining these models to form a complete representation of assessment scoring requires consideration of the final set of tasks administered to an individual examinee (in the case of an adaptive test this may not be known until the student finishes the assessment). Once the complete test form is known, a motif for the assessment can be constructed to represent the full Student Model and all Evidence Models for the tasks used in the assessment form delivered. This is effectively the complete scoring model for the assessment. Fig. 7.8 shows the complete motif for the NetPASS prototype assessment.

The motif shows some things that are not apparent from the Student Model alone. First, it can be observed which nodes from the Student Model are supported by direct evidence from observations (i.e., there are observable variables that are descendants of the proficiency variables in question). These nodes are connected to an observable outcome variable in the motif. Nodes that are not directly connected to observable outcome variables are only supported by indirect evidence through the relationship among proficiency variables. It is usually desirable to design the assessment so that the key reporting variables are supported by direct evidence.

Another notable aspect of the full motif is which proficiency variables have dependencies induced by the Evidence Models. As far as calculating the size of the largest clique in the graph is concerned, it is as if all of the proficiency variables referenced by a particular Evidence Model were connected (Almond et al., 1999). Depending on the design of the assessment, there can be so many induced dependencies that it as if the Student Model was saturated (completely connected), in which case there is no computational advantage of the Bayes net over brute force techniques.

Finally, it is noteworthy to point out the various variables of convenience that have been included in the model to facilitate the modeling process. These include the "context" effect variables that are intended to represent the influence of conditional dependencies induced among observable outcome variables as a result of co-occurrence in a common task. These also include variables of convenience that help distinguish the influence of interaction effects (e.g., "DK & Troubleshooting T1" to represent the influence of the domain knowledge, thus "DK", and troubleshooting proficiency variables from the context effect variable influence on observable outcome variables for Task 1, thus "T1").

CONSTRUCTING A BAYESIAN NETWORK

In order for Bayesian networks to function as a scoring methodology, they must be constructed to meet the intent of the assessment. This Bayes net design for educational measurement generally begins with the identification of relevant Student Model and Evidence Model variables. Bayes net modeling proceeds by building graphical representations of the structure and nature of variable interrelationships, purposely seeking out and representing conditional dependence relationships and structural modifications (e.g., adding variables) to improve efficiency. The process concludes with the specification of conditional probability distributions. Once pretest data become available, they can be used to refine the model, both in terms of structure and in the parameters of the model (the conditional probability distributions). This section briefly discusses these basic Bayes net construction steps, illustrated with examples from NetPASS.

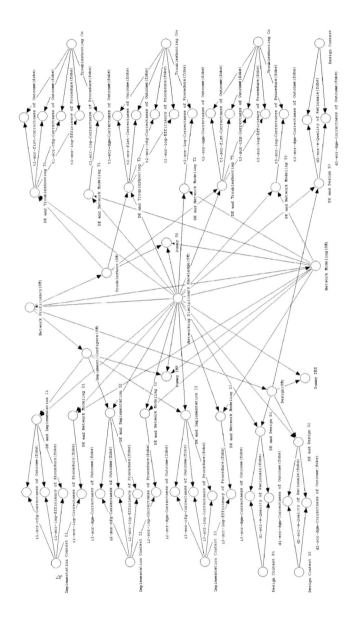

FIG. 7.8. Full NetPASS Model Structure.

229

SPECIFYING MODEL STRUCTURE

The first, and possibly most important, step in building a Bayesian network is identifying the variables. Many resources are typically available to inform this process, including prior research, curriculum, SMEs and other resources, and one of the challenges is sorting through all of the published analyses of the domain and deciding on the most appropriate variables for the goals of the assessment (Mislevy, Steinberg, & Almond, 2002). One method of identifying cognitive variables for inclusion in the network is through cognitive task analysis (CTA); a principled study of cognitive characteristics contributing to differential performance in a domain (see Williamson et al., 2004, for a description of this process for the NetPASS prototype assessment). In the case of NetPASS, these investigations ultimately resulted in the adoption of the Student Model variables represented in Fig. 7.2. This process of domain analysis also serves to identify observable variables for use in Evidence Models. These are derived from domain work that is considered exemplarily of valued work in the domain and that distinguishes between key groups of interest (e.g., competent from beginner or expert from novice). The final determination of the variables to be included in the mode is typically an iterative process and the initial list of potential variables is often too large. Therefore, it is common to review, revise, and redefine the set of variables to reduce the total number to a number appropriate for the planned length, scope and purpose of the assessment. An example of this thinning process was described earlier in the design of NetPASS moving from the initial to the final Student Model (Fig. 7.2 to Fig. 7.3). The initial or full Student Model reflected much of the curriculum in the Cisco Networking Academy Program. The refined Student Model more narrowly reflects the purpose of NetPASS in targeting those parts of the Student Model that are most essential to the domain and least well measured by the existing assessments. The result is that skills like troubleshooting, which are difficult to assess in multiple-choice settings, were maintained, while skills that lend themselves to being addressed well through existing multiple-choice assessments appear only indirectly through their relationship to the "Network Disciplinary Knowledge" skill.

The final Student Model is shown again as Fig. 7.9. This version of the model adds icons (the square boxes) to represent the probability distributions that must be specified. (Technically, these boxes are *directed hyperedges* that join multiple parent nodes to a single child node, and only the variables are "nodes" in the graph, which is technically referred to as a *hypergraph*.)

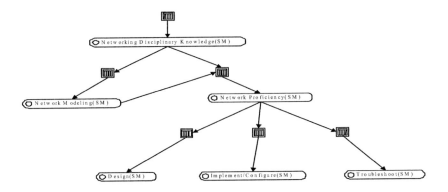

FIG. 7.9. Student Model with distributions.

SPECIFYING PROBABILITY TABLES

Once the structure of the Proficiency and Evidence models are established, the values of the probability tables must be specified. Associated with each variable is a conditional probability table that specifies its distribution given the values of its parents, represented in Figs. 7.7 and 7.9 as squares with vertical lines. Note that there is exactly one distribution square for each variable in the model (for the Proficiency variables, that square exists only in the Student Model). The arrows coming into any given square are connected from the parents of the variable the distribution describes. Thus, the boxes correspond to the factors in the recursive definition of the joint probability distribution of all variables (see Equations 3 and 4).

An example of such a conditional probability table for the NetPASS Network Proficiency variable is provided as Table 7.1. This table provides the states (Novice through Semester 4) for the two parents of Network Proficiency (Network Modeling and Network Disciplinary Knowledge) and the probability of the state of Network Proficiency based on the joint values of the two parent variables. For example, if a student were at the Semester 3 level of Network Modeling and the Semester 4 level of Network Disciplinary Knowledge they would have a .73 probability of being at the Semester 4 level of Network Proficiency. Note also that there are several ones and zeros in the table. These represent logical restrictions on the space of possible combinations. In this case, the SMEs indicated that the state of Network Proficiency could never exceed the level of Network Disciplinary Knowledge. Thus, when Network Disciplinary Knowledge is *Novice* then Network Proficiency must also be *Novice* with probability one. When Network Disciplinary Knowledge is *Semester 1* then there are two possible values for Network Proficiency and all of the others have a probability of zero.

The rows of such tables represent conditional probability distributions, for reasoning deductively: If one knows the values of the parent variables, the corresponding table column gives the probabilities of different possible outcomes for the child. The columns represent likelihood functions, for reasoning inductively: If the value of the child variable were ascertained, the columns represent the likelihood of various configurations of explanatory variables.

Initially, the probabilities that populate the conditional probability tables can be based on estimates from SMEs, who have a substantial understanding of the knowledge structures contributing to domain performance (and are often involved in the model development process). This is typically performed in partnership with statisticians who can assist with the conceptualization of probability distributions. These initial expert-based distributions can then be adjusted based on empirical observation once sufficient examinee data is collected for calibration. The graphical representation also serves as a valuable tool for the representation of structural independence assumptions and for the communication of important ideas with SMEs who can advise and refine model structure in preparation for, or in conjunction with, the specification of the joint distribution of probabilities. This structuring, making full use of conditional independencies, makes the associated probabilities easier for experts to specify since (Hill, 1993):

- The expert only has to consider the distribution of one variable at a time.

- The conditioning of a variable is dependent only on the parents that influence it.

- The experts may consider the conditioning events as fixed scenarios when considering the probabilistic values of the variable.

In practice, the elicitation of conditional probability tables from SMEs is a difficult task. Even sophisticated SMEs have difficulty conceptualizing and consistently applying principles of multiple simultaneous probabilistic relationships between multiple parent and child variables. Furthermore, experts who are not experienced in expressing their judgments as conditional probabilities are subject to heuristic biases during the elicitation process (Kahenman, Slovic, & Tversky, 1982). Difficulty understanding the probabilistic nature of some variables, difficulty considering appropriate probabilities for rare combinations of parent variables, the need for normalization, and the sheer number of such probability judgments all conspire to make specification difficult even for small networks with relatively few states for each variable. As a result, it is not uncommon for SME-specified probabilities to be inconsistent with the intended relationships among variables at first, requiring multiple consistency checks to ensure that the model relationships are functioning as desired.

One tool available for checking the probability specifications is the motif, consisting of the Student Model plus one of the Evidence Models, described earlier. This Bayesian network can be used to evaluate the modeled relationships and conditional probabilities. The process begins by having SMEs state expectations about the value of a target variable based on known values of other variables. The motif can then be used to establish these values and propagate evidence to the other variable in the network. If the posterior distribution for the variable of interest is similar to the expectations of the SMEs, then the model is internally consistent with SME opinion. If this is not the case, further refinement of the specified relationships among variables in the model is required. As this act of using known values of some variables to estimate and then confirming values of related domain variables is often very similar to what SMEs do in practice, the process should produce values that are less subject to inconsistencies between the model parameters and belief about the interaction between domain variables than model parameters derived purely through empirical processes (Kadane, 1980). This kind of checking helps ensure that the model is specified in a rational way that is consistent with the structure of the domain.

One difficulty of SME-based model specification is the sheer number of probabilities that must be specified. Table 7.1 contains 25 rows and five columns for a total of 125 values that must be specified. The fictitious data method[2] of elicitation requires the expert to think about a large number of highly constrained subpopulations, many of which are rare in the population (if the skill variables are moderately correlated). This fact not only makes it hard for the experts to reliably assess those probabilities, it makes it difficult to find data to validate the probability judgments for every possible combination of values of parent variables.

---

[2] This process asks SMEs to imagine, for example, a group of 100 students who are at *Semester 4* level in Network Disciplinary Knowledge, but only at *Semester 2* level in Network Modeling and to estimate the proportion of this group that would be in each of the five possible categories for Network Proficiency.

TABLE 7.1.
An Example of a Conditional Probability Table for Network Proficiency

Network Modeling	Network Proficiency				
	Novice	Semester 1	Semester 2	Semester 3	Semester 4
Network Disciplinary Knowledge = Novice					
Novice	1	0	0	0	0
Semester 1	1	0	0	0	0
Semester 2	1	0	0	0	0
Semester 3	1	0	0	0	0
Semester 4	1	0	0	0	0
Network Disciplinary Knowledge = Semester 1					
Novice	0.269	0.731	0	0	0
Semester 1	0.119	0.881	0	0	0
Semester 2	0.047	0.953	0	0	0
Semester 3	0.018	0.982	0	0	0
Semester 4	0.007	0.993	0	0	0
Network Disciplinary Knowledge = Semester 2					
Novice	0.119	0.381	0.500	0	0
Semester 1	0.047	0.222	0.731	0	0
Semester 2	0.018	0.101	0.881	0	0
Semester 3	0.007	0.041	0.953	0	0
Semester 4	0.002	0.016	0.982	0	0
Network Disciplinary Knowledge = Semester 3					
Novice	0.047	0.222	0.462	0.269	0
Semester 1	0.018	0.101	0.381	0.500	0
Semester 2	0.007	0.041	0.222	0.731	0
Semester 3	0.002	0.016	0.101	0.881	0
Semester 4	0.001	0.006	0.041	0.953	0
Network Disciplinary Knowledge = Semester 4					
Novice	0.018	0.101	0.381	0.381	0.119
Semester 1	0.007	0.041	0.222	0.462	0.269
Semester 2	0.002	0.016	0.101	0.381	0.500
Semester 3	0.001	0.006	0.041	0.222	0.731
Semester 4	0.000	0.002	0.016	0.101	0.881

One method of reducing the burden of probability specification is to use parameterized models. Almond et al. (2001) introduce a set of such parameterized models based on Samejima's graded response model. These models have one parameter (corresponding to an IRT discrimination or slope parameter) for each parent variable and an overall difficulty parameter. The elicitation technique for these models is much simpler, and begins with the SME assessing the fundamental manner in which parent variables interact to produce the observed outcome. Some commonly used patterns are:

- Compensatory—having more of one skill will compensate for having less of another,

- Conjunctive—both skills are necessary to do well on the task,

- Disjunctive—either (any) of the skills can be used to do well on the task, and

- Inhibitor—a minimum threshold of one skill is necessary to solve the problem but is thereafter irrelevant (e.g., a minimum amount of language skill is necessary to solve a math word problem, but after the threshold is met then the math skills predominate).

Once the nature of the relationship is specified, then the SME is asked to rate the relative importance of each of the parent variables (giving the discrimination parameter) and the average level of difficulty. Often these are provided as descriptors that are translated into numeric values by the analyst.

The final step is to assess the SME uncertainty about the parameters. Although this is not strictly necessary for scoring using Bayes nets, assuming no further refinement or empirical modification of conditional probability distributions from SME estimates would be done, it is necessary if the parameters are to be later learned or critiqued on the basis of empirical observations from assessment data. The technique used for NetPASS elicitation was fictitious data. The experts were also asked to represent the degree of confidence in the accuracy of their opinion, as indicated by the number of "students" their estimates represent from their own experience. These are translated into a data point valuation system for later use in weighting the value of SME estimates, in terms of data points, with the data collected from assessment administrations for empirical parameterization. These ratings can be translated into variances for the SME-based parameters. Another technique is for the analyst to judge the variances of the parameters based on the consistency of ratings between the experts.

LEARNING FROM DATA

Regardless of the method and the tools that facilitate specification, the resulting distributions are still based purely on the expertise of a relatively limited number of SMEs working in committee. One of the advantages of working with a full probability model is that there is a built-in mechanism for improving the model from data. Specifically, for any sample of examinees, the model predicts the likelihood of every possible configuration of observed outcomes. If the resultant observed configuration of outcomes (observable variable values) is surprising (relative to alternative configurations), then the model becomes suspect. In such cases, it may be advisable to consider ways to improve the model.

The most straightforward way to adjust a suspect model is by changing the probabilities expressing the relationships between variables. From the Bayesian perspective, uncertainty about the parameters of the model can be expressed with a prior distribution. Therefore, Bayes theorem can be used to update the distributions for model parameters from empirical data. This Bayesian approach to learning model parameters from data contributes to the popularity of the method. Heckerman (1995) provides a tutorial on Bayesian techniques for learning models from data. The general process is outlined below.

The first step in learning models from data is to express uncertainty about the parameters of the model as probability distributions. In a Bayesian network, each row of a conditional probability distribution representing the parameters of the model can be regarded as a multinomial distribution. The Dirichlet Distribution, as the natural conjugate of the multinomial distribution, is useful in specifying the parameters of a Bayesian network model. An independent Dirichlet prior is specified for each row of each conditional probability distribution, referred to as the *hyper-Dirichlet* prior (Spiegelhalter & Lauritzen, 1990). The conjugacy between the multinomial and Dirichlet distributions allows this prior to be expressed in terms of fictitious data for the multinomial distribution. That is, expressing these distributions in the form of fictitious data allows for a characterization of the relative weight, of value, of the SME-specified parameters compared to actual observations in data. For example, Tables 7.2 and 7.3 show hypothetical SME-specified conditional distributions corresponding to the last block of Table 7.1, in which Network Disciplinary Knowledge = Semester 4, that correspond to fictitious examinee sample sizes of 10 and 100 at each combination of values of parent variables.

Markov chain Monte Carlo (MCMC; Gelfand & Smith, 1990; Gilks, Richardson, & Spiegelhalter, 1996; Smith & Roberts, 1993) estimation consists of drawing possibly dependent samples from a distribution of interest and as such provides an appropriate framework for computation in Bayesian analyses (Brooks, 1998; Gelman et al., 1995). Briefly, MCMC estimation consists of drawing values for the model parameters and variables from a series of distributions using rejection sampling techniques such that in the limit the

TABLE 7.2.
An Example of a SME-Specified Conditional Probability Table for Network
Proficiency Based on 10 Fictitious Examinees for Each Row

Network Modeling	Network Proficiency				
	Novice	Semester 1	Semester 2	Semester 3	Semester 4
	Network Disciplinary Knowledge = Semester 4				
Novice	0	1	4	4	1
Semester 1	0	0	2	5	3
Semester 2	0	0	1	4	5
Semester 3	0	0	0	3	7
Semester 4	0	0	0	1	9

TABLE 7.3.
An Example of a SME-Specified Conditional Probability Table for Network
Proficiency Based on 100 Fictitious Examinees for Each Row

Network Modeling	Network Proficiency				
	Novice	Semester 1	Semester 2	Semester 3	Semester 4
	Network Disciplinary Knowledge = Semester 4				
Novice	0	10	40	40	10
Semester 1	0	5	20	50	25
Semester 2	0	2	10	38	50
Semester 3	0	0	5	20	75
Semester 4	0	0	2	10	88

procedure is equal to drawing from the true posterior distribution (Gilks et al.,
1996). That is, to empirically sample from the posterior distribution, it is
sufficient to construct a Markov chain that has the posterior distribution as its
stationary distribution. An arbitrarily large number of iterations may be
performed resulting in values of the unknown parameters and variables that
form an empirical approximation to the posterior distribution

As a result BUGS was the software of choice for Levy and Mislevy (2004)
in calibrating the NetPASS model. The model specification included
parameterizations of the conditional probabilities in terms of Samejima's graded
response model, including compensatory and conjunctive relations. Restrictions
were placed on the conditional probabilities in accordance with the hypothesized
relations among the variables in the Student Model and in the Evidence Models.

As discussed earlier in the context of Table 7.1, these hypothesized relations manifested as structural zeros in the conditional probability tables. Such restrictions were not part of the origins of the graded response model, though they are compatible. The estimation of the model complete with complex relationships, though far from standard, is not beyond the flexibility and power of MCMC.

With even a modest sample size, Levy and Mislevy (2004) were able to demonstrate that model calibration can support (a) learning about parameters that govern the conditional distributions in the Student Model and Evidence Models, (b) evaluation of expert expectations of task difficulty, and (c) inferences regarding an examinee's proficiencies on the basis of the final state of their Student Model. As this last purpose is ancillary to model calibration, it should be performed with due caution. Larger sample sizes would afford further opportunities for learning about model parameters, and facilitate model criticism.

In addition to using data to learn model parameters, such data can also be used to learn about the structure of the model. One approach is to employ diagnostic statistics to indicate whether alternative models might fit the data better. Spiegelhalter, Dawid, Lauitzen, and Cowell (1993) described three different kinds of applications for model misfit measures: parent–child measures, node measures, and global measures. The intent is to apply model criticism indices to these targets as the basis for critiquing and selecting models for implementation. The fact that Student Model variables are inherently latent poses some interesting challenges for these model criticism techniques. Williamson, Almond, and Mislevy (2000) conducted a simulation study that successfully employed variations on those techniques to detect model misfit. Sinharay (in press) and Sinharay, Almond and Yan (2004) approached the problem from a graphical modeling perspective.

Development and refinement of model criticism techniques may ultimately lead to fully automated model search strategies that attempt to select the model structure (and parameters) which best fit the data. (Heckerman, 1995, provided a starting point for learning about model search strategies.) In the educational measurement application, however, fully automated strategies have two fundamental problems to overcome: the number of latent variables; and the question of interpretation. With respect to the latent variable problem, there is a tension between the number of latent variables that may be desirable to include in support of an educational measure and the number that can be reasonably supported from data. Furthermore, the very fact that the variables are latent undermines the ability of many current methods of model criticism, and therefore model search, for Bayesian networks. With respect to the interpretation problem, good proficiency variables must satisfy three criteria: (1) they must be clearly defined (so that tasks can be coded as to whether or not the proficiency is used), (2) they must be measurable (in the sense that good information can be obtained about them from the proposed test design, and (3) they must be instructionally relevant (i.e., instructors must be able to choose appropriate actions based on their values). It is difficult to imagine that a statistical algorithm alone could ensure that these criteria are satisfied and hence, it is likely that model building and refinement will always be a collaborative effort between SMEs and psychometricians.

OPERATION OF NETPASS

This section illustrates the use of Bayes nets and other automated scoring concepts just presented by following a portion of NetPASS administration through the four-process model (see chap. 2, "Evidence-Centered Design," this volume). This begins with the activity selection process and proceeds through the presentation process, evidence identification, and evidence accumulation, with an emphasis on the role of Bayes nets in this process.

ACTIVITY SELECTION PROCESS

Because NetPASS supports learning rather than high-stakes decision-making, students are free to select assessment activities based on their own perceived needs and guidance from classroom instructors. This is in contrast to high-stakes testing environments, in which tasks are typically selected to meet particular criteria (e.g., domain sampling, adaptive testing).

Once a student obtains a logon identifier, logs onto the NetPASS system, and initializes the assessment, he or she is presented with a scenario navigation screen, an example of which is shown in Fig. 7.10. The scenario navigation screen permits the student to choose the type of assessment scenario (design, implementation, or troubleshooting) and a level of difficulty (here, difficulty is defined relative to the targeted population of students in the 3rd semester of the CNAP curriculum). For this example, let us assume that the student is interested in working through the medium-difficulty troubleshooting scenario.

The second stage of the activity selection process for this example brings the student to the activity selection screen. The first third of this screen was previously shown in Fig. 7.5. The remaining two thirds of the screen, providing instructions and scheduling information, is shown in Fig. 7.11. This screen presents the fundamental network situation and represents the troubleshooting problem the student must solve.

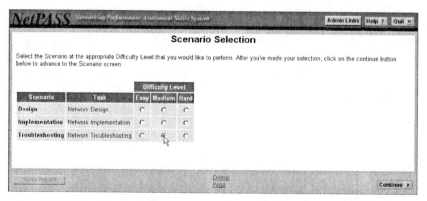

FIG. 7.10. NetPASS Scenario navigation interface.

From this screen (see Fig. 7.11) the student may select any of a variety of work activities by clicking on the appropriate button. These work activities include the completion of a *network diagram* that represents the student's perception of the components, structure, and intended function of the network (by clicking on the "Begin" button to the right of "Create Network Diagram"); the initialization of the interface for interacting directly with the malfunctioning network (by clicking on the "Begin" button to the right of "Troubleshoot Network"); and the ability to complete a *faultlist* in which the student indicates the network faults that were identified during the troubleshooting, and the location of these faults in the network (by clicking on the "Begin" button to the right of "List Faults").

Although the student is free to undertake these activities in any sequence, to skip some activities entirely, or to complete a portion of an activity before going to another activity and returning to complete the original activity later, the nature of the activities suggest a logical sequence: The network diagram is useful to prepare an approach to troubleshooting that would target the most likely sources of malfunction in the network once the student begins working directly with the network components. Similarly, there is little utility from attempting to complete the list of identified faults and their locations before first directly investigating the network through the network interface activity.

For this example, let us assume that the student forgoes producing a network diagram (which can be a common occurrence for some students confident in their ability to understand and manipulate the network), and proceeds directly to interacting with the network through the command interface (by selecting the "Begin" button to the right of "Troubleshoot Network"). With this selection made, the system proceeds to the presentation process, to present the selected activity to the student for completion.

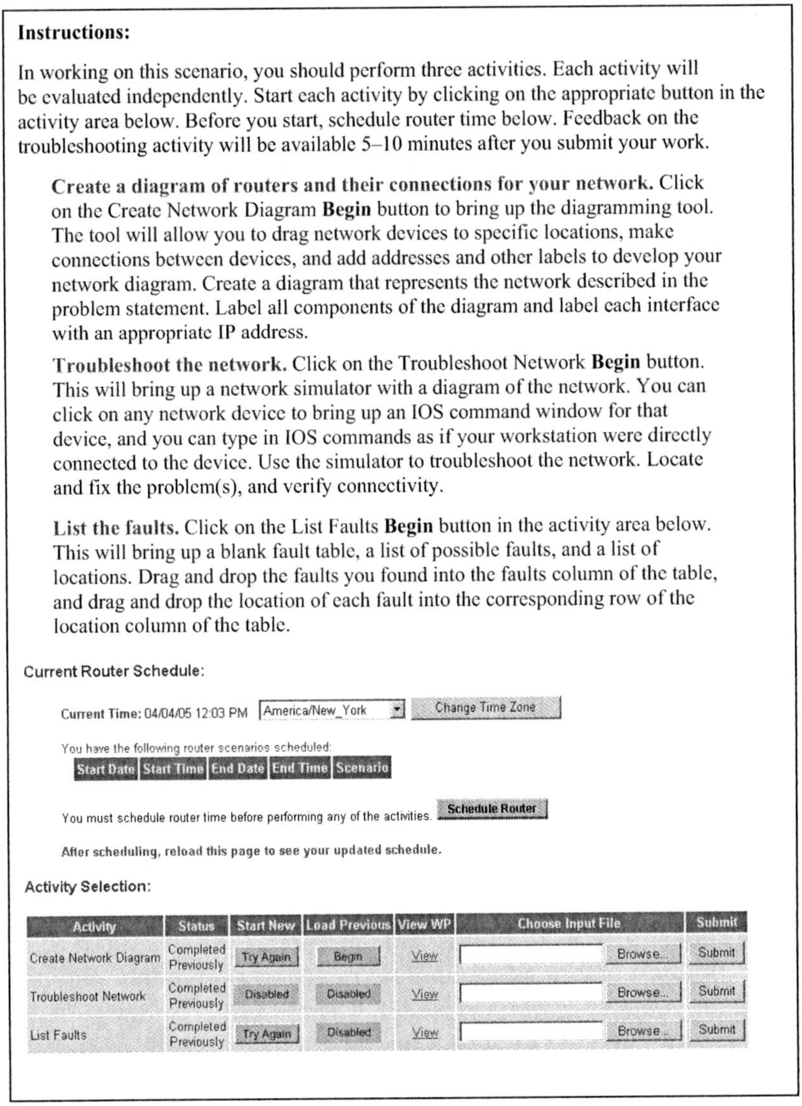

Instructions:

In working on this scenario, you should perform three activities. Each activity will be evaluated independently. Start each activity by clicking on the appropriate button in the activity area below. Before you start, schedule router time below. Feedback on the troubleshooting activity will be available 5–10 minutes after you submit your work.

Create a diagram of routers and their connections for your network. Click on the Create Network Diagram **Begin** button to bring up the diagramming tool. The tool will allow you to drag network devices to specific locations, make connections between devices, and add addresses and other labels to develop your network diagram. Create a diagram that represents the network described in the problem statement. Label all components of the diagram and label each interface with an appropriate IP address.

Troubleshoot the network. Click on the Troubleshoot Network **Begin** button. This will bring up a network simulator with a diagram of the network. You can click on any network device to bring up an IOS command window for that device, and you can type in IOS commands as if your workstation were directly connected to the device. Use the simulator to troubleshoot the network. Locate and fix the problem(s), and verify connectivity.

List the faults. Click on the List Faults **Begin** button in the activity area below. This will bring up a blank fault table, a list of possible faults, and a list of locations. Drag and drop the faults you found into the faults column of the table, and drag and drop the location of each fault into the corresponding row of the location column of the table.

Current Router Schedule:

Current Time: 04/04/05 12:03 PM America/New_York ▾   Change Time Zone

You have the following router scenarios scheduled:

Start Date	Start Time	End Date	End Time	Scenario

You must schedule router time before performing any of the activities. Schedule Router

After scheduling, reload this page to see your updated schedule.

Activity Selection:

Activity	Status	Start New	Load Previous	View WP	Choose Input File	Submit
Create Network Diagram	Completed Previously	Try Again	Begin	View	[ ] Browse...	Submit
Troubleshoot Network	Completed Previously	Disabled	Disabled	View	[ ] Browse...	Submit
List Faults	Completed Previously	Try Again	Disabled	View	[ ] Browse...	Submit

FIG. 7.11. Medium difficulty Troubleshooting Scenario navigation screen.

PRESENTATION PROCESS

Because the Task Models are designed to permit several types of student choice—including choice of scenario, choice of task within the scenario, and choosing to omit certain aspects of scenario performance—all have direct implications for the presentation processes in delivering the assessment. At the beginning of each scenario the simulator must be able to automatically load the initial configuration file associated with the scenario and provide a command window (see Fig. 7.12) from which students can interact with the network, thus allowing students to perform all reasonable actions that could be performed on a real network. Furthermore, the presentation process for these scenarios must save all interactions with the system in a log file that can be accessed by other software for scoring.

An example of this interactive command window, with some commands and system response already entered, is shown in Fig. 7.12. As the student interacts with the command window, all commands and responses are saved to the log file for subsequent scoring. Once the student has completed interacting with the command language interface, he or she can continue with other work activities or leave the scenario and submit it for scoring and feedback. For this example, let us assume that the student completes the work with the command window interface and exits the scenario without completing the other work activities. When the student is finished, the presentation process sends two work products on to the Evidence Identification Process: the *log* file—a complete list of actions and system responses—and the *configuration file*—the final state of the computer network that the student left in place upon exiting.

EVIDENCE IDENTIFICATION PROCESS

The raw responses (work product) from the NetPASS task are too large and unwieldy to be directly interpreted as evidence. The role of the Evidence Identification Process is to identify from the work product the key observable outcome variables that provide evidence for inferences reported to the student. There are two kinds of feedback that the student receives as a result of these interactions with the NetPASS tasks. *Task-based diagnostic* feedback is based solely on the observed performance outcomes for a single task, whereas the *summary* feedback is based on the accumulation of evidence across tasks and is based on the results of the Evidence Accumulation Process, which is based on the cumulative *observed* outcomes from each of potentially many assessment tasks.

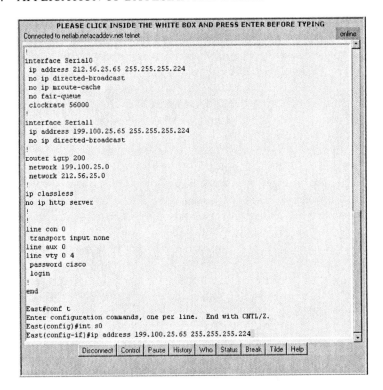

FIG. 7.12. Command language interface with simple input for the medium Troubleshooting Scenario.

Although there is overlap between the data collected for summary score reporting and the data used in determination of the diagnostic feedback variables, the diagnostic feedback is not a simple restatement of the observed outcomes sent to the Evidence Accumulation Process. Rather, the diagnostic feedback observables report on performance elements with specific anticipated educational benefits for students, rather than the more general summaries of ability that are provided from Student Model variables as part of summary score reporting. The values of these task feedback variables are tied to behavior-specific feedback that is provided to students who complete the tasks. This task-level feedback informs students about difficulties and specific misconceptions they may have had with each task, and enables them to take efforts to improve their performance on future tasks.

The Evidence Models used in NetPASS imposed several requirements for the Evidence Identification Process. Evidence Identification must identify observables to be used for summary scoring as well as those used in the selection of task-level feedback. Conceptually, two distinct Evidence Identification processes are applied to each work product: one producing scoring observables and the other producing diagnostic observables. For this example, the evidence used to inform the Student Model variables (and subsequently, the variables used for score reporting) is discussed.

The log file that was produced from the interface presented in Fig. 7.12 is submitted for parsing. That is, the first stage of evidence identification requires the automated scoring algorithm to identify and codify the complete log file transaction of commands and system responses. This parsing process is rule-driven and searches for classes of commands and associated system responses and summarizes them as the relevant evidence that is used to update the Evidence Model portion of the Bayesian network. An example of the rule structure that summarizes evidence from the work product is provided below for the Correctness of Procedure analysis of the log file work product described above, which is also represented as one of the variables in the Evidence Model represented in Fig. 7.7.

CORRECTNESS OF PROCEDURE FROM LOG FILE WORK PRODUCT

The Correctness of Procedure for the log file is a summary evidence variable for observables from the log file work product. It is one of two summary evidence variables derived from the log file work product. Each of these observables is comprised of subcomponent variables as presented in Fig. 7.13. As an illustration of how these observables combine to be summarized as Correctness of Procedure, let us first consider the Sequence of Actions under Procedural Sequence Logic. It was determined that an optimal sequence of actions when conducting troubleshooting activities is to (1) query the network to identify faults, (2) perform actions on the network to remedy identified faults, and (3) confirm that the actions had the desired effects in fixing the network faults. One of the roles of the parsing process in evidence identification is to determine whether each command entered by the student is a *query* of the system, an *action* on the system intended to implement some change to the network, or a *confirmation* of the system to ensure that an implemented change has had the desired effect. Through this identification and codification process the algorithms can identify patterns of performance to determine if they are consistent with the overall pattern of *query*, *action*, and *confirmation*. Additional

a) Correctness of Procedure (Procedural Sequence Logic)
  (1) Sequence of targets
  (2) Sequence of actions
b) Efficiency of Procedure
  (1) Help usage
  (2) IOS syntax
  (3) Volume of actions

FIG. 7.13.   Hierarchy of Log File evidential variables for log file work product.

evidence identification rules combine the information on appropriate Sequence of Actions with information on the sequence of targets addressed in troubleshooting to form an evaluation of overall Procedural Sequence Logic, which is represented in the Evidence Model as Correctness of Procedure.

In this example let us assume that the Correctness of Procedure in the Log File work product was High and that the Efficiency of Procedure was evaluated as Medium (both variables can take on the values of High, Medium, and Low). In addition, because the actions taken on the network result in a new configuration for the computer network, the final configuration file is an additional work product that provides the Correctness of Outcome variable from the Configuration File. Let us assume that the Correctness of Outcome based on the configuration file is Medium. The three Evidence Model observables, Correctness of Procedure (Log File work product) Efficiency of Procedure (Log File work product) and Correctness of Outcome (Configuration File work product) have now been identified and are submitted as evidence for the evidence BIN accumulation process updating the values of Student Model variables.

EVIDENCE ACCUMULATION PROCESS

The Evidence Model previously presented as Fig. 7.6 is presented again here as Fig. 7.14, this time without the probability distributions explicitly represented and with the probabilities *initialized*, that is, with the Bayesian network updating active and without any evidence entered into the network. All variables are treated as unobserved. (For convenience of presentation, the distributions in Fig. 7.14 are marginalized over the intermediate variables in Fig. 7.7.) The probability distributions resulting from system initialization are represented next to each variable in the network. In the absence of any evidence from work product performance (any observations for the five observable variables), these

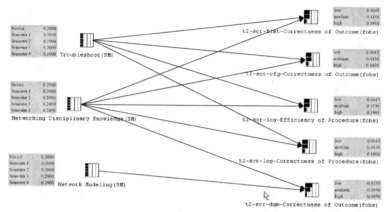

FIG. 7.14. Initialized Evidence Model for medium troubleshooting sans evidence.

probability distributions represent the performance expectations from the target population of third semester students in the CLI computer network curriculum. Note that the prior distributions for the ability variables are uniform, indicating that there is currently no preponderance of evidence for belief about a student's status on these proficiencies. The distributions for the observable variables, however, are informative and reflect the difficulty of the observables for the target population.

Given the previously described evaluation of the log work product as having high Correctness of Procedure, medium Efficiency of Procedure, and medium Correctness of Outcome from the configuration file, with no observations for the two remaining observable variables in the network, these observations are entered into the Evidence Model and the evidence propagated to the other network variables. The updated Evidence Model is provided as Fig. 7.15.

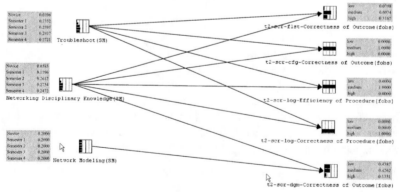

FIG. 7.15. Evidence Model with three observables entered.

Note that the three observed variables are now known values and the probability distributions of the remaining variables in the network have been updated to reflect the propagation of this evidence throughout the Evidence Model. The Student Model variables reflect the new belief about the student based on their performance on the task. In addition, the probability distributions for the neighboring observable variables have also been updated, reflecting the new belief about the expected level of performance on these activities given the level of performance observed from the log file and the configuration file.

The updated probability distributions of the Student Model variables present in the Evidence Model also influence the probability distributions of the other Student Model variables. When the evidence contained in the individual Evidence Model is "docked" with the full Student Model the evidence propagates to the other Student Model variables. The updated Student Model, after observing this evidence presented above, is provided as Fig. 7.16. Note that there are several patterns of probability updating occurring when the Evidence Model is docked with the full Student Model. Most obvious is the change in posterior distributions directly associated with tasks that have been observed. However, note that the posterior probabilities for the variables directly linked to observables differ in Figs. 7.15 and 7.16. This illustrates the influence of the structure of the Student Model variables on belief about the values of these variables. Specifically, Fig. 7.15 illustrates the posterior distributions under the assumption of a reduced set of independent Student Model variables whereas Fig. 7.16 illustrates the influence of the interdependencies of the full Student Model under conditional independence assumptions. The other changes in posterior distribution are the result of indirect evidence propagation through the network. For example, in Fig. 7.16 the network modeling variable has changed from a uniform prior to an informative one as a result of the indirect evidence propagated through the network proficiency variable. This, in turn, propagated through to provide a new set of posteriors for the observable task variables that have not been observed in the assessment. If no further tasks were taken by the student these would remain as the best estimates of the student ability given the evidence provided. Otherwise, if the student completes additional tasks this cyclical process of activity selection, presentation, evidence identification, and evidence accumulation would continue. The complete NetPass model, combining the Student Model variables and the multiple Evidence Models is provided as Fig. 7.8.

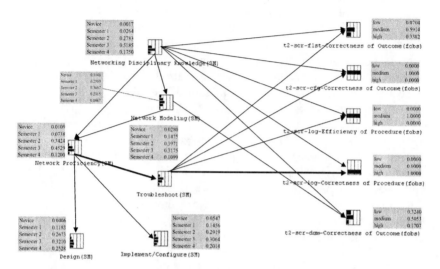

FIG. 7.16. Student Model updated with evidence from the medium difficulty
Troubleshooting Scenario.

SCORE REPORTING

The NetPASS design calls for two different kinds of score reporting: summary
score reporting and task-based feedback. Summary Score reports are provided
by the Evidence Accumulation and describe the final estimates of student ability
from their assessment performance (Bayes net representing current beliefs about
the student's proficiencies). The task-based feedback comes from the Evidence
Identification process and is based solely on student performance within a
particular task. Task-based feedback is directly tied to what the student did
during the assessment, and hence is generally more immediate and accessible.
Summary score feedback incorporates evidence from all of the tasks and is
generally more reliable. The summary score also tends to address skills at a
higher, more abstract level, whereas the task-based feedback tends to address
skills at a finer grain size. Both types are described in the following section.

SUMMARY SCORE REPORTING

The Student Model provides the basis for summary reporting, with each of the
proficiencies in the Student Model serving as reporting variables. Reporting
variables are structured to meet requirements for making specific claims about
the student and to fulfill the reporting intent of the assessment design. These

Student Model variables are updated for a student via the statistical model as the evidence is accumulated across tasks during the assessment. Each Student Model variable is distinguished at five levels: novice, first semester, second semester, third semester, and fourth semester of the CCNA curriculum. For each proficiency variable, the student is described in terms of probabilities of having the networking ability typical of students at a particular level (novice through fourth semester). These levels, and the rationale behind the probabilistic values associated with them, are associated with the claims to be made on the basis of the assessment. Although summary reporting can be generated at the completion of any number of tasks, the higher the number of tasks completed, the more accurate the resultant estimates of ability. Students and teachers can use these reports to target gaps in students' knowledge and abilities and focus their learning activities.

TASK LEVEL FEEDBACK

Although the summary score incorporates evidence from many tasks, the task-based feedback uses only observables from a single task. The observable used in task-level feedback, calculated during Evidence Identification, may or may not be the same as the observables sent to the Evidence Accumulation process. Often they are at a finer grain size, and consist of intermediate variables used in determining the values of observables sent to Evidence Accumulation. Occasionally, they are extra observables defined specifically for the purposes of reporting task-based feedback. For example, students receive feedback for troubleshooting problems on the following aspects of their solutions:

- The efficiency of their performance in terms of the volume of actions, their use of help, and their degree of difficulty using IOS commands.

- The degree to which they followed reasonable troubleshooting sequences of gathering information to identify faults, fixing faults, and testing the network.

- The faults they correctly identified, faults they missed, and parts of the configuration where they mistakenly identified faults that did not exist.

- Errors they made that are task specific.

Generally, the task-level feedback is implemented by having alternative versions of the feedback text that are selected on the basis of the values of the feedback observables. If desired, excerpts from the student's performance can be included. By giving feedback with a close connection to the actual work, this helps the student gain an appreciation for what is important in the domain. Wilson and Sloane (2000) pursued this approach by presenting and discussing the rubrics used for Evidence Identification with the students. In both cases, by gaining a better understanding about what makes a good performance, the student can apply this knowledge towards improving future performance.

In pilot testing with students, the NetPASS task-level feedback was judged to be very successful. The summary score feedback was less successful, in part because the students rarely had a chance to complete more than one or two tasks, but primarily because students did not readily understand score reports presented to them as probability distributions over ability categories.

SPECIAL CONSIDERATIONS FOR HIGH STAKES ASSESSMENT

The development considerations for Bayesian networks described earlier are relevant to both high-stakes and low-stakes assessment. However, many of the design decisions depend on the purpose of the assessment, therefore the final assessment design and scoring models from this process may be very different depending on assessment purpose. High-stakes assessment also brings an increased need for test security, including multiple forms for which results must be comparable. This section briefly touches on three issues that change as the stakes change: reliability, validity, and linking multiple forms.

RELIABILITY AND GRAIN SIZE

The type of inferences that will be made about the examinee largely determines the grain size used in the Student Model. With the purpose of the assessment clearly established the goal is to avoid collecting data that provide little value as evidence about the targeted inferences (e.g., Messick, 1989, on construct underrepresentation and construct-irrelevant variance). If the purpose of the assessment is purely for summary selection and evaluation the Student Models should be more coarsely grained than in applications for which the purpose is tutoring, detailed diagnosis, or instructional. Consequently, high-stakes assessments typically have fewer variables in the proficiency variables representing higher level skills (or else fewer proficiency variables are used for reporting). The assessment tasks tend to be focused less on a thorough assessment of nuances of cognitive understanding and more on repeated, and therefore presumably more reliable, evidence about the cognitive elements critical to the classification purposes of the assessment.

The higher stakes also increase the need for reliability (in the sense of repeatability) of the test scores. As with classical test theory, the reliability of a Bayes net-based assessment depends primarily on the length of the test; or more importantly the amount of direct evidence about each of the reporting variables. This also tends to push the Student Model towards fewer variables, as it is typically possible to measure only a few parts of the domain well under the typical constraints of high stakes tests.

VALIDITY

In low-stakes educational implementation (such as for NetPASS) if elements of the Student Model and the resultant diagnostic feedback are not completely valid the negative consequences are fairly limited, being restricted to a particular tutoring element either presented to a student who would not benefit (time cost) or not presented to a student who would benefit (educational cost). Due to the lower impact of errors in the Student Model for such systems the construction of the Student Models, and the corresponding Bayesian networks, in these systems has often been initially rather ad hoc and with relatively low precision in the selection of instructional actions (Chipman, Nichols, & Brennan, 1995). In contrast, for high-stakes assessment for licensure or certification the negative impact may be severe, including restriction of an otherwise qualified candidate from practicing in their field, with the accompanying loss of income and opportunity, or the licensure of an individual who presents a danger to the public. The implications of this difference in importance of Student Model accuracy, and thus the ability of the assessment to make appropriate inferences, is that for high-stakes assessment there must be greater rigor in the construction of Student Models, more care in task construction, and empirical confirmation of the model through pretesting.

Of course, validity is not a fixed and singular entity but is rather a consideration of a variety of sources of evidence that lend credence to the processes and outcomes of assessment. Or, as defined by Messick (1989):

> Validity is an integrated evaluative judgment of the degree to which empirical evidence and theoretical rationales support the adequacy and appropriateness of inferences and actions based on test scores or other modes of assessment. ... What is to be validated is not the test or observation device as such but the inferences derived from test scores or other indicators—inferences about score meaning or interpretation and about the implications for action that the interpretation entails. (pp. 13–14)

Therefore, it is not only the inferences resulting from the assessment which are subject to validation research but the Student Models themselves that must be a focus of efforts to confirm their adequacy as representations of cognitive structures and strategies. As a result the importance of validity evidence for cognitive assessment becomes more critical as the validity of the Student Model itself must be monitored as well as the relationships to variables outside of the Student Model (Almond & Mislevy, 1999). For example, model criticism tools and studies, such as the Williamson et al. (2000) investigation of the impact of missing Student Models, are needed.

Towards this end the Cognitive Task Analysis provides an elaborated form of construct validation (Embretson, 1983; Messick, 1989) for the assessment when the Student Model underlying the assessment is constructed from the empirical findings of the CTA (Snow & Lohman, 1993). The CTAs undertaken for the development of cognitive assessments, then, ensure that the construct validity of an assessment is built into the foundations of test construction rather than being the hoped-for result of a vaguely defined process. With regard to the CTA, which underlies the development of cognitive assessments, Messick (1989) wrote: "Possibly most illuminating of all [evidence of validity] are direct probes and modeling of the processes underlying test responses, an approach becoming both more accessible and more powerful with continuing developments in cognitive psychology" (p. 17). Therefore the increased importance of validity evidence for high-stakes cognitive assessment serves to increase the importance of the CTA as a major contributor of evidence of construct validity.

The Evidence-Centered Design process (Mislevy, Steinberg & Almond, 2003; Mislevy, Steinberg, Almond, & Lukas, chap. 2, this volume) often uses a CTA as a starting point for domain definition. In many respects a CTA helps make the validity argument of the assessment central to the construction of the model. In the case of NetPASS, a CTA was conducted as part of the design process, the results of which are presented in Williamson et al. (2004). As the previous discussion shows, the use of Bayesian network measurement models is complementary to the ECD process. In particular, the graphs used in the Bayes nets provide a natural description of the evidentiary relationships between proficiency variables and observed outcomes.

The importance of validity evidence for the process and inferences of cognitive assessment are amplified due to the fact that the evidence supporting the construct validity also provides evidence for the validity of the Student Model as a representation of cognition. This underscores the importance of methods of model criticism not only as a statistical modeling tool, but as a validity mechanism for the underlying cognitive theory driving the statistical model. After all, any omission of important nodes from the statistical model, for example, could be indicative of construct underrepresentation in the design of the assessment. Therefore, it is not merely the assessment itself but also the cognitive model that becomes the focus of validation efforts, which has subsequent implications for the way in which cognitive understanding and learning are conceptualized for the domain and for related fields. In the process of collecting evidence of construct validity through the construct representation phase of assessment design it is important to use a clear method of comparing alternative theories of task performance (Embretson, 1983). One such method is to operationalize the competing theories in quantitative models and to compare the subsequent model fits between the competing models (Embretson, 1983).

LINKING

With the high stakes also comes the need to produce multiple forms of an assessment that are, in some sense, comparable. These multiple forms must somehow be linked to a common scale (this "linking" is "equating" in a weak sense of the word). Fortunately, the same procedure described above for calibrating the assessment model to pretest data can be used to link across multiple forms. As long as there is an anchor test of sufficient size, or else an anchor population, calibration can be used to link multiple forms in a manner analogous to the use of calibration to link forms in Item Response Theory. Mislevy et al. (1999) demonstrated this with a small example.

CONCLUSION

This chapter has focused on the development and implementation of Bayesian inference networks as a probabilistic scoring methodology for automated scoring of complex data. The application of BNs to automated scoring, although requiring expertise in probabilistic methods and an understanding of their implications, isn't really about the numbers. Instead, as Glenn Shafer emphasized (quoted in Pearl, 1988, p. 77), it is a formal mechanism for representing our best reasoning in making inferences about ability from evidence collected from student interactions with complex computerized simulations.

As we increase our understanding of the capabilities of the BN approach to structure of reasoning and build new assessments that inform an understanding of best practices, we will expand our ability to reason rigorously about the relationship between proficiency and task performance. This capability will in turn support a growing body of knowledge about methods and applications of automated scoring for complex data.

REFERENCES

Ackerman, T. A., & Smith, P. L. (1988). A comparison of the information provided by essay, multiple-choice, and free-response writing tests. *Applied Psychological Measurement, 12*(2), 117–128.

Almond, R. G. (1995). *Graphical Belief Modeling*. London, UK: Chapman and Hall.

Almond, R. G., DiBello, L., Jenkins, F., Mislevy, R. J., Senturk, D., Steinberg, L. S., & Yan, D. (2001). Models for conditional probability tables in educational assessment. In T. Jaakkola & T. Richardson (Eds.), *Artificial Intelligence and Statistics 2001* (pp. 137–143). San Francisco, CA: Morgan Kaufmann.

Almond, R. G., Herskovits, E., Mislevy, R. J., & Steinberg, L. S. (1999). Transfer of information between system and evidence models. In D. Heckerman & J. Whittaker (Eds.), Artificial Intelligence and Statistics 99 (pp. 181–186). San Francisco, CA: Morgan Kaufmann.

Almond, R. G., & Mislevy, R. J. (1999). Graphical models and computerized adaptive testing. *Applied Psychological Measurement, 23*, 223–237.

Bradlow, E. T., Wainer, H., & Wang, X. (1999). A Bayesian random effects model for testlets. *Psychometrika, 64*, 153–168.

Brooks, S. P. (1998). Markov chain Monte Carlo method and its application. *The Statistician, 47*, 69–100.

Brown, J. S., & Burton, R. R. (1978). Diagnostic models for procedural errors in basic mathematical skills. *Cognitive Science, 2*, 155–192.

Chase, W. G., & Simon, H. A. (1973a). The mind's eye in chess. In W. G. Chase (Ed.), *Visual information processing*, (pp. 215–281). New York: Academic Press.

Chase, W. G., & Simon, H. A. (1973b). Perception in chess. *Cognitive Psychology, 4*, 55–81.

Chi, M. T. H., Feltovich, P., & Glaser, R. (1981). Categorization and representation of physics problems by experts and novices. *Cognitive Science, 5*, 121–152.

Chipman, S. F., Nichols, P. D., & Brennan, R. L. (1995). Introduction. In P. D. Nichols, S. F. Chipman, & R. L. Brennan (Eds.) *Cognitively diagnostic assessment* (1–18). Mahwah, NJ: Lawrence Erlbaum Associates.

Clauser, B. E., Subhiyah R. G., Nungester R. J., Ripkey D. R., Clyman S. G., & McKinley D. (1995). Scoring a performance-based assessment by modeling the judgments of experts. *Journal of Educational Measurement, 32*, 397–415.

Cliff, N. (1983). Some cautions concerning the application of causal modeling methods. *Multivariate Behavioral Research, 18*, 115–126.

Collins, A. (1990). Reformulating testing to measure learning and thinking. In N. Frederiksen, R. Glaser, A. Lesgold, & M. G. Shafto (Eds.), *Diagnostic monitoring of skill and knowledge acquisition* (pp. 75–87). Hillsdale, NJ: Lawrence Erlbaum Associates.

Corbett, A. T., Anderson, J. R., & O'Brien, A. T. (1995). Student modeling in the ACT Programming Tutor. In P. D. Nichols, S. F. Chipman, & R. L. Brennan (Eds.) *Cognitively diagnostic assessment* (19–41). Hillsdale, NJ: Lawrence Erlbaum Associates.

De Groot, A. D. (1965). *Thought and choice in chess*. The Hague: Mouton.

Dempster A. P. (1990) Bayes, Fisher and belief functions. In S. Geisser, J. Hodges, S. J. Press, & A. Zellner, (Eds.) *Bayesian and Likelihood Methods in Statistics and Econometrics: Essays in Honor of George A. Barnard* (pp. 35–47). New York: North-Holland.

Derry, S. J., & Hawks, L. W. (1993). Local cognitive modeling of problem-solving behavior: An application of fuzzy theory. In S. P. Lajoie & S. J. Derry (Eds.), Computers as Cognitive Tools (pp. 107–140). Hillsdale, NJ: Lawrence Erlbaum Associates.

Edwards, W. (1998). Hailfinder: Tools for and experiences with Bayesian normative modeling. *American Psychologist, 53*, 416–428.

Embretson, S. (1983). Construct validity: Construct representation versus nomothetic span. *Psychological Bulletin, 93,* 179–197.

Fiske, E. (1990, January 31) But is the child learning? Schools trying new tests. *The New York Times,* pp. A1, B6.

Frederiksen, N. (1984). The real test bias: Influences of testing on teaching and learning. *American Psychologist, 39,* 193–202.

Frederiksen, J. R., & Collins, A. (1989). A systems approach to educational testing. *Educational Researcher, 18(9),* 27–32.

Gelfand, A. E., & Smith, A. F. M. (1990). Sampling-based approaches to calculating marginal densities. *Journal of the American Statistical Association, 85,* 398–409.

Gelman, A., Carlin, J. B., Stern, H. S., & Rubin, D. B. (1995). *Bayesian data analysis.* London: Chapman & Hall.

Gilks, W. R., Richardson, S., & Spiegelhalter, D. J. (Eds.). (1996). *Markov chain Monte Carlo in practice.* London: Chapman & Hall.

Gitomer, D. H., Steinberg, L. S., & Mislevy, R. J. (1995). Diagnostic assessment of troubleshooting skill in an intelligent tutoring system. In P. D. Nichols, S. F. Chipman, & R. L. Brennan (Eds.), *Cognitively diagnostic assessment* (pp. 73–102). Hillsdale, NJ: Lawrence Erlbaum Associates.

Gitomer, D. H., & Yamamoto, K. (1991). Performance modeling that integrates latent trait and class theory. *Journal of Educational Measurement, 28 (2),* 173–189.

Glymour, C., Scheines, R., Spirtes, P., & Kelly, K. (1987). *Discovering causal structure.* San Diego: Academic Press.

Good, I. J. (1950). *Probability and the weighing of evidence.* London: Charles Griffin and Co. Ltd.

Greeno, J. (1989). Situations, mental models, and generative knowledge. In D. Klahr & K. Kotovsky (Eds.), Complex Information Processing, (pp. 285–318). Hillsdale, NJ: Lawrence Erlbaum Associates.

Heckerman, D., Breese, J. S., & Rommelse, K. (1994a). *Troubleshooting under uncertainty.* Technical Report MSR–TR–94–07. Redmond, WA: Microsoft Research.

Heckerman, D. (1995) *A tutorial on learning with Bayesian networks.* Technical Report MSR–TR–95–06, Microsoft Research, March, 1995 (revised November, 1996). Retrieved from ftp://ftp.research.microsoft.com/pub/tr/tr-95-06.pdf.

Hill, B. M. (1993). Parametric models for A n: Splitting processes and mixtures. *Journal of the Royal Statistical Society, B 55,* 423–433.

Howard, R. A., & Matheson, J. E. (1984). Readings on the principles and applications of decision analysis, Vol. 2. Menlo Park, CA: Strategic Decisions Group.

Irvine, S. H., & Kyllonen, P. C. (Eds.). (2002). *Item generation for test development.* Mahwah, NJ: Lawrence Erlbaum Associates.

Jensen, F. V. (1996). *An introduction to Bayesian Networks.* New York, NY: Springer-Verlag.

Kadane, J. B. (1980). Predictive and structural methods for eliciting prior distributions. In A. Zellner (Ed.), Bayesian Analysis and Statistics (pp. 89-93). Amsterdam: North Holland.

Kahneman, D., Slovic, P., & Tversky, A. (1982). Judgment under uncertainty: Heuristics and biases. Cambridge, UK: Cambridge University Press.

Lauritzen, S. L., & Spiegelhalter, D. J. (1988). Local computations with probabilities on graphical structures and their applications to expert systems. *Journal of the Royal Statistical Society, B, 50* (2), 154–227.

Lesgold, A. M., Feltovich, P. J., Glaser, R., & Wang, Y. (1981). *The acquisition of perceptual diagnostic skill in radiology* (Technical Report No. PDS-1). Pittsburgh, PA: University of Pittsburgh, Learning Research and Development Center.

Levy, R., & Mislevy, R. J (2004). Specifying and refining a measurement model for a computer-based interactive assessment. *International Journal of Testing, 4,* 333–369.

Masters, G. N., & Mislevy, R. J. (1993). New views of student learning: Impliations for educational measurement. In N. Frederiksen, R. J. Mislevy, & I. I. Bejar (Eds.), *Test theory for a new generation of tests* (pp. 41–71). Hillsdale, NJ: Lawrence Erlbaum Associates.

Messick, S. (1989). Validity. In R. L. Linn (Ed.), *Educational measurement* (3rd ed., pp. 13–103). New York: Macmillan.

Mislevy R. J. (1994). Evidence and inference in educational assessment. *Psychometrika, 59 (4),* 439–483.

Mislevy, R. J. (1995). Probability-based inference in cognitive diagnosis. In P. D. Nichols, S. F. Chipman, & R. L. Brennan (Eds.) *Cognitively diagnostic assessment* (pp. 43–72). Hillsdale, NJ: Lawrence Erlbaum Associates.

Mislevy, R. J. (1996). Test theory reconceived. *Journal of Educational Measurement, 33,* 379–416.

Mislevy, R. J., Almond, R. G., Yan, D., & Steinberg, L. (1999). Bayes nets in educational assessment: Where the numbers come from. In K. B. Laskey & Prade, H. (Eds.), *Uncertainty in Artificial Intelligence '99* (437—446). San Francisco, CA: Morgan Kaufmann

Mislevy, R. J., & Gitomer, D. H. (1996). The role of probability-based inference in an intelligent tutoring system. *User Mediated and User-Adapted Interaction, 5,* 253–282.

Mislevy, R. J., Steinberg, L. S., & Almond, R. G. (2003). On the structure of educational assessment (with discussion). *Measurement: Interdisciplinary Research and Perspective. 1*(1) 3–62.

Mislevy, R. J., Steinberg, L. S., Breyer, F. J., Almond, R. G., & Johnson, L. (1999). A cognitive task analysis, with implications for designing a simulation-based assessment system. *Computers and Human Behavior, 15*(3): 335-374.

Neapolitan, R. E. (2004) Learning Bayesian Networks. Englewood Cliffs, NJ: Prentice Hall.

Nesher, P. (1986). Learning mathematics: A cognitive perspective. *American Psychologist, 41,* 1114–1122.

Newell, A. (1990). *Unified theories of cognition.* Cambridge, MA: Harvard University Press.

Newell, A., & Simon, H. A. (1988). The theory of human problem solving. In A. M. Collins & E. E. Smith (Eds.), *Readings in cognitive science: A perspective from psychology and artificial intelligence* (pp. 33–51). San Francisco, CA: Morgan Kaufmann.

Pearl, J. (1982). Reverend Bayes on inference engines: A distributed hierarchical approach. In D. Waltz (Ed.), *Proceedings of American Association for Artificial Intelligence National Conference on AI, Pittsburgh,* (pp. 133–136). Menlo Park, CA: AAAI.

Pearl, J. (1988). *Probabilistic reasoning in intelligent systems: Networks of plausible inference* (2nd ed.). San Francisco, CA: Morgan Kaufmann.

Rubin, D. B. (1984). Bayesianly justifiable and relevant frequency calculations for the applied statistician. *Annals of Statistics, 12,* 1151–1172.

Schum, D. A. (1987). *Evidence and inference for the intelligence analyst.* Lanham, MD: University Press of America.

Shachter, R. D. (1986). Evaluating influence diagrams. *Operations Research, 34,* 871–882.

Shafer, G. (1996). The art of causal conjecture. Cambridge, MA: MIT Press.

Sinharay, S. (in press). Assessing item fit of Bayesian networks using the posterior predictive model checking method. *Journal of Educational and Behavioral Statistics.*

Sinharay, S., Almond, R. G., & Yan, D. (2004). Model checking for models with discrete proficiency variables in educational assessment. *ETS Research Report,*RR-04-07. Princeton, NJ: Education Testing Service.

Smith, A. F. M., & Roberts, G. O. (1993). Bayesian computation via the Gibbs sampler and related Markov chain Monte Carlo methods. *Journal of the Royal Statistical Society, B, 55,* 3–23.

Snow, R.E., & Lohman, D.F. (1993). Cognitive psychology, new test design, and new test theory, an introduction. In N. Frederiksen, R.J. Mislevy, & I. Bejar (Eds.), *Test theory for a new generation of tests.* Hillsdale, NJ: Lawrence Erlbaum Associates.

Spiegelhalter, D. J., Dawid, A. P., Lauitzen, S. L., & Cowell, R. G. (1993). Bayesian analysis in expert systems. *Statistical Science, 8*(3), 219–283.

Spiegelhalter, D. J., & Lauritzen, S. L. (1990). Sequential updating of conditional probabilities on directed graphical structures. *Networks, 20,* 579–605.

Spiegelhalter, D. J., Thomas, A., Best, N. G., & Lunn, D. (2003). *WinBUGS version 1.4: User manual.* Cambridge Medical Research Council Biostatistics Unit. Retrieved from http://www.mrc-bsu.cam.ac.uk/bugs/

Steinberg, L. S., & Gitomer, D. H. (1993). Cognitive task analysis and interface design in a technical troubleshooting domain. *Knowledge-Based Systems, 6,* 249–257.

Thissen, D., & Wainer, H. (Eds.) (2001). *Test scoring.* Mahwah, NJ: Lawrence Erlbaum Associates.

VanLehn, K., & Martin, J. (1998) Evaluation on an assessment system based on Bayesian student modeling. *International Journal of Artificial Intelligence and Education, 8*(2), 179–221.

Ward, W. C., Frederiksen, N., & Carlson, S. B. (1980). Construct validity of free-response and machine-scoreable forms of a test. *Journal of Educational Measurement, 17,* 11–29.

Williamson, D. M., Almond, R. G., & Mislevy, R. J. (2000). Model criticism of Bayesian networks with latent variables. In C. Boutilier & M. Goldzmidt (Eds.), *Uncertainty in artificial intelligence: Proceedings of the sixteenth conference* (pp. 634–643). San Francisco, CA: Morgan Kaufmann.

Williamson, D. M., Bauer, M. I., Steinberg, L. S., Mislevy, R. J., & Behrens, J. T. (2004). Design rationale for a complex performance assessment. *International Journal of Testing, 4*(4), 303–332.

Wilson, M., & Sloane, K. (2000). From principles to practice: An embedded assessment system. *Applied Measurement in Education , 13,* 181–208.

8

Artificial Neural Networks

Ronald H. Stevens
UCLA IMMEX Project

Adrian Casillas, MD
UCLA Med-Clinical Immunology and Allergy

> *What we call chaos is just patterns we haven't recognized. What we call
> random is just patterns we can't decipher. What we can't understand we call
> nonsense.*—Chuck Palahniuk; retrieved January 30, 2006, from
> http://rss.brainydictionary.com/quotes/quotes/c/chuckpalah201092.html

INTRODUCTION: BACKGROUND

Digital technologies, when appropriately embedded within the context of a
discipline and a curriculum, can begin to address some of the issues of authentic
assessment which is repeatedly cited as an overarching problem in U.S.
secondary and post secondary education (Pellegrino, Chudowsky, & Glaser,
2001). As a result of advancements in hardware, software and connectivity,
computer simulations for teaching and learning are becoming more common,
and while earlier complex computer simulations required decades of
programmer years to develop, times can now be shortened to as little as several
months, making them candidates for assessments.

Simulations[1], appropriately designed, implemented, and evaluated, can
create environments for active involvement that can promote learning by
including many opportunities to solve problems and examine phenomena across
contexts and perspectives in engaging and challenging ways (Bransford, Brown,
& Cocking, 1999). They can provide experiences that are too risky or expensive
to otherwise implement (Lane, Slavin, & Zie, 2001), and can support decision-
making, systems thinking, and perspective taking that are hard to provide in

---

[1] The term *simulations* can broadly refer to games, models, and immersive and manipulated
environments in computer and non-computer environments. Simulations, as referred to here, are
online scenarios where participants adopt a functional role in a simulated environment where a
problem exists, and search and data interpretation is required to resolve the issue(s).

259

other ways (Resnick, 1994). With the increased use of simulations for learning, it is also likely that the dimensions of assessment will begin to change and the data collection and reporting capabilities of simulations will greatly enhance an educator's ability to personalize learning and provide incremental, targeted (and most likely immediate) formative and summative feedback to multiple audiences (Pellegrino et al., 2001).

Frameworks for the design of these simulations are being refined and guided less by the limitations of the presentation media and more by cognitive analyses (Mislevy, Steinberg, Breyer, Almond, & Johnson, 1999). These frameworks structure an understanding of the goals of the tasks (licensing, learning, low/high stakes testing, etc.), the needs and abilities of the students and the decision outcomes that are needed by the intended audience (Stevens & Palacio-Cayetano, 2003).

Outcome measures such as student efficiency and effectiveness (a completed simulation, a correct response, time measures, etc.) can be addressed statistically and, when used in combination with Item Response Theory (IRT) tools, have been useful for validating the simulation, for determining isomorphic equivalence of tasks, and for initial accumulation of evidence regarding student performance. These are also useful for relating the simulation results to other student traits (gender, SES) or measures (standardized tests).

As analyses become more complex and the degree of cognitive complexity and granularity being studied increases, the number and nature of performance categories and the boundaries of category membership become less clear. This is especially likely where the real-world challenges of using technology in the classrooms would be expected to influence the quality of the student performance data obtained for subsequent scoring These challenges include: (1) access to hardware and software, (2) connectivity, (3) student and teacher experience and attitudes with using technology, (4) curricular time, etcetera. Given these complexities, a reasonable *a priori* assumption would be that the performance data obtained would be messy, noisy, perhaps incomplete and rich in outliers, properties that artificial neural networks are especially flexible at dealing with (Principie, Euliano, & Lefebvre, 2000).

This chapter begins with an overview of IMMEX, an online classroom learning/assessment system for investigating the use of strategies during scientific problem solving, and then follows with the features of artificial neural networks that make them an attractive candidate on which to build an automated scoring system. Next, details are presented on the student and task models and the identification and accumulation of evidence. This is followed by a series of validation studies and closes with a discussion on open issues and areas for future research.

The sample problem set[2] highlighted throughout this chapter is a series of genetics cases called *True Roots* involving a case of uncertain parenthood. We highlight this problem set as it has been particularly informative about how students develop strategic thinking skills. Similar analyses have been performed for other IMMEX problem sets focusing on qualitative chemical analyses (Vendlinski & Stevens, 2001), math cases based on the SAT (Paek, 2002), forensic sciences, genetics (Stevens, Johnson, & Soller, 2005), asthma, and immunology (Kanowith-Klein, Burch, & Stevens, 1998), as well as social science (Stevens & Dexter, 2003).

IMMEX: AN EXAMPLE OF A COMPLEX SIMULATION WITH COMPLICATED STUDENT PERFORMANCE PATTERNS

Motivation

For the past 12 years, the IMMEX Project at UCLA has been developing technologies around the broad model of problem solving to probe the development of student understanding in multiple domains (Palacio-Cayetano, Allen, & Stevens, 1999; Stevens, 1991; Stevens & Najafi, 1993; Underdahl, Palacio-Cayetano, & Stevens, 2001). Although originally designed for intranet delivery, IMMEX cases are now delivered via the Internet (http://www.immex.ucla.edu) making them widely available to diverse audiences worldwide.

This software platform was originally motivated by the need to assess the development of medical students' diagnostic skills. The original approach taken was to present a simulated patient with a clinical immunology disorder, and then provide sets of essential and non-essential laboratory data that the students can select in any order of their choosing to efficiently and effectively diagnose the patient's problem. This approach has been successfully expanded to K–16 education by extending the fundamental cognitive paradigm of problem solving and search to other sciences, and engaging in an aggressive program of community engagement and outreach (Palacio-Cayetano, Allen, & Stevens, 1999). While differences of course exist in the student models across this broad spectrum of students and disciplines (as well as levels of expertise), the evidence identification and accumulation process has nevertheless been remarkably robust, and our central goal of providing real-time information to students and

---

[2] A *problem set* is a series of simulation tasks that share the same problem space, yet contain different data and possible solutions to the case.

teachers regarding problem-solving performance and progress to accelerate learning and the understanding of complex subjects has remained the same.

From a research perspective, the IMMEX Project has focused on refining the ability to extract meaningful cognitive behaviors relating to student performance from the sequence of student actions within simulations. Our rationale extends from the observation that while much of human thinking and reasoning appears to occur in parallel, most intentional human acts are sequential; a decision is made, a hypothesis is modified, a problem is solved, etcetera. From the perspective of developing an assessment, this would suggest that the sequence of intentional acts (i. e., the work product) may contain evidence of human cognition. The challenge is to find the natural cognitive structure(s) and behaviors inherent in this stream of intentional actions. IMMEX approaches these challenges through a process approach to influence learning (e. g., by identifying the analytical sequences of problem solving as a process, making inferences about the cognitive strategies being used, and determining the educational interventions on the basis of these processes), by sorting the many different sequences into classes of performance via artificial neural network analysis and drawing cognitive inferences from class membership.

In the terminology of evidence-centered assessment design (ECD; Mislevy, Steinberg, Almond, & Lukas, chap. 2, this volume), the artificial neural network is an evidence identification process, or task-level scoring. A preliminary phase of evidence identification is the identification of lower-level features of a student's solution, such as ordered sequences of problem-solving moves. The output of the neural net is a classification into an empirically-derived class, which is interpreted in terms of the level or style of problem-solving that was exhibited. This classification is an observable variable that summarizes performance on the task. As such, it can be used for immediate feedback to the student, serve as input to an evidence accumulation or test-level scoring process, or serve as data for further research. These individual ANN performance classifications are then extended by Hidden Markov Modeling (HMM) to develop progress models of experience.

Design

There are three broad design frameworks for the IMMEX problem-solving environment that support this approach: (1) the design of the Task Model through the definition of the problem spaces, (2) the accumulation, aggregation and reporting of evidence of student proficiencies, and (3) optimizing the presentation process for the realities of K–16 science classrooms. Our overall development approach follows the model of evidence-centered assessment design (Mislevy, Steinberg, Almond, Breyer, & Johnson, 2001; Mislevy, Steinberg, Breyer, Almond, & Johnson, 1999) where the models of the knowledge and skills that we hope students to learn or have learned (Student Models) are mapped onto behaviors and performance indicators that provide evidence of these constructs (Evidence Models) which are then designed into tasks that will provide that evidence (Task Models). In response to the realities of developing and implementing problem-solving software for diverse settings we have streamlined the Assembly and Delivery System Models by involving teachers in many aspects of the project including design, development, implementation and analysis (Palacio-Cayetano, Allen, & Stevens, 1999; Underdahl et al., 2001). In addition, given the breadth of the project's coverage, we have explored Measurement Models for inductively deriving/defining Evidence Models of student proficiency from the online Work Products collected.

IMMEX problem solving Tasks follow the hypothetical-deductive learning model of scientific inquiry (Lawson, 1995; Olson & Loucks-Horsley, 2000), where Student Model Variables include the abilities to frame a problem from a descriptive scenario, judge what information is relevant, plan a search strategy, gather information, and eventually reach a decision that demonstrates understanding (http://www.immex.ucla.edu). An example of an existing IMMEX problem set that provides evidence of the ability of students to conduct a genetic investigation is shown in Fig. 8.1.

True Roots was designed and created by a team of biology teachers and university faculty to assess high school student's understanding of genetics (Palacio-Cayetano, 1997). In the problem[3] posed, students are introduced to Leucine, a young girl, who fears that she is a victim of "baby swapping" at birth and begins to conduct a genetic investigation to discover which of five sets of possible parents are truly hers. The students conducting the online investigation can order tests for blood type, DNA restriction mapping, karyotype, fingerprints, and pedigree charts for both Leucine and each set of parents. For students new to this process, the IMMEX Presentation Material also provides students with library resource guides and expert advice that scaffold student's content knowledge. These dictionary and library resources are available at no cost to encourage students to develop self-learning habits. There is often extensive use

---

[3] In this paper we refer to specific simulations, problems, or cases as equivalent forms. The term *simulation* draws from the computer science literature, *problems* from the cognitive science literature, and *cases* from the case-based reasoning literature.

of these items on the early cases of a problem set, but by the third case most, but not all, students no longer access these items. These strategic transitions are explored later.

For *True Roots*, and other IMMEX problem sets, a Domain Analysis was conducted to document the content, cognitive skill requirements, pedagogies, standards alignment and potential implementation issues for this problem set (http://www.immex.ucla.edu/docs/subjectheading/hazmat.htm). To make the cases interesting to students, the simulations portray realistic scenarios, and to ensure that students gain adequate experience, the problem sets contains multiple cases (5-60+) that can be performed in class, assigned as homework, or used for testing. These cases are of known difficulty from IRT analysis, allowing teachers to select "hard" or "easy" cases depending on the ability of their students.

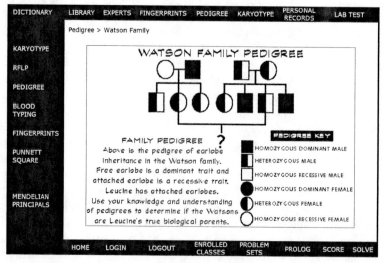

FIG. 8.1. Sample screen from IMMEX problem, True Roots. The major categories of test items available are arranged on the top of the workspace and become amplified on the left. Each selection presents a single piece of information that requires student interpretation. If the student is not familiar with the content, supporting information is available in the Dictionary/Library resources. The bar at the lower portion of the screen contains buttons for navigating the IMMEX user space.

Work Products

The work product produced by a student and captured by the IMMEX presentation process is a trace of all of the problem-solving actions a student takes in the course of solving the problem. That is, not only which actions have been taken, but the timing and order in which they occurred, are captured. This section describes representations of the IMMEX work product, and notes reports that are generated from it at the levels of individual students and groups of students.

Through the capture and modeling of these intentional student acts in the IMMEX environment, we have developed Reporting Rules, and automated Score Reporting tools to predicatively model student learning and understanding. These tools allow both real-time and off-line reports of how students solve a particular case, as well as how student ability changes over time (Pellegrino et al., 2001; Vendlinski & Stevens, 2000; Vendlinski & Stevens, 2002). These reports provide: (a) Immediate online feedback of class and student performance that can link problem-solving efficiency to other metrics (AP scores, course grades; Paek, 2002); (b) Maps of students' search of the problem space that help visualize problem-solving approaches, and reveal improvement of strategies over time (Stevens, 1991); (c) Neural net analysis of student data that reveals clusters of common problem solving strategies for large numbers of students (Casillas, Clyman, Fan, & Stevens, 2000; Hurst, & Casillas, 1997; Stevens & Najafi, 1993; Stevens, Lopo, & Wang, 1996); and (d) Hidden Markov Models of classroom progress that provide probabilistic inferences about trajectories of student progress, suggest points of intervention, document their effects, and allow comparison of problem solving progress across diverse educational settings (Stevens, Soller, Cooper, & Sprang, 2004; Vendlinski & Stevens, 2003).

Solving IMMEX problems requires an integration of domain knowledge and cognitive process skills, and evaluations have shown that they provide rich cognitive environments (Chung, deVries, Cheak, Stevens, & Bewley, 2002) that also results in the collection of complicated performance data. While such complex data can be modeled in many ways, one of our initial approaches to examining a new dataset is to visualize the sequence of actions that individual students and groups of students took while engaged on IMMEX simulations. This builds a graphical representation of the student's Work Product from case presentation through solution and reveals the complicated and complex paths students chose to solve cases. This representation is called a *search path map* (SPM) and initially consists of a template representing all possible information items available (as menu items/buttons) to the student in her or his search for a case solution (Fig. 8.2). For *True Roots*, this template contains 54 data items available to the students as menu items or buttons.

For this problem set, the Task Model Variables (menu items) are arranged and color coded onscreen into: (1) *Reference information* (top center) which helps students to define and interpret concepts and results; (2) *Advice from "experts"* (upper right) which is neutral in content, but may provide contextual information; and (3) *Research data* (lower half) that provide the necessary interpretative data. These research items consist of different sets of laboratory results from blood typing, Restriction Fragment Length Polymorphism (RFLP; commonly known as DNA fingerprinting), and chromosomal karyotype tests, as well as pedigree charts for earlobe attachment inheritance, and Punnett squares for analyzing the inheritance of fingerprints.

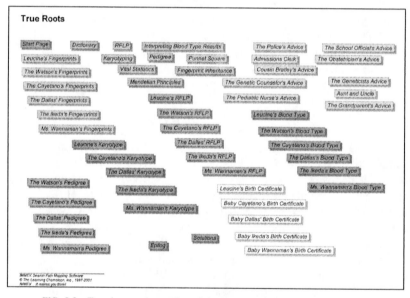

FIG. 8.2. Template representation of the True Roots problem space. Search path map templates facilitate the construction of visual representations of the problem space upon which student performances can be overlaid. In this representation, the library resource and expert help items are arranged at the top of the template. Each of the major categories of test items (e. g., Fingerprints, RFLP, Blood Typing, etc.) are uniquely color-coded, with each of the submenu items (e. g., Leucine, Watsons, etc.) arranged in the order they would be found in the different menus within the IMMEX problem space. Multiple template representations are possible, as the items could also be arranged according to possible parent groups, or arranged with regard to the most relevant items for each case.

The search path map displays the items that the student selected and in addition, IMMEX inserts a line between each rectangle indicating the order in which the student selected the information, while also recording how much time a student spent on each item before moving on to their next step (Fig. 8.3). The combination of choices available to a student while solving a case is large. For *True Roots*, a student has 2,862 choices when moving from one of the 54 menu items to another one (e. g., N^2-N menu items).

The data complexity becomes apparent when the maps are aggregated, for instance, at the level of a classroom of student performances (Fig. 8.4). Here, the more common sequences of item selections are shown by thicker lines, and more common patterns of search begin to emerge. It is apparent, however, that significant heterogeneity in student test selection is occurring. This becomes even more apparent when the performances are visualized across different classes.

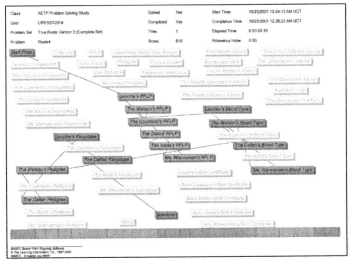

FIG. 8.3. Sample search path map (SPM). The performance of student CRESST2014 has been overlaid on the True Roots template with lines connecting the sequence of test selection. The lines go from the upper left hand corner of the "from" test to the lower center of the "to" test. Items not selected are shown in transparent gray. At the top of the figure are the overall statistics of the case performance. At the bottom of the figure is a timeline where the colors of the squares link to the colors of the items selected and the width of each rectangle is proportional to the time spent on that item. These maps are immediately available to teachers and students at the completion of a problem.

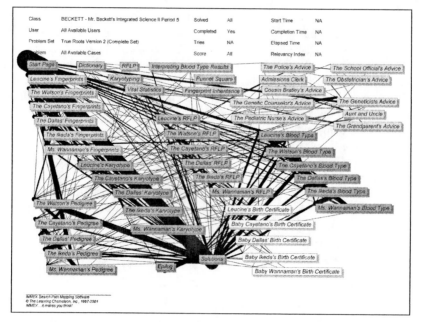

FIG. 8.4. A group composite search path map for one classroom. The True Roots performances of 25 high school students on cases were aggregated and displayed on the template, with the thickness of the lines being proportional to the number of students making a particular selection.

Evidence

The complexity of the IMMEX work product suggests the need for higher order data aggregation and organizing principles. Several approaches are possible. One approach is to aggregate strategies predicted from the cognitive requirements identified during the construction of the task model. For *True Roots*, these are defined by the criteria in Table 8.1.

A second approach relies more on the inherent structure in the data that becomes possible following extensive testing. For this we use unsupervised artificial neural networks as described later. Ideally, the two approaches should be complementary and lead to a unified and refined model. We contrast these two approaches later in the chapter and show that they are in fact consistent and complementary.

TABLE 8.1
Task Model Strategy Definitions

Strategy Type	Description
Prolific	Categorized by a thorough search of the problem space including the five relevant concept/data domains, as well as resource and conjecture menu items.
Redundant	Show an elimination of resource conjecture items but maintain a comprehensive search of the data domains. Reordering tests for parents who have already been eliminated by prior testing is also characteristic of this type of search.
Efficient	Depict searches which access only that information which is necessary to solve, without ordering tests for parents who have been eliminated through prior test results.
Limited Guessing	Demonstrate premature closure of the problem as indicated by not gathering enough information to conclusively solve the case, or evidence of guessing.

OVERVIEW MODEL: EVIDENCE IDENTIFICATION AND ACCUMULATION

A single level of analysis is unlikely to be useful to all audiences. Parents and the community are most interested in student understanding and progress, whereas teachers and students, and researchers in particular, often require data of finer granularity. A summary schema for our collection, aggregation, and reporting of strategic performance data through generic IMMEX tasks is shown in Fig. 8.5. The collection of evidence begins with the recording of each Action Option[4] selected (Fig. 8.5.A) by students as they navigate the problem space in response to the problem posed. From the theories of strategy selection, the micro-information of student's individual choices during problem solving would be expected to contain strategic information, and in fact, when combined with time latencies this information also provides information about the distribution

---

[4] The actions available to students for problem-solving are sometimes referred to as "task variables" in other IMMEX presentations. We are using the term "action options" to describe them here in order to avoid confusion with the ECD term "task model variables." ECD task model variables refer to salient features of the task environment and stimulus materials, and the list of action options available to a student in a given IMMEX problem could, in fact, be cast as one of possibly many task model variables in this sense.

IMMEX Performance Reporting Constructs	
A. Item Selection	*Examples*
Significance Students solving cases spend 35% more time on the first step than students missing cases. **Data Source/Criteria** Problem framing times, problem solving times.	
B. Completed Performance	
Significance Students approach cases in many ways, progress at different rates and respond differently to feedback. **Data Source/Criteria** Sequence of test selections, hypothesis generation/revision.	
C. Strategy	
Significance Common performance groupings indicating preferred problem-solving approaches **Data Source/Criteria** Neural network clustering of similar performances, inter-network reliabilities, validation of clustering with search path maps.	
D. Strategic Transitions	
Significance Predictive, longitudinal models of individual and group learning trajectories. **Data Source/Criteria** Sequential Performance of a series of problem instances.	

FIG. 8.5. Summary stages of evidence identification and accumulation.

of effort during the problem-solving episode. For instance, Paek (2002) demonstrated that on a series of IMMEX mathematics problems, students solving these cases spent 35% more time on the first step of the problem than those students who missed the problems. This is analogous to the finding that experts spend proportionally more time in framing a problem than do novices (Baxter & Glaser, 1997).

Although a single student action during the performance is occasionally informative for making claims of strategic proficiency in IMMEX problem-solving (such as "guessing" when a student chooses to solve a case as an initial move and without viewing any information), experience suggests that a series and/or sequence of actions is more consistently revealing. These series are seldom random and while students may eventually look at all the information contained in a problem space, they will often view menu items sequentially along pathways that share some common features rather than following entirely haphazard approaches. We believe that the paths that students employ while completing an IMMEX case provide evidence of a (complex) strategy, which we define as a sequence of steps needed to identify, interpret and use appropriate and necessary facts to reach a logical conclusion or to eliminate or discount other reasonable conclusions.

This sequence and search information is captured in the completed performance (Fig. 8.5.B), which is the next level of data aggregation. Here, students have searched the problem space, made a decision(s) about the embedded problem and have received feedback as to whether or not they were successful. Although this was originally identified by examination of hundreds of search path maps, we now use artificial neural technologies to begin to automate this process. The classifications resulting from the neural network analysis provide the strategic groupings (Fig. 8.5.C)

After each performance is assigned to a cluster they are chronologically ordered for each student providing longitudinal models of student problem solving. Strategies can be dynamically revised or become more persistent when they have proven adequate to repeatedly achieve the goals of the tasks. More advanced students learn how to adapt their strategies and solve the simulations by learning from previous attempts. Less advanced students may adopt a specific strategy early in the course of problem solving and some may retain that specific strategy or a similar strategy type, even if such a procedure repeatedly fails (Fig. 8.5.D).

When viewed individually, strategic transition analysis addresses the progress of each student. Aggregation of these analyses can provide similar information at the classroom or school level and can allow across-school or grade level comparisons of the distribution of strategies used to solve the cases in a problem-set. Moreover, these diagrams can allow cross-classroom modeling not only of the predicted effect of proposed pedagogical interventions, but also how such an intervention might ultimately affect the strategies used by these students.

DATA MINING PROPERTIES OF ARTIFICIAL NEURAL NETWORKS

Rationale

The apparent complexity of the data, combined with the presence of patterns within the data, suggested (Stevens & Najafi, 1993) that artificial neural networks (ANN) might have practical advantages for developing parsing rules for the initial work product modeling, and for providing different perspectives for data already modeled by other approaches described in this volume. Artificial neural networks provide an adaptable pattern recognition system that is able to find inherent patterns in data.

They derive their name and properties from the connectionist literature and share parallels with the theories of predicted brain function (Rumelhart & McClelland, 1986). Although neural networks have been extensively used to investigate and model cognition, including language development (McClelland & Goddard, 1997), the differential diagnosis of autism, and mental retardation (Cohen, Sudhalter, Landon-Jimenez, & Keogh, 1993), they are also versatile and practical for many aspects of pattern recognition, prediction, and estimation and have a demonstrated ability to perform such functions in fields as diverse as education (Stevens & Najafi, 1993), medicine (Casillas, Clyman, Fan, & Stevens, 1999) and business (Koprowski, 2003).

The computational models of artificial neural networks are defined by four parameters: (1) a group of processing units (also called nodes, or neurons[5]); (2) a connectionist architecture consisting of a series of weighted connections (artificial synapses) between the neurons; (3) a learning algorithm for training purposes which is usually either supervised (where the training data contains both the desired input and output vectors) or unsupervised (where only input vectors are supplied); and (4) a recall algorithm (for testing or classifying new data). Unlike conventional programming tools, ANN's are not programmed per

---

[5] The term *neuron* is generally used when discussing the architecture of the artificial neural network, whereas the term *node* generally refers to the locations of the classified performances on the resulting ANN topology after training.

se, but rather develop recognition capabilities through a process of repeated training with hundreds/thousands of exemplar patterns.

A general mathematical model of an artificial neuron is formally described by the properties in Fig. 8.6. They include:

- *Input connections (inputs):* x_1, x_2, x_3.......x_n that receive data from the external environment. The values can be binary, $\{0,1\}$, bivalent, $\{-1,1\}$, continuous $[0,1]$, or symbolic (which become processed into binary formats). There are weights bound to these input connections w_1, w_2, w_3....w_n.

- *The input function f,* calculates the aggregated net input signal to the neuron $u=f(x,w)$ where x and w are the input and weight vectors correspondingly. F is usually the summation function:

$$u = \sum_{i=1}^{n} xi.wi$$

- *An activation (signal)* function s calculates the activation level of the neuron $a = s(u)$.

- *An output function* that calculates the output signal value emitted through the output of the neuron $o = g(a)$ (which is usually assumed to be equal to the activation level of the neuron, that is, $o = a$).

During neural network training, as student's Work Products are repeatedly input, the weights between the inputs and the internal neurons are adjusted using a procedure called back-propagation (Rumelhart & McClelland, 1986), to reflect the relative importance of different patterns of external input or events in the training set. In effect, the weights come to represent the differential experience

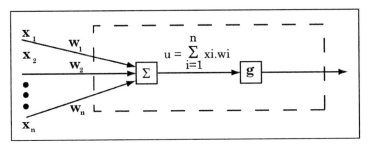

FIG. 8.6. A model of an artificial neuron.

and the effects of learning. The activation value of each input is multiplied by the weight of each connection, and the activation value of the internal neuron is the sum of these products. Within these neurons, the activation value is then adjusted by the summation (or transfer) function, which modifies the activation value and this transformed value becomes the output. There may be different types of transfer functions including a sigmoid function, a step function, a linear function, and variations of each. The transfer function regulates the output of the internal neuron, keeping it within mathematically defined limits. After some flexible number of cycles, the trained system generates multiple outputs that classifies aspects of problem-solving behavior such as strategy selection and use.

When appropriately trained, neural networks can generalize the patterns learned during training to encompass new instances, and predict the properties of each exemplar. Relating this to student performance of online simulations, if a new performance (defined by sequential test item selection patterns) does not exactly match the exemplars provided during training, the neural networks will extrapolate the best output according to the global data model generated during training. For performance assessment purposes, this ability to generalize would be important for "filling in the gaps" given the expected diversity between students with different levels of experience. The ability of ANN's to produce meaningful classifications also only degrades slowly with increasing amounts of missing data. Again, as individuals with different experiences will process data differently, it is likely that there would be a significant amount of missing data as performances are collected from diverse audiences.

The groups of neural network architectures we have been most interested in, termed *unsupervised neural networks*, extract dominant features of the dataset as training progresses, and share properties with other clustering algorithms. Of the multiple clustering approaches available (Valafar, 2002) including hierarchical clustering, k-means clustering, Bayesian clustering, and artificial neural networks, the self-organizing artificial neural network mapping procedures (SOMS), first described by Kohonen (Kohonen, 1990, 2001) have been our methods of choice (Stevens, Lopo, & Wang, 1996).

The goal of the SOM, is to find prototype vectors that represent the input data set and at the same time realize a continuous mapping from input space to an output matrix. SOMS have a number of features that make them well suited to clustering and analysis of student performance sequences. First, they have good computational properties and are easy to implement, reasonably fast and scalable to large data sets, all useful properties for an automated scoring system. Second, they have been well studied and empirically tested on a wide variety of problems where there are noisy data, outliers, and non-uniform data density distributions (Mangiameli, Chen, & West 1996). Third, consistent with our goals, they also help insert an objective step into the category generating process as the data is for the most part uncompressed and unbiased by other performance indicators.

This, in part, results from properties that may allow them to represent and present the nature of the performance data better than the other clustering methods. For instance, the agglomerative hierarchical clustering approach, which fuses single member clusters into bigger and bigger clusters, results in a phylogenic tree whose branch lengths represent the degree of similarity between the sets. This is well suited to situations of true hierarchical descent (such as evolution of species), but may not be the most suitable for grouping the multiple distinct ways that students approach and solve problems. The deterministic nature of this pair wise clustering can also cause points to be grouped based on local decisions, with no opportunity to reevaluate the clustering, potentially locking in accidental features, especially if the data is expected to be "messy".

Similarly, k-means clustering, while useful when one knows how many distinct performance patterns to expect, results in a collection of clusters that is unorganized, and not conducive to higher-level organizational interpretation. Also, given the inductive approach IMMEX explores for extracting performance models, this approach could be constraining during the "discovery" phase of modeling. Bayesian clustering (see Chapter 7 in this volume), another powerful clustering approach is perhaps more appropriate at later stages of modeling when a strong prior distribution on the data is available. As discussed later, Bayesian networks may be a particularly powerful approach for formalizing our strategic transition analysis.

In SOM, like k-means clustering, the data is assigned to a predetermined set of clusters that have been randomly chosen. Unlike k-means clustering, what follows is an iterative process where the performance vectors in each cluster are trained to find the best distinctions between the different clusters imposing a partial structure on the data. During the training process, through repeated comparison with the dataset, the nodes change in a way that captures the distribution of variability of the data set. In this way, similar performance patterns map close together in the network, and as far as possible from the different patterns. At the end of the training process, the neurons of the SOM grid have clusters of patterns assigned, and the trained neurons represent an average pattern of the cluster of data that map onto it, effectively reducing the data space. The result is a topological ordering of the neural network nodes according to the structure of the data where geometric distance becomes a metaphor for strategic similarity.

The SOM results from the combination of three processes: competition, cooperation, and adaptation (Fig. 8.7).

- *Competition*: For a given input pattern, all the neurons compute an activation function and the neuron with the largest activation is declared a winner. To begin, each neuron in a SOM is assigned a weight vector with the same dimensionality N as the input space (which, in IMMEX, would be the number of items available, plus additional efficiency or latency information). Any given input pattern is then compared to the weight vector of each neuron and the neuron that is closest (generally a Euclidean distance) is declared the winner.

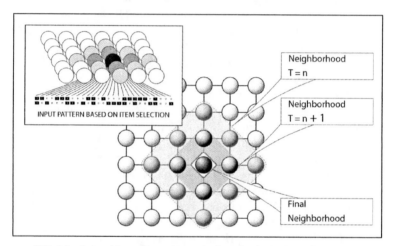

FIG. 8.7. Competition, cooperation, and adaptation in SOM. In the first step (insert), an input pattern consisting of 54 1's and 0's, which represent the menu items that a student chose while solving a case, are evaluated by each of the 36 neurons that comprise the neural network. The neuron whose randomized weight most closely matches the input vector (illustrated in black) is declared the winner and its weights are updated to more closely match the input pattern. The neurons in the immediate vicinity (neighborhood) of the winning neuron also update their weights, although not as much as the winner. This process continues repeatedly for each exemplar in the dataset. As training proceeds and the neurons are reorganizing around data clusters, the size of the neighborhood slowly decreases until at the completion of the training process each neuron has its own unique neighborhood. Details are described in the text.

- *Cooperation*: In order to stimulate a topological ordering, the winner spreads its activation over a neighborhood of neurons in the map. The activation of the winning neuron is spread around neurons in the immediate neighborhood so that topologically close neurons will become sensitive to similar patterns. The neighborhood of the winner is determined from the topology of the lattice (often a square or diamond organization) and is a function of the number of lateral connections to the winner. The size of the neighborhood is initially large to preserve the topology, but shrinks over time (T_1....T_n) to allow neurons to specialize in the latter stage of training.

- *Adaptation*: The winner and neighboring neurons adapt their activation function in order to become more sensitive to that particular input pattern. During training the winner neuron and its topological neighbors are adapted to make their weight vectors more similar to the input pattern that caused the activation. The neurons that are closer to the winner adapt more heavily than neurons that are further away and neurons are moved a bit closer to the input pattern. The magnitude of the adaptation is controlled with a learning rate that decays over time to ensure convergence of the SOM.

These properties are established by:

- A learning rate decay rule (Equation 1)

$$\eta(t) = \eta_0 \left(-\frac{t}{T_1} \right)$$ (1)

- A neighborhood kernel function (Equation 2),

$$h_{ik}(t) = \exp\left(-\frac{d_{ik}^2}{2\sigma(t)^2} \right)$$ (2)

where d_{ik} is the lattice distance between w_i and w_k, and;

- A neighborhood size decay rule (Equation 3).

$$\sigma(t) = \sigma_0 \exp\left(-\frac{t}{T_2} \right)$$ (3)

Procedurally, the training occurs through the following steps:

1. Initialize weights to some small, random values
2. Repeat until convergence{

a.   Select the next input pattern $x^{(n}$ from the database

   i. Find the unit w_j that best matches the input pattern $x^{(n)}$ (Equation 4)

$$i(x^{(n)}) = \frac{\arg\min}{j} \|x^{(n} - w_j\| \tag{4}$$

   ii. Update the weights of the winner w_j and all its neighbors w_k
     (Equation 5)

$$w_k = w_k + \eta(t) \cdot h_{ik}(t) \cdot (x^{(n} - w_k) \tag{5}$$

   }

b.   Decrease the learning rate $\eta(t)$

c.   Decrease the neighborhood size $\sigma(t)$

In this way, the best-matching model vectors tend to fire when the winning model vector fires. In an attempt to improve competition, there are methods that are employed to prevent excessive winning by one set of neurons, leaving other neurons to continually lose and play no role in the adaptation process. Here, conscience is employed to regulate the times that a neuron can win. When a neuron's weight vector is not close to a data cluster, it will fail to win the competition resulting in loss of that neuron in the adaptive process. Such nodes are not contributing to the solution and are thus "dead" neurons. To circumvent this problem and utilize the entire output space, a conscience factor can be applied so that a winning node can be "penalized" if it wins the competition more than a certain number of times. Consequently, neurons that lose are helped to win. The number of wins is estimated by the inverse of the number of neurons in the output space, and each neuron's win frequency is represented by

$$c_i(n + 1) = c_i(n) + \beta(o_i(n) - c_i(n)) \tag{6}$$

where $o(n)$ is 1 (winner) or 0 (loser) and β (the conscience factor) is a predetermined constant that the user can specify. Values that have been used typically range from 0.0001 to 0.01. In our current examples, the larger β value was used. Each time a neuron wins, the estimate of its winnings is increased. Each neuron updates its own fractional percentage of wins or losses as a way to bias its penalty for winning too often or reward for not winning enough by:

$$\beta_i = \gamma(1/N - c_i) \tag{7}$$

where γ is a constant, again determined by the user. This penalty term has ranged from 0 to 0.3 in our current examples. The bias term can then be subtracted from the Euclidean distance before a winner is selected. The bias term will be positive if the neuron is losing or negative if it is winning often. A positive bias will result in decreasing the distance to the cluster with the neuron's weight making an impact on the updated weights. If the bias term is negative, the distance is increased resulting in less impact of the neuron's weight and a decreased chance that the neuron will win repeatedly.

LIMITATIONS OF ARTIFICIAL NEURAL NETWORKS

Although artificial neural networks are effective pattern recognizers, and the design is cognitively plausible and can be understood by users, they are not a black-box into which one can put data and expect an easily interpretable answer. They require careful inspection of the output to check that they have performed correctly and usually will need tweaking, adjustment, and a number of runs to get a valid answer. Another limitation is that they suffer from a certain lack of precision. For instance, ANN's lack algorithmic clarity and it can be difficult to explain "how" a trained network arrived at a prediction. It is not always clear what specific criteria are being iteratively optimized in training, and, to some extent, this has to be directed during training (i. e., by choosing to train with sequences of items, or just the presence/absence of an item choice). However, we do not view this as a major obstacle as we are more interested currently in inductively determining strategy types (i. e., discovering structure) and changes in strategy types with experience, than we are in deriving and understanding a particular classification model.

Finally, there are practical issues to consider such as number of neurons, the topology of the training architecture, learning rates and conscience, etc that can often be defined only empirically as they relate closely to the data being investigated. These are discussed in detail later in this chapter.

STUDENT MODELS: SELECTION AND USE OF STRATEGIES

Student strategies, whether successful or not, are aggregates of multiple cognitive processes including comprehension of the material, search for other relevant information, evaluation of the quality of the information, the drawing of appropriate inferences from the information, and the use of self-regulation processes that help keep the student on track. Documenting student strategies at various levels of detail can therefore not only provide evidence of a student's changing understanding of the task, but can also provide experimental evidence of the relative contribution of different cognitive processes to the strategy.

Strategies used by students can then become a phenotype, or a proxy so to speak, of the working state of a student's knowledge.

Student Model Variables

The Student Model representing the strategic proficiencies important as students engage in IMMEX problem solving is shown in Figure 8.8.

Effective problem-solving strategies in science result from a combination of general science principles, domain-specific knowledge, and procedural knowledge and skills. For each IMMEX problem set, these proficiencies are composed of smaller sets of proficiencies that become mapped onto the tasks.

Most generally, IMMEX investigates proficiencies associated with knowledge/skills common to science such as design of experiments, graphical representations of data, systematic investigation of the causal relevance of different variables, etcetera. From a strategic perspective, evidence as to the presence/level of these skills in *True Roots* would for example, be the development of an effective elimination strategy for Leucine and the potential parents, or not retesting individuals for whom data is already available. Next, there are the domain-specific knowledge/skills of genetics and associated

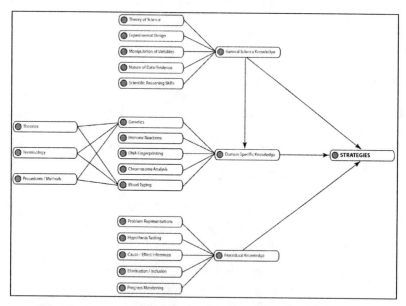

FIG. 8.8. A model of student proficiencies for True Roots assessment.

disciplines contained within the problem set. These are related to the familiarity with the language of the discipline (terminologies), the expected outcomes from manipulation of different variables (theories), and the procedures that provide the interpretative evidence to conduct the investigation (methods). IMMEX probes these proficiencies by tracking the use of the library and associated resources, by inferential modeling of students understanding of items within the context/sequence of other item selections, and by the solutions to the cases. Finally, there are the procedural and regulatory skills that influence the time on task, the initial strategies selected, etcetera.

Purpose Definition: Student's Selection and Use of Strategies

The theoretical design the IMMEX™ Project uses for creating the Task and Evidence Models for investigating students' selection and use of strategies during scientific problem solving is based on extensive work by others (Haider & Frensch, 1996; Schuun, Lovett, & Reder, 2001; Schuun & Reder, 2001; VanLehn, 1996) and can be organized around the following principles:

- Principle 1: Each individual selects the best strategy for them on a particular problem, and individuals might vary because of learning in the domain and/or process parameter differences;

- Principle 2: People adapt strategies to changing rates of success. Note that the base rate of success is not the same for all people on a task or for an individual on different tasks;

- Principle 3: Paths of strategy development emerge as students gain experience; and,

- Principle 4: Improvement in performance is accompanied by an increase in speed and reduction in the data processed.

We believe that the paths that students employ while navigating an IMMEX task provide evidence of a strategy, which we define as a sequence of steps needed to identify, interpret, and use appropriate and necessary facts to reach a logical conclusion or to eliminate or discount other reasonable conclusions. From these strategies a student demonstrates understanding by consistently, and efficiently deriving logical problem solutions.

The knowledge needed to solve problems in a complex domain such as biology or chemistry is composed of many principles, examples, technical details, generalizations, heuristics and other pieces of relevant information. From a cognitive perspective, these components can be broadly grouped into factual (declarative), reasoning (procedural), and regulatory (metacognitive) knowledge/skills (Anderson, 1980), and each play complementary roles in the construction of such science knowledge. Declarative knowledge is characterized by knowledge that people can report (knowing that) and facilitates the construction of organized frameworks of science concepts providing scaffolding for the acquisition of new concepts (Novak & Gowin, 1984). Teacher-centered instructional practices are the most effective at developing declarative knowledge and benefit students who require a more structured-learning approach (Von Secker & Lissitz, 1999).

Procedural knowledge is characterized by knowledge that appears in a performance but cannot be easily reported (knowing how) and along with regulatory skills, manifests itself as strategy selection and utilization mechanisms associated with hypothesis-driven (Lawson, 2000) and goal-oriented situations. In scientific reasoning the declarative and procedural knowledge exist as a continuum from domain general skills (for instance, how to graph results) and domain specific components (how to analyze flow cytometry graphs). These continually help distinguish the relative levels of professional expertise that different users bring to the simulations.

These reasoning skills are important for achievement in science (Krijik & Haney, 1987; Staver & Halsted, 1985), and students may require extended experience for maximum effects on achievement (Renner, & Lawson, 1973). For instance, Johnson & Lawson (1998) have shown that reasoning abilities accounted for more achievement variance in a community college biology course than did either prior knowledge or the number of biology courses taken. Improvement in reasoning skills has also been shown to occur as a result of prolonged instruction and can lead to long-term gains in science achievement (which may exhibit transfer to other disciplines) (Shayer & Adey, 1993). This indicates that duration and intensity of exposure to reasoning situations are important factors for the development of reasoning skills and more individually targeted interventions that may enrich/personalize the process. This suggests the need to provide students with diverse, continual and prolonged problem-solving experiences; others (Pellegrino et al., 2001) would also argue the need to begin routinely assessing students in such formats.

Instructional practices for developing scientific reasoning skills take many forms, including laboratory, inquiry-based science, and increasingly, computer simulations, but generally share the properties of being student-centered, socially interactive (Brown, Collins, & Duguid, 1989), and constructivist, involving many opportunities to gather evidence to support claims, analyze data quantitatively, and construct explanations. Problem-solving approaches provide such rich reasoning environments and have been used as effective instructional strategies in professional schools for some time (Elstein, 1993; Kolodner, 1993;

Schank, Kozma, Coleman, & Coppola, 2000). These approaches have been attractive and effective, not only for the motivational and realistic contexts that they provide, but also for the balance of knowledge styles needed during the problem solving tasks and the different perspectives they reveal about student learning (Barrett & Depinet, 1991). Along with case-based reasoning, these approaches are grounded in the belief that real-life reasoning and problem-solving behavior is almost never original, and that solutions to new problems are adoptions of previous problem solutions (Kolodner, 1997). Whether this is through the recall of exemplar cases (either representative or contradictory; Berry & Broadbent, 1988), or by mental model generalizations (Johnson-Laird, 1983), or scripts (Hudson, Fivush & Kuebli, 1992) across a number of cases is less clear as some aspects of strategic reasoning may involve the use of compiled knowledge or implicit memory, that is, for the most part, unconscious (Reder, Nhouyvanisvong, Schunn, Ayers, Angstadt et al., 2000).

The details of the problem solving approach are often described in terms of the hypo-deductive learning cycle where explanations of phenomena are investigated and refined.[6] From a cognitive perspective, there is a starting condition, a goal condition, and resources to transit between these two cognitive states. In most situations this is an iterative process where intermediate goals (hypotheses) are confirmed/rejected based on the latest information available. If a student were pursuing a particular hypothesis or line of reasoning, the goal of acquiring additional information would be to increase the confidence in the validity of this reasoning chain. Conflicting data, if obtained, would instead decrease the confidence in the current hypothesis and result in the initiation of a modified search of the problem space. An important aspect of this model is that students engaged in such activities continually select and revise strategies to optimize the outcomes.

Evidence Accumulation: Refinement of Strategies

Changes in the use of the Student Model components can also be dynamically investigated by evidence accumulation across a series of cases. Individual IMMEX cases are usually part of a problem set where there are shared information items, but the data details presented with each item are quite different depending on the case. These parallel forms have the advantages of (1) providing multiple perspectives of a problem space, (2) giving students multiple opportunities to practice their problem solving, (3) reducing discussion among

---

[6] For a historical perspective on learning cycles, see Lawson (1995; pp. 155–169).

students during assessment episodes and, most importantly, (4) providing evidence of strategic progress as students continually test and refine strategies. A number of informal and graphical methods of accumulating evidence across tasks are routinely used in IMMEX applications. (The final section of this chapter looks ahead to a more formal probability-based evidence-accumulation process based on hidden Markov models.)

Typically, students who are being introduced to a new IMMEX problem-solving environment begin with a broad investigation of relevant and irrelevant information coupled with recognizing and/or learning key concepts. This often occurs in the first case, though occasionally performers who are unsure of their interpretations continue to use this approach on the second case. When students become able to distinguish between relevant and irrelevant information, they begin to revisit content domains which they are most comfortable negotiating. This explicit demonstration of a problem-solving approach is termed *strategy adoption* and is usually visible by the third case of a problem set. At this juncture, performers of multiple IMMEX Tasks often exhibit persistence at this strategy and effectively transit from content novice to content competent strategies within a span of several cases; and, with enough repetition at expert level strategies, the problem-solving process once again becomes more implicit for these students. A major challenge arises when students adopt and persist with an ineffective and unproductive strategy. Effective student modeling at this stage could be used to suggest targeted interventions.

TASK MODELS: SPECIFICATIONS FOR DESIGNING IMMEX PRESENTATION MATERIAL

There are six specifications that we use for designing the IMMEX Presentation Material. These specifications are crafted in response to the Student Model principles of strategy selection that suggest that there is significant strategic information in the way students perceive and approach a problem and a problem space. To ensure that meaningful strategic evidence is captured from the initial and subsequent encounters, it is important that the Task Model carefully considers (1) the content and pedagogy embedded (domain analysis); (2) the composition of the problem space (to reveal observable behaviors); (3) the cognitive complexity of the problems; (4) the provision for repeat experiences (evidence accumulation); (5) the constraints placed on the problem space (presentation material specifications); and (6) the capture of meaningful information (evidence identification).

Although *True Roots* was designed for a high school level understanding of basic genetics principles, it has also been used extensively in the community college and university environments and we have recorded nearly 8,000 performances from these groups (Palacio-Cayetano, Allen, & Stevens, 1999). The overall percentage of *True Roots* cases in this data that were solved was 75.6%.

Domain Analysis: Document the Embedded Content and Pedagogy

During the initial design and at different stages during the Assembly cycle, domain analyses of the problem spaces and the problems are conducted to ensure that the content being presented is accurate and appropriate for the intended audience, and that the cases are pedagogically sound and align with relevant instructional and content standards. Teams of teachers, content experts, and educators perform these mappings, often with the input from students. Next, the scenarios should portray reality; some collaborators use these simulations to provide real-world, yet virtual experiences where students can become familiar with the discipline and practice decision making in a low-stakes environment. Third, the data must be consistent throughout the case in that the different items point to the same case result. Finally, in science problem sets, each menu item on its own often has inherent value (i. e., the molecular weight of a compound, a method for investigating molecular signaling, etc.), and these should be contemporary and supported by background information for students who are less familiar with this information. These mappings are being formalized into online searchable XML documents that provide the detailed dimensions of content, standards alignment, and cognitive skills within and across the discipline. The goal of this documentation is to supplement the Dublin Core and Gateway to Educational Materials (Andresen, Baker, Bearman, Caplan, Cathro, Childress, et al., 2000) meta-language qualifiers with discipline-specific hierarchies of subject headings to create, descriptive XML documents that can satisfy the needs of teachers and researchers alike.

Reveal Observable Behaviors

This specification addresses the quantity and quality of action options that constitute and structure the problem space (or search space) so that many strategic approaches can be accommodated. To avoid linear solutions/thinking and to not limit the diversity of strategies, the problem space should contain many action options (30–100). Within this problem space sufficient information, library resources, expert opinions, hints, etcetera should also be present to support students with weaker content knowledge and to keep them engaged. To promote integrative thinking, no one action option should provide an unambiguous solution to the case. Finally, if at all possible, most of the information a student would need to solve the problem should be present in the problem space.

Efficient student performance and progress in the *True Roots* environment requires that students:

- Develop an elimination strategy where Leucine is tested for a trait (such as blood typing) and then different parents are eliminated via discordant parent results.

- Reduce their use of redundant data, that is, if Parent Set 1 has been eliminated by RFLP, they shouldn't re-test them.

- Optimize their strategies on repeat performances of similar cases by reducing reliance on library material, expert help, etcetera.

While these strategies seem intuitive, in reality, the observable behaviors of students on these cases are highly diverse, and show different trajectories towards becoming efficient problem solvers.

Provide and Document Cognitive Complexity

Specifications 1 and 2 help developers make a "best guess" about the construction of a particular problem space. Once student performance data is obtained, it becomes possible to derive a more refined perspective through research studies.

Given problem spaces of a sufficient size and scope, problem solving in this environment should require an integration of domain knowledge and cognitive process skills, and research studies have shown that IMMEX provides a rich cognitive environment for problem solving. For instance, in a large study of undergraduate students, concurrent verbal protocol analysis has indicated that more than 90% of student verbalizations while solving a typical IMMEX case could be mapped into 12 distinct cognitive and metacognitive processes including the need for accurate cause-effect inferences, accurate evaluation of information, clarification of gaps in knowledge, monitoring of problem solving behavior, etcetera. (Chung et al., 2002). As expected, outside evaluators have also documented that students and teachers perceive problem sets like *True Roots* more as a tool for reasoning and integrating information than as a system for learning new facts (Chen, Chung, Klein, de Vries, & Burnam, 2001).

Accumulate Evidence

The second and third principles of strategy selection and use also suggest that with time, either within the first simulation or through multiple performances of parallel tasks, students should be able to learn which strategies are "best" and modify their initial approaches as needed. This implies that opportunities should be available for students to improve and that these changes (or lack thereof) in the weights of evidence should be updated to the Student Model to document when and under what conditions these changes occur. As noted earlier, informal and graphical, rather than psychometric, evidence accumulation procedures are employed in most IMMEX applications, in line with the primary role of cases as learning experiences. The hidden Markov models addressed in the final section address more formally the patterns of performance and learning across cases.

IMMEX addresses this need by designing problem sets that contain between 5 and 50 different instances (or clones) of a problem that share the same problem space but contain different solutions and different data. As part of the Activity Selection Process, these cases can be sequenced by the teachers either randomly or by level of difficulty previously established. Eventually cases may be automatically staged in response to the current strategic model of the student obtained from prior problem performances. These parallel forms have the further advantages of providing multiple perspectives of a problem space, and reducing discussion among students during learning and/or assessment episodes.

The provision for repeat problem solving experiences can also be extended to a larger design principle that addresses the construction of integrated curricula. The literature suggests the importance of prolonged time/experience with scientific reasoning activities for maximum effect on student performance (Shayer & Adey, 1993). To provide such year-round coverage of problem-solving scenarios, we have begun to develop integrated curricular problem sets in chemistry, molecular biology, and biology, each with 6–8 different problem sets (with each containing 20+ cases). Such curricula have provided students with over 100 problem-solving experiences over a 9-month period (Stevens, Sprank, Simpson, Vendlinski, Palacio-Cayetano, et al., 2001).

Presentation Material Specifications: Constrain and Extend the Problem Space

For strategic improvement, some measure(s) of success must be a component of the task (Strategic Principle 2), and although such measures can be diverse (a score, a solution, successfully stabilizing a simulation, submitting an essay to be scored, personal feedback, etc.), they should be present. These components fall into the category of constraints, which can have powerful influences on students' strategies, but are perhaps the least well understood of the design specifications.

A common constraint is to include a cost (or risk, or time penalty) for each item requested or for each incorrect "guess" at a solution that helps focus student attention on each decision during the performance. A second constraint is the time allotted to solve a case and this can be naturally encouraged through a 1–2 hour course or lab format, or can be more structured (i. e., solve 3 cases in 60 minutes). Students can also work individually on cases or collaboratively in groups, and evidence from Case et al. (2002) suggests that working in groups not only influences the strategies that students use, but also can jog students out of poor strategies. Finally, it is possible to extend the problems by ending the case in different ways. In most IMMEX cases, students choose an answer from a list. On more sociologically based IMMEX cases, the cases end with the students submitting an online essay to a question posed in the prologue that is also scored online by the faculty (Stevens & Dexter, 2003).

An overall design feature, however, is to not constrain the cases so much, either through hints or by limiting the scope of the question asked, so that the exercise becomes directed and linear.

Evidence Identification: Designs for Capturing Intentional Actions

There are, of course, many inherent challenges in this approach. First, is that intentional acts must be captured. Second, is to determine how human cognition is distributed across the stream of actions, and this relates, in part, to the granularity of the information collected. Third, is how to best process that information.

Other challenges would include the likely difference in approaches by different students according to the theories of strategy selection. One key feature to these challenges is the ability to capture intentional acts. Several IMMEX design features increase the likelihood that intentional acts are being captured. First, limited information is presented on the screen removing ambiguity about what is being viewed. Second, given a cost structure, students must "pay" for each item accessed. Third, these intentional acts are related to a decision regarding the outcome of the case.

RESPONSE SCORING PROCESS

Artificial Neural Network Evidence Identification.

When analyzing the IMMEX performances of students through individual or group search path mapping, the complexity of the task is immediately obvious.

As the number of menu items or action options in an IMMEX problem increases, so too does the way a student might move through the problem space. If one considers the order in which a student viewed different pieces of information, the number of paths through the problem space increases in a factorial manner with each additional item of information. This same magnitude is present even if one only considers what information a student retrieved in arriving at an answer. Such a large number of possibilities makes it almost impossible for humans to consistently find a pattern in student performances and to do so without introducing preconceived biases of how students *should* solve a problem.

Nevertheless, the first phase of evidence identification produces observables variables that are relatively few in number, and include (1) the action options selected, (2) (often) the order of selection, and (3) (occasionally) the latencies between selections. The second phase is accomplished by the ANN. Setting up this evidence identification process continues through the steps of data preprocessing, neural network training, and cluster validation, and then to defining rules for interpreting cluster membership in terms of student model variables.

Data Pre-processing. The data preprocessing begins by identifying all the cases in a problem set that students have completed. Incomplete performances, while perhaps informative of starting schema, provide incomplete representations of strategic knowledge and have not yet been analyzed. The *input structure* used consists of preprocessed data that represents each exemplar (performance) by the type of test item used as the characteristic used or, alternatively, the sequence of steps taken. This type of input representation results in an equal number of inputs used to represent each performance. These inputs are numbered from 1 to 54, indicating that there are 54 possible test items that can characterize a performance without accounting for items that may be repeated. This series of performances will then require 54 input neurons, resulting in an input matrix of n x 54 where n is the number of exemplars in the data set, in this case, $n = 1710$. Each exemplar had 54 inputs, where the value of each input is 1 if the test item was used or 0 if the test item was not used. The group identifiers for these items are shown in Fig. 8.9. For instance, the early items 1-10 represent lookup items in the Library, items 22-25 are fingerprinting analyses, etc.

Neural Network Training Conditions. The *Kohonen layer* is the actual neural network layer that will represent the input and the relationships in that input that will ultimately be projected on a certain output space. The Kohonen layer was structured to have a certain relationship between its neurons such that each neuron has four neighboring neurons. Such a configuration is termed a "diamond" indicating that the neuron, at the center of the 4-pointed diamond, has each of 4 corners as neighbors. This configuration is favored over the square Kohonen, where each neuron has eight neighbors, or the linear Kohonen, where each neuron has only two neighbors. The diamond structure has consistently resulted in a good representation of the input space with adequate data cluster formation in the output space. The conscience is a feature of the Kohonen layer that must be specified. A β factor of 0. 01 with a γ factor of 0.03 was applied to ensure adequate updating of the weights from each of the neurons. The other consideration of the network's design is the scheduling of the rate of decay of the neighborhood size and the size of the step taken to reach the minimum. These factors are scheduled to occur from epoch 50 to 500. This is done to allow cluster centers to become established in the output space before any constraints are placed on the neighborhood size or the step size. Once epoch number 50 is reached, the rate of neighborhood begins to decrease from 4 to 1 and the step size begins to diminish. The scheduling function is linear and preset to a small negative value that is updated at each epoch. The β constant values for the step size and neighborhood decrease are 0.00001 and 0.001 respectively. These values have been derived empirically to ensure continuous, steady decline of both parameters throughout the training period.

The *output* is the space on which the input will be projected. This space is defined as a number of rows and columns which define the output. A 6 x 6 output space is defined by 6 rows and 6 columns. This also implies that the number of outputs form the Kohonen layer is 36 (6 x 6). Furthermore, the output neurons must be configured to reflect the desire to one winner per update (only one neuron wins each time). This architecture requires a "winner-take-all" type of neuron, but one must recall that the conscience factors have been adjusted to allow losing neurons to win depending on the fraction of wins or losses as described earlier. As discussed in the section on Outstanding Issues, different output spaces serve different purposes depending on the granularity of the analysis desired.

For the following studies, self-organizing Kohonen neural networks were trained with 1710 student performances from high school and community college students and freshman students from two major universities. The neural network consisted of a 6 x 6 neuron grid trained in a diamond configuration.

Cluster Validation. Designing neural networks that find known data clusters in representative data (for instance, expected strategies defined during the Task Analysis) and that produce useful results are two useful methods for validating the resulting clusters. As discussed later, this validation of evidence continues by analyzing representative group and individual search path maps to determine whether the clusters "make sense" from both a content and pedagogy perspective. These validations direct an iterative process for determining whether the number of categories obtained by the training process are too few (as shown by an individual cluster having many diverse problem-solving approaches) or too many (as shown by multiple clusters containing similar search path map patterns). Estimating the reliability of category clustering is an additional validation step and a guiding approach we have used is directed by inter-network reliability. Here, parallel (between three and five) neural networks are trained with the preprocessed datasets and estimates of the degree of co-clustering of cluster members across the different networks are generated. For problem sets such as *True Roots*, the co-clustering of members across at least two of three independent neural networks approaches 98%, with 44% co-clustering across the three networks. Those that are clustered together across all three networks are termed Class 1, those that cluster on two of three trained networks Class 2, and those uniquely clustered across the networks are termed Class 3. Some nodes have a higher than expected number of Class 1 performances, whereas other nodes are enriched in Class 2 performances. There is no apparent topology to the nodes with the different classes of performances, but the nodes containing the lower numbers of performances are often enriched in Class 2 performances. Further validation continues through the research process when cluster membership is analyzed across different classrooms and becomes linked with other student performance data.

Defining Properties of Clustered Performances

After training, the performances clustered at each neuron were analyzed for (1) the frequency of selection of individual menu items, (2) the percentage of cases solved, (3) the total number of performances at each neuron, and (4) the internetwork training reliability. Fig. 8.9 shows such an analysis for two representative neurons where there has been either an indiscriminate and prolific selection of items (Neuron 6), or a more refined sequence of test selections focusing on pedigree and RFLP and blood typing (Neuron 13).

In these figures, the individual menu items are organized sequentially according to different categories of research and resource items available. These are labeled according to the templates in Fig. 8.1 and 8.2. The performances clustered at Neuron 6 reveal a prolific approach to test selection, which is often

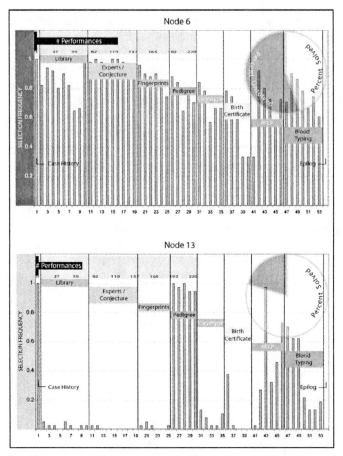

FIG. 8.9. Sample nodal analysis. Each nodal analysis diagram provides four pieces of information regarding the performances at each node. First, there is a histogram showing the frequency with which each test was selected by performances at the particular node. These can be identified by the labels for the 54 possible tests. This is useful to determine the test ordering characteristics of the performances at a particular node, and the relation of these performances with those of neighboring neurons. These histograms display the entire range of frequency data, and occasionally it is more appropriate to apply a "threshold mask," perhaps at .3 or .4, to better highlight the most frequent tests. Next, in the upper right hand corner is a pie chart indicating the percent of cases that were correctly solved by students. At the top of each chart is a bar graph of the total number of performances clustering at the particular neuron, and lastly, the highlighting on the Y axis indicates whether a neuron contained mainly Class 1 performances (dark gray), Class 2 performances (light gray), or Class 3 performances (white).

a preferred initial approach for students on IMMEX cases as they explore the problem space. Given the apparent lack of test selectivity, the frequency of solving the case (upper right hand corner) is not surprisingly low. Neuron 13 clusters student performances where the main category of information was pedigree with secondary categories of genetic fingerprinting (RFLP) and blood typing. As expected from the more refined search strategy of these students, the percentage of cases solved at this neuron is high.

A similar analysis of the composition of the entire 36 neuron set is shown in Fig. 8.10. The performances were uniformly distributed across the neural networks with the exception of a valley of performances near the upper portion of the network, suggesting the network architecture and training protocols were not over or under-constrained.

As expected from the properties of self-organizing networks and the organization of the input data (for these studies, the selection of an item), the performance data shows topological ordering across the network. The most obvious feature is based on the quantity of items selected with very prolific performances clustering on the right portions of the map while the very limited performances are more to the left. Moving down the topological map, there is a reduction in the use of library resource items on the right side. Some nodes, like 7, 15, and 25 contain test selections from a single menu category (Pedigree, RFLP, and Blood Typing respectively). Other neurons contain particular combinations of repeated items. Node 20, for example, is enriched for performances where RFLP, Blood Typing, and Karyotype data predominates, whereas Node 32 contains performances enriched for Pedigree, RFLP, and Blood Typing.

We define the categories resulting from the above neural network processing as *strategies* as they represent general approaches to a problem solution used by many students. Although most members of a cluster have a unique performance sequence, they share common items/sequences. Fig. 8.11, for example, shows four representative examples of performances at Node 20. Here the core test items are RFLP (center), blood typing (right) and some variable elements of karyotype (left).

Across the neural network topology, there was variability in the frequency of the cases solved with lower percentages around the right and bottom portions of the topological map, and a higher solution frequency in the middle and upper left portions of the map suggesting that different strategies have different degrees of success for students (Fig. 8. 10). While some of the strategies routinely seem to allow a student using the strategy to solve a problem (neurons

13, 19, 20, 33, etc.), other strategies seldom produce that result (neurons 3, 11, 12). These latter strategies are generally those of the non-efficient type as described in Table 8.1. Efficiency and effectiveness can therefore begin to be associated with a strategy. As this information was not included in the training parameters, it is not surprising that there is no obvious topological ordering with regard to the solved frequency.

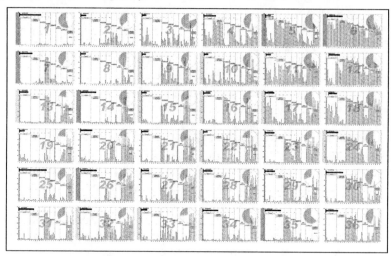

FIG. 8.10. Complete *True Roots* neural network output map. See Fig. 8.9 for details.

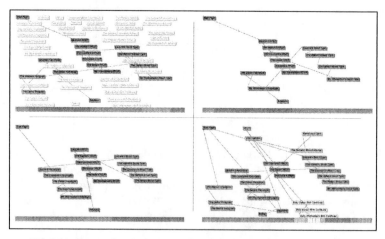

FIG. 8.11. Four performances grouped at Node 20.

Dynamics of Strategy Changes

The dynamic changes in the use of the predicted strategies in Table 8.1 as students perform the five cases in the *True Roots* problem sets are detailed below.

Prolific Strategy Type. Typically, students who are being introduced into a new IMMEX problem-solving environment begin with a broad investigation of relevant and irrelevant information coupled with the recognition and/or learning of key concepts. It is not unusual for students to use this strategy on the first case of a problem set as they are exploring and defining the problem space, collectively called *framing*. However, if learning is occurring, then with practice on multiple cases, task relevant items will be separated from task redundant information and the most relevant aspects of the task will become focused on (Haider & Frensch, 1996). This should result in the abandonment of the prolific strategy, an increase in the solved rate, and a decrease in the amount of time spent per case. As shown in Fig. 8.12, most students began with a prolific strategy type and, on subsequent cases, the use of this strategy type declined. By the fourth case, the students still using this strategy were particularly at risk for missing the solution.

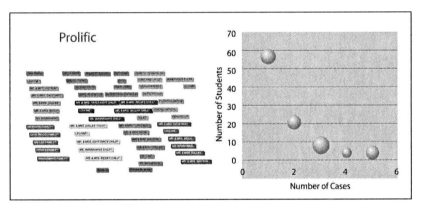

FIG. 8.12. Dynamics of prolific strategy type. The number of students using the prolific strategy type (Y-axis) is plotted vs. the case performed. The size of the circles is proportional to the solution frequency.

Redundant Strategy Type. When students can distinguish relevant and irrelevant information, they selectively revisit the content areas on subsequent cases where they are most comfortable negotiating to eliminate possible parents. Here it is not unusual for students to start developing favorite sets of test items, such as blood typing or fingerprinting, that they will consistently embed into their strategies. This complex selection of a repertoire of test selection protocols is at least in part influenced (according to verbal protocols) by familiarity with the terms from prior experiences (TV, newspapers, science courses) and/or by the format in which the data is displayed. For instance, pattern matching between RFLP digests seems easier for some students than does antibody agglutination that has more complex fundamentals.

The redundant strategy type appears to be an intermediate stage in the development of efficient strategies in that the student understands the need for comparing the child Leucine with the different parents across a particular test group (i. e., blood typing or RFLP) to eliminate possible parents. The strategy is not optimized, however, as the same parents are often retested multiple times with different laboratory tests even though they should have been eliminated.

As shown in Fig. 8.13, the redundant strategy was the second most frequent starting strategy and initially had a relatively poor rate of success. The frequency of use of this strategy increased on the second case (with a corresponding decrease in the prolific strategy), and then progressively declined.

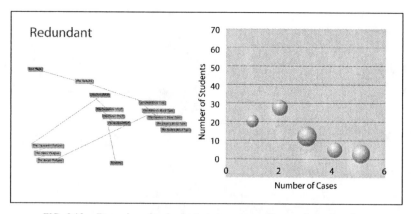

FIG. 8.13. Dynamics of redundant strategy type. The number of students using the prolific strategy type (Y-axis) is plotted vs. the case performed. The size of the circles is proportional to the solution frequency.

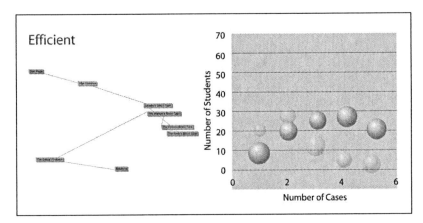

FIG. 8.14. Dynamics of efficient strategy type. The number of students using the prolific strategy type (Y-axis) is plotted vs. the case performed. The size of the circles is proportional to the solution frequency.

Efficient Strategy Type. As shown in Fig. 8.14, the solve rate for the efficient strategy type is high (80%) and consistent, although few students in this test set understood the problem space well enough on the first case to employ an efficient strategy. The use of this strategy slowly increased with each case attempted peaking at Case 4. The decrease of all the numbers on the fifth case in is due to students not completing the 5 problem sets in the allotted time.

Limited Strategy Type. The limited strategy type identifies students who are attempting to solve the case with insufficient information (at least on the early problem sets). The frequency of this strategy is highly implementation site dependent, with some high school classes showing a preponderance of guessing strategies. In this tightly controlled experimental situation with more advanced students, few initially used a limited strategy. Paradoxically, the use of this strategy increased on subsequent cases and was accompanied by a high solution frequency. Retrospective analysis of their verbal protocols indicated that some of the students were going outside the scope of the problem space and learning a higher strategy (i. e., knowing there are only five parents and knowing which ones they had before). Following this result, we recommend a minimum of 10+ cases in a problem set to restrict the use of this alternative strategy.

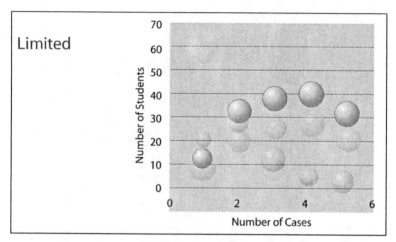

FIG. 8.15. Dynamics of limited strategy type. The number of students using the limited strategy type (Y-axis) is plotted vs. the case performed. The size of the circles is proportional to the solution frequency.

While the previous figures were representative of more than 100 community college students, Fig. 8.16 shows the details of such strategic transitions over a series of five *True Roots* cases by a single student. On the first performance, the student performed a thorough exploration of the problem space, spending a bit over 31 minutes on the case. As expected from the topology of the trained neural network, this performance was clustered at neuron 6 (Fig. 8.10), which is characterized by extensive test ordering. On the second case, the student no longer required the library and expert resources, but still engaged in an extensive data search. This performance was successfully completed in 6 minutes. The neural network recognized the abandonment of the library resources and clustered this performance at neuron 24. Over the next three performances (which required 4, 2, and 3 minutes respectively), the student continued to refine his/her strategy from a redundant strategy (neuron 27), to a limited strategy (neuron 19), to an efficient strategy (neuron 26). These latter three performances were more closely topologically ordered with each other than with the first two performances, suggesting a strategic transition occurred between the second and third case. Such strategic transitions may be important indicators of the evolution of a student's understanding and can possibly serve as loci for targeting interventions.

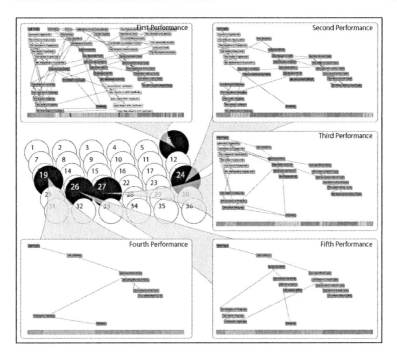

FIG. 8.16.   Sample of an individual student's progress on five True Roots cases. The search path maps of student 2044's performances are shown with the corresponding classification of these performances by the trained ANN. Note the shifting in the classification topology between performances two and three.

VALIDATING THE CONSTRUCTS OF STRATEGIES AND STRATEGY TYPES

Previous validation studies have shown that IMMEX in general (and *True Roots* in particular) is:

- Cognitively complex;
- Engaging and motivating for students and teachers;
- Capable of being implemented in a wide number of disciplines and settings.

We have also shown that it is possible to create cases with the same level of difficulty (as measured by Item Response Theory), as well as with predictable levels of difficulty (Vendlinski & Stevens, 2002).

The following studies were conducted to examine whether the *True Roots* problem set behaved in a predictable way when developed and analyzed according to the above framework. Our hypotheses were (1) that students of different abilities would approach and solve these cases with strategies consistent with these abilities; and (2) that students with higher measures of scientific reasoning would employ more effective strategies. These studies address the concurrent validity (the ability to distinguish between groups it should theoretically be able to distinguish between) and convergent validity (the degree to which the operationalization converged on other operationalizations).

Relating Ability to Problem Solving Strategic Approaches

Two student populations that could potentially provide varying degrees of problem-solving ability were recruited from a university freshman class (n = 94), and entering students from a nearby community college (n = 105). By tapping two different levels of the institutionalized selection process, we gain the maximum variability within the 17–18 year old range to link to the previous strategic trends.

The ability of the two groups of students was first significantly different on the task itself: the university students were above (82%) the average solution frequency of the 8000+ performances of *True Roots* in our database (76%), while the community college students were below this average at 67% (p<0.001). Differences were also seen in the way that the students approached the cases. The community college students accessed significantly more resource (p < .001) and conjecture (p < .001) items than did the university level students.

A more detailed indicator of ability level differences between the community college level and university participants involved the linkage between what students *said* during the concurrent verbalization and what they *did* simultaneously on the IMMEX task (Chung et al., 2002). The community college students used more "simple statements" (repeating of text from the item ordered indicative of non-analysis; (p < .001), had fewer "correct cause and effect" statements (p = .014), were less able to evaluate information correctly (p = .003), and asked fewer questions during decision making (p = .026), which suggests lack of hypothesis building. Moreover, the university students were more likely to make statements that clarified gaps in knowledge (p = .012) and articulated judgments of information relevancy (p < .001), while the community college students verbalized more awareness of task goals and their progress—or lack thereof—toward achieving those goals (p < .001).

While both university and community college students used all four strategy types defined in Table 8.2 across the five cases, the university students used a higher proportion of Efficient strategies while the community college students used more Prolific and Limited strategy types (Pearson Chi-Square = 44.2, p<0.001).

The dynamic changes use of prolific and efficient strategies, which showed the greatest disparity between the community college and university students, were then examined across the five cases. As shown in Fig. 8.17, the university students appeared to be a step ahead of the community college students in the abandonment of prolific and redundant strategies, and between one and two steps in the adoption of efficient strategies.

To provide supporting evidence of the difference in student ability, both student populations completed the Classroom Test of Scientific Reasoning (CTSR) (Lawson, 1995) as an independent measure of scientific reasoning ability level. The modified version of the CTSR (22 multiple-choice items) was designed to assess a student's ability to separate variables, to conserve weight and volume, and to use proportional logic as well as combinational reasoning and correlations. The university students had a mean score of 71% whereas the community college students had a mean score of 49%, and this disparity was significant ($t = 7.844$; $p < .001$).

Next, the students' use of different strategy types was measured as a function of their CTSR scores. As shown in Table 8.3, those students who scored on the lower end of the CTSR used more Prolific, Redundant, and Limited strategies while those students who scored on the upper end of the CTSR used more Efficient strategies than expected.

TABLE 8.2
Strategy Type Use by University and Community College Students

			Ability Level		Total
			University	Community College	
Strategy Type	Prolific	Count	58	98	156
		Expected Count	73.8	82.2	156.0
	Redundant	Count	91	105	196
		Expected Count	92.7	103.3	196.0
	Efficient	Count	218	181	399
		Expected Count	188.7	210.3	399.0
	Limited	Count	34	63	97
		Expected Count	45.9	51.1	97.0
Total		Count	401	447	848
		Expected Count	401.0	447.0	848.0

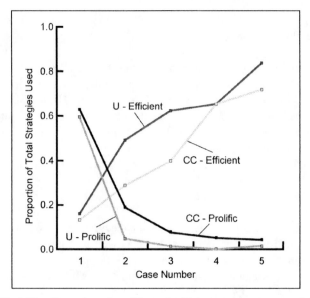

FIG. 8.17.   Dynamics of prolific and efficient strategy type used by community college and university students. The proportion of performance characterized as either prolific or efficient strategies is plotted vs. the case performed.

TABLE 8.3
Strategy Type Use by Students with Different CTSR Scores

			100–80	79–60	59–50	49–30	29–0	Total
Strategy Type	Prolific	Count	31	46	31	34	26	168
		Expected Count	40.1	51.2	29.2	29.4	17.9	168.0
	Redundant	Count	24	48	20	28	21	141
		Expected Count	33.7	43.0	24.5	24.7	15.1	141.0
	Efficient	Count	129	140	78	61	26	434
		Expected Count	103.7	132.3	75.5	76.1	46.4	434.0
	Limited	Count	15	20	16	23	16	90
		Expected Count	21.5	27.4	15.7	15.8	9.6	90.0
Total		Count	199	254	145	146	89	833
		Expected Count	199.0	254.0	145.0	146.0	89.0	833.0

Strategic Transitions and Trajectories

The studies just described demonstrate our ability to relate the observations of student's strategy selection and use with their educational experience and reasoning skills, both important aspects of potential automated scoring systems. The evidence also indicates that there are selective starting and ending strategies across sequences of problem-solving episodes, and that students tend to make progress along partially defined trajectories. In this section we explore extensions to the Evidence Accumulation Process that begin to formally describe these transitions and trajectories and suggest linkages with other automated scoring approaches in this volume.

Fig. 8.16 provided the fundamentals for this evidence accumulation process, which helps define the experience-driven refinements in problem-solving strategy development. From an automatic scoring perspective, the important components of this process are both the positions of each performance on the neural network topological map, as well as the transitions between neurons as performances are accumulated, as these help define the current state of a student's strategic knowledge and the possible trajectories of future learning. For instance, on student 2044's first performance, nearly all 54 available items were tested; on the second performance, there was a reduction of library resources, but still extensive examination of the data items. This was followed by a progressive refinement of efficient data driven approaches on performances 3 to 5. These changes in strategy were accompanied by changes in the nodal classification on the ANN topology map, effectively creating a performance trajectory.

This approach of tracing trajectories across the neural network topology space can be expanded to encompass a class, all the students of a particular teacher, groups with different levels of experience, etcetera, to help refine the performance and summary scoring model.

A visual representation of such a transition analysis is shown in Fig. 8.18, and displays all the transitions (213 total) made by two classes of high school students (with the same teacher). Similar to our search path mapping procedure described earlier, the lines connect the neuronal from-to transitions associated with a performance, again going from the upper left corner of the "from" neuron to the center of the "to" neuron. The thickness of the lines represents the number of performances, highlighting the major transitions and showing the diversity of learning trajectories in classroom settings. In these aggregated transition maps, the peaked arrows, most noticeably at neurons 25 and 31, indicate the repeat use of strategies. The students in these classes showed preferential use of strategies mapping to the lower left of the neural network topology map, representing those that rely extensively on two content/test areas, blood typing and pedigree. The thicker lines from *Start* leading to this area suggest that these topics were included in the initial starting strategies of this group of students. Studies are underway to begin to relate starting and dominant strategies to curricular content

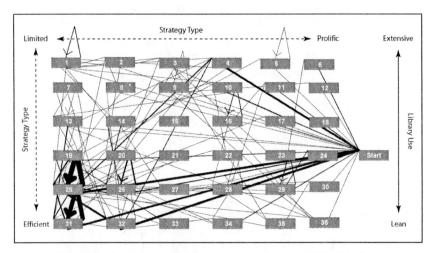

FIG. 8.18. Group Transition Map on a 6 x 6 Neuron ANN. This figure illustrates the performance transitions students (55 students, 213 performances) make as they move from case to case in the five case *True Roots* problem set. The lines emanating from the left-most box (Start) indicate the first performance. The thickness of these and subsequent lines is proportional to the number of students making a particular transition, and the "peaked hats" indicate repeat transitions. The performance characteristics at each neuron are shown in Fig. 8.10 and are broadly defined with regard to strategy type and the use of the library resources by the figure axes.

coverage and classroom practice and early results suggest that the classroom/section environment and/or the way the task is represented in each environment is of primary significance (Stevens, Johnson, & Soller, 2005).

One approach to dynamically modeling this information would be to probabilistically link the transitions. However, with 1296 possible transitions in a 36-neuron map, such models would likely lack predictive power. In a previous study we used Markov Chain analysis for modeling student's adoption of particular strategies and showing the persistent use of selected strategies. Recently we have used Hidden Markov Modeling to extend these preliminary results to more predicatively model student learning pathways (Stevens et al, 2004). Markov models are used to model processes that move stochastically through a series of predefined states (Rabiner, 1989). The states are not directly observed, but are associated with a probability distribution function.

The set of parameters that specify a HMM include:

- The set of states $S=\{s_1, s_2, \ldots s_n\}$

- The state sequence $Q=\{q_1, q_2, \ldots q_k\}$ q_k S

- The *prior probabilities* are the probability distribution of q_i being the first state of a state sequence.

- The *transition probabilities* are the probability to go from a state i to a state j, i.e. $P(q_i \mid q_j)$. They are stored in a matrix (A) where each term a_{ij} denotes a probability $P(q_i \mid q_j)$.

- The *emission probabilities* are the probability distribution functions that characterize each state q_i i.e., $p(x \mid q_i)$.

In our studies, the observed emissions are the neural network nodes at which each performance in a sequence of performances is clustered. So for student 2044 (Fig. 8.16), this sequence would be [6 24 27 19 26]. Based on our previous results, we postulated that a 5-state model might be appropriate given the strategy types (Prolific, Redundant, Efficient, Limited, Guessing) previously defined by the cognitive task analysis (Table 8.1), and confirmed through the inspection of the data (Figs. 8.12–8.15).

The HMM classification procedure is a supervised machine learning algorithm that requires training to generate useful transition and emission matrices. During the HMM training phase, 908 performance sequences were presented to the HMM modeling software (MatLab, The Math Works, Natick, MA) and during training, the transition matrix between the states is updated to most closely match the sequence transitions in the data. The process is analogous to the updating of the weights in an ANN described earlier, and the model reached a convergence threshold of 1e-4 after 64 epochs. The result was a state transition matrix and an emission matrix that indicated the probability of each emission at each proposed state.

The emission probabilities for each of the 36 neural network nodes, is plotted for each of the five states in Fig. 8.19 A–E. Most of the neural network nodes were preferentially associated with a single state, although some duplication existed for some of the nodes with higher numbers of performances such as 25 and 30. When the topology of the states was overlaid on the 6 x 6 neural network grid, each state (Fig. 8.19 F), represented topology regions of the neural network that were often contiguous and were earlier defined as being prolific, efficient, redundant, or limited by both the task analysis (Table 8.1) and the manual inspection of the topology space that was used for the earlier validation studies.

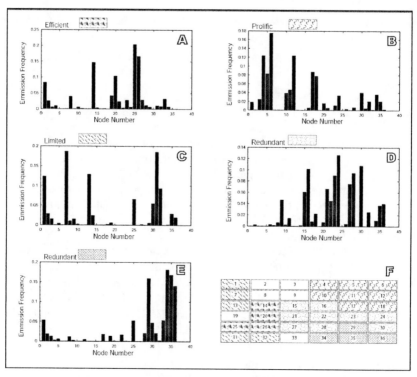

FIG. 8.19. State information for the trained HMM. A 5-state HMM was trained with 908 exemplars containing sequences of between one and five performances. Following training, the probability of emitting a particular neural network node at a particular state was plotted vs. the node number (Fig. 8.19 A-E). In Fig. 8.19 F, the major nodes emitted at each state are overlaid on the ANN topology map from Fig. 8.10.

A more dynamic correspondence between the states defined by Hidden Markov Modeling and those earlier defined by visual inspection is shown in Fig. 8.20 that compares the kinetics of the prolific and efficient strategies of university and community college students. Comparison of this figure with Fig. 8.17 demonstrates similar kinetics, with the community college students switching from the prolific strategy and adopting the efficient strategy more slowly than the undergraduate students. Combined, these data suggest that HMM may provide a reliable method for extraction of information from sequences of performances that compares well with the results obtained by visual inspection by investigators.

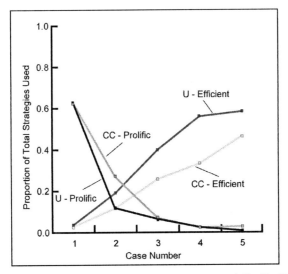

FIG. 8.20. Dynamics of prolific and efficient strategy type, defined by HMM, used by community college and university students. The proportion of performance characterized as prolific and efficient strategies by HMM modeling is plotted vs. the case performed. Compare with Fig. 8.17.

A further advantage of a HMM is that it allows predictions to be made regarding the student's learning trajectory. This was explored in the following way. First, a "true" mapping of each node and the corresponding state was conducted for each performance of a performance sequence. For each step of each sequence (i. e., going from performance 2 to 3, or 3 to 4, or 4 to 5), the posterior state probabilities of the emission sequence (nodes) were calculated to give the probability that the model is in a particular state when it generated a symbol in the sequence, given that the sequence was emitted. For instance, sequence [18 36 29] mapped to states 4 5 5.

This "true" value was then compared with the most likely value obtained when the last sequence value was substituted by each of the 36 possible emissions, for instance [18 36 X] where X = 1 to 36. The best predicted value for X was the emission with the maximum likelihood, given the HMM, and the best predicted state was the state with the maximum likelihood for that sequence.

Comparing the "true" node and state values with the predicted values gives an estimate of the predictive power of the model (Table 8.4). From this table, the

TABLE 8.4
Predictive Abilities of the Trained HMM

Performance	Case 1 to 2	Case 2 to 3	Case 3 to 4	Case 4 to 5
% Predicted Nodes	11%	14%	14%	11%
% Predicted States	66%	71%	78%	82%

n = 708 sequences of performances (between 2 and 5 cases long)

predictability of the individual nodes was difficult (but 4 to 5 fold better than random), but predicting across states achieved a prediction accuracy of over 80%. It also appeared that as the performance sequence increased, the prediction rate also increased, probably reflecting that by performance 3, 4, and 5, students are more likely to use repeated strategies.

While we have focused on a single IMMEX problem set in genetics for this review, these studies have been confirmed with a high school/university problem set termed Hazmat and extended to show strategic differences across gender and whether students are working individually or in groups (Stevens et al., 2004; Stevens & Soller, 2005).

ACKNOWLEDGMENTS

Supported in part by grants from the National Science Foundation (NSF-ROLE 0231995, DUE Award 0126050, ESE 9453918, HRD-0429156), the PT^3 Program of the U.S. Department of Education (Implementation Grant, P342A-990532), and the Howard Hughes Medical Institute Precollege Initiative. The authors particularly thank Dr. Amy Soller for advice on HMM modeling, and John Stallings for editorial and illustration support. Artificial neural network and hidden Markov modeling software were developed using Matlab (The Mathworks, Natick, MA).

REFERENCES

Anderson, J. R. (1980). *Cognitive psychology and its implications*. San Francisco: W.H. Freeman.
Andresen, L., Baker, T., Bearman, D., Caplan, P., Cathro, W., & Childress, E. (2000). Dublin Core Qualifiers Available at http://www.dublincore.org/documents/2000/07/11/dcmes-qualifiers/
Barrett, G. V., & Depinet, R. L. (1991). A reconsideration of testing for competence rather than for intelligence. *American Psychologist. 46*(10) 1012-1024.
Baxter, G. P., & Glaser, R. (1997). *An approach to analyzing the cognitive complexity of science performance assessments*. Los Angeles, CA: National Center for Research on Evaluation,

Standards and Student Testing (CRESST), Center for the Study of Evaluation. University of California, Los Angeles.

Berry, D. C., & Broadbent, D. E. (1988). Interactive tasks and the implicit-explicit distinction. *British Journal of Psychology, 79*, 251–272.

Bransford, J. D., Brown, A. L., & Cocking, R. R. (1999). *How people learn: Brain, mind, experience, and school.* Washington, DC: National Academies Press.

Brown, J. S., Collins, A., & Duguid, P. (1989). Situated cognition and the culture of learning. *Educational Researcher 18*(1), 32–42.

Case, E. L., Cooper, M., Stevens, R., and Vendlinski, T. (2002, April). Using the IMMEX system to teach and assess problem solving in general chemistry. ACS Annual Meeting Presentation, Orlando, Florida. Available at http://www.acs.org/portal/PersonalScheduler/EventView.jsp? paper_key=200723&session_key=34422

Casillas, A. M., Clyman, S. G., Fan, V. Y., and Stevens, R. (1999). Exploring alternative models of complex patient management with artificial neural networks. *Advances in Health Sciences Education 1*, 1–19.

Casillas, A., Clyman, S., Fan, Y., and Stevens, R. (2000). Exploring Alternative Models of Complex Patient Management with Artificial Neural Networks. *Advances in Health Sciences Education 5*, 23–41. Netherlands: Kluwer Academic Publishers.

Chen, E., Chung, G., Klein, D., de Vries, L., and Burnam, B. (2001). How Teachers Use IMMEX in the Classroom. *CSE paper.* Los Angeles: University of California, National Center for Research on Evaluation, Standards, and Student Testing (CRESST). Available at http://www.immex.ucla.edu/docs/publications/pdf/evaluationforteachers.pdf

Chung, G. K. W. K, deVries, L. F., Cheak, A. M., Stevens, R. H., & Bewley, W. L. (2002). Cognitive process validation of an online problem solving assessment. *Computers and Human Behavior, 18*, 669.

Cohen, I. R., Sudhalter, V., Landon-Jiminez, D., & Keogh, M. (1993). A neural network approach to the classification of autism. *Journal of Autism and Developmental Disorders, 23*, 443–466.

Elstein A. S. (1993). Beyond multiple-choice questions and essays: The need for a new way to assess clinical competence, *Academic Medicine.* 68:244–249.

Greeno, J. G., Collins A. M., & Resnick, L. B. (1996). Cognition and learning. In D. Berliner & R. Calfee (Eds.), Handbook of Educational Psychology (pp. 15–46). New York, NY: Simon & Schuster Macmillan.

Haider, H., & Frensch, P. A. (1996). The role of information reduction in skill acquisition. *Cognitive Psychology, 30*, 304-337

Hudson, J., Fivush, R., & Kuebli, J. (1992). Scripts and episodes: The development of event memory. *Applied Cognitive Psychology, 6*, 625–636.

Hurst, K., & Casillas, A. (1997). Exploring the dynamics of complex problem-solving with artificial neural network-based assessment systems. *CSE Technical Report No. 387.* Los Angeles: University of California, National Center for Research on Evaluation, Standards, and Student Testing (CRESST).

Johnson, M. A., & Lawson, A. E. (1998). What are the relative effects of reasoning ability and prior knowledge on biology achievement in expository and inquiry classes? *Journal of Research in Science Teaching, 35*(1), 89–103.

Johnson-Laird, P. N. (1983). *Mental models.* Cambridge, UK: Cambridge University Press.

Kanowith-Klein, S., Burch, C., & Stevens, R. (1998). Sleuthing for science. *Journal of Staff Development, 9*(3), 48–53.

Kohonen, T. (1990). The self-organizing map. *Proceedings of the Institute of Electrical and Electronics Engineers, 78*(9), 1464–1480.

Kohonen, T. (2001). *Self organizing maps.* (3rd ed.) Springer Series in Information Sciences, *30*, Heidelberg, Germany: Springer.

Kolodner, J. L. (1993*). Case-based reasoning.* San Francisco, CA: Morgan Kaufmann.

Kolodner, J. L. (1997). Educational implications of analogy: A view from case-based reasoning. *American Psychologist, 52,* 57–66.

Koprowski, G. J. (2003). Neural-network technology moves into the mainstream. Available at TechNewsWorld, http://www.technewsworld.com/perl/story/31280.html.

Krijik, J., & Haney, R., (1987). Proportional reasoning and achievement in high school chemistry. *School Science and Mathematics, 70,* 813–820.

Lane, L., Slavin, S., & Zie, A. (2001). Simulation in medical education: A review. *Simulation and Gaming, 32*(3), 297–314.

Lawson, A. E. (1995). *Science teaching and the development of thinking.* Belmont, CA: Wadsworth Publishing Company.

Lawson, A. E. (2000). Classroom test of scientific reasoning [Multiple choice version]. Based on the development and validation of the classroom test of formal reasoning. *Journal of Research in Science Teaching, 15,* 11–24.

Mangiameli, P., Chen, S. K., & West, D. A comparison of SOM neural network and hierarchical clustering methods. *European Journal of Operational Research, 93*(2), 402–417.

McClelland, J. L., & Goddard, N. H. (1996). Considerations arising from a complementary learning systems perspective on hippocampus and neocortex. *Hippocampus, 6,* 654–665.

Mislevy, R. J., Almond, R. G., Yan, D., & Steinberg, L. S. (1999). Bayes nets in educational assessment: Where do the numbers come from? In K. B. Laskey & H. Prade (Eds.), Proceedings of the Fifteenth Conference on Uncertainty in Artificial Intelligence, (pp. 437–446). San Francisco: Morgan Kaufmann.

Mislevy, R. J., Steinberg, L. S., Breyer, F. J., Almond, R. G., & Johnson, L. (1999). A cognitive task analysis, with implications for designing a simulation-based assessment system. *Computers and Human Behavior, 15,* 335–374.

Mislevy, R. J., Steinberg, L. S., Almond, R. G., Breyer, F. J., and Johnson, L. (2001) Making Sense of Data From Complex Assessments. *CSE Technical Report 538.* Los Angeles: University of California, National Center for Research on Evaluation, Standards, and Student Testing (CRESST).

Murphy, K. (1998). Hidden Markov Model (HMM) toolbox for Matlab. Available at http://www.ai.met.edu/~murphyk/Software/HMM/hmm.html.

Novak, J. & Gowin, D. (1984). *Learning how to learn.* New York: Cambridge University Press.

Olson, A., & Loucks-Horsley, S. (Eds.). (2000). *Inquiry and the National Science Education Standards: A guide for teaching and learning.* Washington, DC: National Academy Press.

Pack, P. (2002). *Problem solving strategies and metacognitive skills on SAT mathematics items.* Unpublished thesis, University of California, Berkeley.

Palacio-Cayetano, J. (1997). Problem solving skills in high school biology: The effectiveness of the IMMEX™ problem solving assessment software. *Dissertation.* University of Southern California

Palacio-Cayetano, J., Allen, R. D., & Stevens, R. (1999) Computer-assisted evaluation—the next generation. *The American Biology Teacher, 61*(7), 514–522

Palacio-Cayetano, J., Kanowith-Klein, S., & Stevens, R. (1999). UCLA's outreach program of science education in the Los Angeles schools. *Academic Medicine, 7*(4), 348–351.

Pellegrino, J., Chudowsky, N., & Glaser, R. (2001). *Knowing what students know: The science and design of educational assessment.* Washington DC: National Academies Press.

Plunkett, K., & Sinha, C. (1992). Connectionism and developmental theory. *British Journal of Developmental Psychology, 10,* 209–254.

Principie, J., Euliano, N., & Lefebvre, W. C. (2000) *Neural adaptive systems.* NY: Wiley.

Rabiner, L. (1989). A tutorial on Hidden Markov Models and selected applications in speech recognition. *Proceedings of the Institute of Electrical and Electronics Engineers, 77,* 257–286.

Reder, L., Nhouyvanisvong, A., Schunn, C., Ayers, M., Angstadt, P., & Hiraki, K. (2000). A mechanistic account of the mirror effect for word frequency: A computational model of remember-know judgments in a continuous recognition paradigm. *Journal of Experimental Psychology: Learning, Memory, and Cognition, 26*(2), 294–320.

Reder, L., & Schunn, C. (1996). Metacognition does not imply awareness: Strategy choice is governed by implicit memory and learning. In L. M. Reder (Ed.), *Implicit Memory and Cognition,* (pp. 45–77). Mahwah, NJ: Lawrence Erlbaum Associates.

Renner, J. W., & Lawson, A. E. (1973). Promoting intellectual development through science teaching. *Physics Teacher, 11*(5), 273–276.

Resnick, M. (1994). *Turtles, termites and traffic jams: Explorations in massively parallel microworlds.* Cambridge, MA: MIT Press.

Rumelhart, D. E., Hinton, G. E., & Williams, R. J. (1986) Learning internal representations by error backpropagation. In D. E. Rumelhart, J. L. McClelland, and the PDP Research Group (Eds.), *Parallel distributed processing: Explorations in the microstructure of cognition. Volume 1* (pp. 318–362). Cambridge, MA: MIT Press.

Rumelhart, D. E., & McClelland, J. L. (1986). *Parallel distributed processing: Explorations in the Microstructure of Cognition. Volume 1: Foundations.* Cambridge, MA: MIT Press.

Schank, P., Kozma, R., Coleman, E., & Coppola, B. (2000). Promoting representational competence to facilitate understanding and epistemological thinking in chemistry. *REPP Project Second Year Report* (National Science Foundation# REC-9814653). Menlo Park, CA: SRI International.

Schunn, C. & Anderson, J. R. (2002). The generality/specificity of expertise in scientific reasoning. *Cognitive Science, 2,* 162–179

Schunn, C., Lovett, M. C., and Reder, L. (2001). Awareness and working memory in strategy adaptivity. *Memory & Cognition, 29*(2); 254–266.

Schunn, C., & Reder, L. (2001). Another source of individual differences: Strategy adaptivity to changing rates of success. *Journal of Experimental Psychology: General, 130,* 59–76.

Scott, G. (1997) Toward an understanding of middle school students' problem-solving strategies: Establishing a foundation for teacher inquiry. *Dissertation.* School of Education, University of California, Los Angeles.

Shayer, M., & Adey, P. (1993). Accelerating the development of formal thinking in middle and high school students. IV: Three years after a two-year intervention. *Journal of Research in Science Teaching, 30,* 351–366.

Soller, A., & Lesgold, A. M. (2003). A computational approach to analyzing online knowledge sharing interaction. Proceedings of the 11th International Conference on Artificial Intelligence in Education (AI-ED, 2003), Sydney, Australia.

Staver. J., & Halsted, D., (1985). The effects of reasoning, use of models, sex type, and their interactions on posttest achievement in chemical bonding after constant instruction. *Journal of Research in Science Teaching, 22,* 437–447.

Stevens, R. H. (1991). Search Path Mapping: A versatile approach for visualizing problem-solving behavior. *Academic Medicine, 66*(9), S72–S75.

Stevens, R. H., & Dexter, S. (2003 April). *Developing teachers decision making strategies for effective technology integration: Design frameworks.* Presentation at the 2003 American Educational Research Association Symposium, Chicago, Il.

Stevens, R. H., Ikeda, J., Casillas, A. M., Palacio-Cayetano, J., & Clyman, S. G. (1999). Artificial neural network-based performance assessments. *Computers in Human Behavior, 15*, 295–314.

Stevens, R. H., Johnson, D. F., & Soller, A. (2005) Probabilities and predictions: Modeling the development of scientific competence. Cell Biology Education. *The American Society for Cell Biology, 4*, 52–65.

Stevens, R. H., Kwak A. R., & McCoy J. M. (1992). Solving the problem of how medical students solve problems. *M.D. Computing, 8*(1), 13–20.

Stevens, R. H., Lopo, A., & Wang, P. (1996). Artificial neural networks can distinguish novice and expert strategies during complex problem-solving. *Journal of the American Medical Informatics Association, 3*(2), 131–138.

Stevens, R. H., & Najafi, K. (1993). Artificial neural networks as adjuncts for assessing medical students' problem-solving performances on computer-based simulations. *Computers and Biomedical Research, 26*(2), 172–187.

Stevens, R. H., & Palacio-Cayetano, J. (2003). Designing technology environments for accelerating strategic skill development. *Cell Biology Education, 2*, 162–179.

Stevens, R. H., & Soller, A. (2005). Machine learning models of problem space navigation: The influence of gender. *Computer Sciences and Information Systems.* ComSIS Consortium, *2*(2), 83–98.

Stevens, R. H., Soller, A., Cooper, M., & Sprang, M. (2004) Modeling the development of problem solving skills in chemistry with a web-based tutor. *Intelligent Tutoring Systems.* In J. C. Lester, R. M. Vicari, & F. Paraguaca (Eds). Heidelberg, Germany: Springer-Verlag. 7th International Conference Proceedings (pp. 580–591).

Stevens, R. H., Sprang, M., Simpson, E., Vendlinski, T., Palacio-Cayetano, J., & Pack, P. (2001, April). *Tracing the development, transfer and retention of problem–solving skills.* Presentation at the American Educational Research Association Symposium. Seattle, Washington.

Underdahl, J., Palacio-Cayetano, J., & Stevens, R. H., (2001). Practice makes perfect: Assessing and enhancing knowledge and problem-solving skills with IMMEX software. *Learning and Leading with Technology. 28*, 26-31.

Valafar, F. (2002). Pattern recognition techniques in microarray data analysis: A survey. *Annals of the New York Academy of Sciences* (980) 41–64.

VanLehn, K. (1996). Cognitive skill acquisition. *Annual Review of Psychology, 47*, 513–539.

Vendlinski, T., & Stevens, R. H. (2000). The Use of Artificial Neural Nets (ANN) to Help Evaluate Student Problem Solving Strategies. In B. Fishman & S. O'Connor-Divelbiss (Eds.), *Fourth International Conference of the Learning Sciences* (pp. 108-114). Mahwah, NJ: Lawrence Erlbaum Associates.

Vendlinski, T. & Stevens R. H. (2002). A Markov model analysis of problem-solving progress and transfer. *The Journal of Technology, Learning and Assessment, 1*(3), 1–20.

Von Secker, C. E., & Lissitz, R. W. (1999). Estimating the impact of instructional practices on student achievement in science. *Journal of Research in Science Teaching, 36*, 1110–1126.

9

Strategies for Evidence Identification Through Linguistic Assessment of Textual Responses

Paul Deane
Educational Testing Service

In different non-linguistic contexts, the same linguistic features were perceived in different ways. We think that a reader reading a nominal style in an intrinsically good paper sensed a match between an abstract, i.e., educated or mature, style and clear thinking; a competent reader reading nominal style in an intrinsically bad paper responded to the abstract style as an attempt to cover up with turgid language an absence of careful thought.—
Joseph Williams (1982, p. 423)

It is hardly possible to overstate the importance of textual material in assessment. Most assessments are presented in textual form, and commonly include tasks with a significant textual component, such as writing, verbal comprehension, or verbal reasoning. However, when assessments require textual responses from students—whether short sentence-length answers or full-length essays—manual scoring has been the norm, with all the issues that arise from human rather than automated scoring (cf. Bejar, chap. 3, this volume, for a discussion.) The alternative—automated scoring of free textual responses—has only recently become viable, despite the potential for computer-based scoring demonstrated almost 40 years ago in Page (1966a and b). Within the last several years, a number of automatic scoring methods have been developed with applications not only to essay scoring (cf. Shermis & Burstein, 2003), but also in a variety of other educational settings such as automatic tutoring (Graesser, Wiemer-Hastings, K., Wiemer-Hastings, P., Kreuz, & Tutoring Research Group, 1999). One of the characteristics of text that must be taken into account in any approach to text scoring is the close relationship among different aspects of an assessment model: properties of the prompt; properties of the student response; models of student knowledge and of the task the student is performing and the like. There are often very strong correspondences between particular aspects of the textual product scored and multiple features of an assessment model, so that

313

very similar techniques may often be applied to all three, and the task of disentangling which aspect of the model is being measured directly can become fairly complex.

This chapter presents an overview of the current state of the art in textual response scoring, focusing on surveying evidence identification techniques that support automated scoring (and due to the parallelism just noted, in some cases the same techniques are applicable to characterizations of the student and task model or the work product as well.) The chapter presents and classifies methods based on the type of analytic technique applied and explores the assumptions underlying their development and resulting implications for their use. One of the chief challenges in this area is that there is tension among three poles of analysis: construct representation (the extent to which the measured variables reflect linguistic and cognitive structure), nomothetic span (the relationship with external variables, such as the scores of human graders, cf. Embretson, 1983), and engineering feasibility (the extent to which it is necessary to use heuristics and proxies for the targeted construct in order to enable automatic scoring). The techniques and applications discussed in this chapter vary in how they address this tension, and the variety of ways in which they address it has important implications for how they can be appropriately deployed consistent with Evidence-Centered Design (ECD; Mislevy, Almond, Steinberg, & Lukas, chap. 2, this volume). Neither the techniques nor the procedures discussed in the following sections were designed with ECD in mind, mainly because scoring and related text manipulations are often viewed as independent processes, in isolation from issues of student and task modeling. Indeed, in current applications, automated scoring based on linguistic analyses are tuned to maximize agreement with human raters "operating in factory mode." More careful consideration of the entire evidentiary argument would bring into better focus the correspondence between the evidence sought and extracted from textual responses, and the inferences about the aspects of students' knowledge and skill they are meant to support.

In particular, we are concerned with methods which can be viewed as components to be incorporated in an evidence model for open-ended textual response—specifically, for the phase of *evidence identification*, in which the aspects of a given performance that provide evidence about the student model variables are identified and possibly summarized, though still at the level of the individual task[1]. It is important, however, to be aware not only of the strengths

---

[1] See chapter 2 on the distinction between *evidence identification*, which usually concerns scoring of individual task performances, and *evidence accumulation*, which usually concerns synthesizing information across multiple tasks in a measurement model.

of these methods, but also of their limitations. Human language is among the most complex products of human thought, embodying multiple levels of structure and presupposing a variety of skills and capacities, so that it is critical to be aware of the strengths and weaknesses of particular techniques and to understand in each case which aspects of the human capacity for language are most directly measured.

The importance of taking evidentiary considerations into account is underscored by the complexity of text as a product of human cognition. Consider in particular the sheer size of the problem space for text analysis. A large corpus of English texts typically contains hundreds of thousands of distinct word types. Although only a few tens of thousands appear with any great frequency, the range of alternative word forms available to the writer at any point is at least on the order of thousands; and if a text is of any significant length, the potential number of distinct texts rapidly grows to astronomical size. There are limits on this variety, limits reflecting the constraints of English grammar, of semantic coherence, of rhetorical effectiveness and readability, and within those bounds there are variations reflecting a variety of specific skills and competencies: knowledge of vocabulary, mastery of grammar and discourse structure, argumentative and rhetorical skill, general background knowledge and knowledge of specific subject matters, and so forth. Given the complexities of the linguistic material, techniques for automatic scoring at the task level focus on particular aspects of the text; their effectiveness depends on the extent to which they select appropriate elements for analysis. On the one hand, for purposes of evidence identification it is important to determine whether the scoring algorithm is obtaining evidence of an appropriate linguistic construct; on the other hand, for purposes of evidence aggregation it is important to consider whether the nomothetic span is appropriate and supports valid inferences at the level of the student model.

For some purposes, a very limited view of textual content or responses may suffice, but there are risks associated with restricting the scope of analysis to a small set of relatively abstract features. Such risks are relatively minor if the purpose is to assess a relatively global and stable characteristic, such as the reading ability of students or its textual inverse, the reading difficulty of texts. But in other assessments, only a very close match between measured variables and the underlying cognitive structure will suffice. Consider, for instance, the task of scoring tests that require short verbal responses (in the range from one sentence to a short paragraph. A constructed response assessment of this nature has very strong face validity, as the questions require the test subject to directly verbalize subject matter knowledge. But on the other hand, nearly any slippage from a thorough linguistic analysis is likely to cause problems in an automatic scoring system, as was noted by Bejar (1988) in the context of scoring sentences. If synonyms are missed, correct answers will be scored as incorrect; if details of grammatical structure are ignored, incorrect answers may be scored as correct; and in general, the better the linguistic analysis, the less likely the scoring system is to be misled by the many-to-many mappings from form to content that are typical of natural language.

Automated scoring of textual response thus requires as its fundamental prerequisite a complex of techniques which address the full linguistic structure of texts (and thus the full verbal capacity of test subjects) to a greater or lesser extent, and with greater or lesser inferential complexity. Approaches to the scoring of textual responses to be discussed in this chapter involve three types of linguistic analyses [2]:

- *Linguistic feature-based methods.* In these approaches, specific linguistic features are extracted from target texts and regression analyses are performed to determine their correlation with variables that summarize performance in a task that is conceptually meaningful or that correlates with measures of student proficiency as gauged by a criterion such as human raters or performance on other tasks. In this class of methods, the focus is on both extracting features and summarizing them at the level of individual task performances. The features that are being extracted correspond to construct-level categories, that is, to categories of linguistic structure, such as particular grammatical constructions, particular classes of words, or other construct-level generalizations over language structure.

- *Vector space methods.* These include Latent Semantic Analysis. These approaches construct a vector model over large quantities of linguistic information and use cosine distance (or some other metric on the vector space) as the basis of an empirically derived predictive model. In this class of methods, the focus is on a mathematical summary of features, where features may be as simple as the vector of counts of words used. Such methods can be distinguished from feature-based methods in that they employ no direct representation of construct-level categories. Generalizations about construct structure emerge from the mathematical summary of the features and not from the features themselves.

- *Linguistic structure analysis.* In these approaches, natural language processing techniques are applied to build a (partial) model of the mental representations associated with task-relevant constructs, and these representations are used in turn to predict task-relevant constructs. The natural language processing techniques can vary from relatively simple information extraction techniques, where the focus is on

---

[2] These are general methods for analyzing text quite independent of automated scoring, but provide a useful framework for distinguishing the means by which different scoring techniques achieve results.

identifying recurrent patterns, to full sentence and discourse parsing with semantic interpretation. What distinguishes linguistic analysis of this sort from simpler methods is that the analysis extracts a structure, a set of elements and their relations, rather than simple quantifiable properties such as word counts or the frequency of construct categories.

Use of these methods is not mutually exclusive. Thus, of the current automatic essay scoring systems, Project Essay Grade (PEG, cf. Page, 1994; Page, 2003) primarily uses feature-based methods (with some use of linguistic methods to identify features); the Intelligent Essay Assessor (IEA, cf. Landauer, Laham, & Foltz, 2003; Foltz, Laham, & Landauer, 1999a) primarily uses Latent Semantic Analysis, and E-rater (Burstein, 2003; Burstein, Kukich, Wolff, Lu, Chodorow et al., 1998a) uses a combination of feature analysis, vector space methods, and linguistic analysis.

The methods described here are not solely applicable to scoring. They represent general methods for identifying linguistically significant aspects of textual data. The same techniques can often be deployed directly as part of a scoring method or less directly to characterize aspects of the work product, the student model, or the task model. It will be important to keep this in mind in the discussion that follows, because some of the methods to be discussed have been employed most typically outside an assessment context, and their application to assessment requires an intelligent assessment of the nature of the evidence that they provide for each aspect of an ECD model.

Given the strong interaction between the method used and the assessment purposes for which each method is most appropriate, the remainder of this chapter is organized in terms of the general methods used, with specific applications of each method being discussed in context, as explained in the following paragraphs.

Feature-based methods include simple lexical statistics, such as word frequency, number of words per sentence, and other word-based text statistics; features based on lists of words belonging to particular semantic or discourse-functional classes, along with features extracted by more sophisticated linguistic algorithms, such as counts of tagged grammatical categories, cues for specific grammatical structures, and so forth. In addition to the use of features in the PEG and E-rater essay scoring systems, similar features are employed in genre analysis (cf. Biber, 1998; Biber, Reppen, Clark, & Walter, 2001) and in certain natural language processing (NLP) methods for text categorization. Feature-based methods are most useful when there are strong task-model justifications for the correlation between identified feature and the construct to be measured. Where this justification is weak or lacking, there is the danger that performance on the assessment will be relatively easy to coach, leading to the potential for controversies such as have attended the introduction of automated essay scoring systems (cf. Page, 1996; Powers, Burstein, Chodorow, Fowles, & Kukich, 2001).

Vector space methods have a number of advantages for scoring system development. They require only a text corpus large enough to provide useful co-occurrence information (i.e., counts of how frequently one word or other linguistic element appears in the presence of another) and they do not require an independent regression on large numbers of features. Their key feature is providing relatively robust models of textual content, which makes them particularly useful for applications where determining identity of general subject matter is most important. Latent Semantic Analysis is the most popular vector space method (see Landauer & Dumais, 1997, for an overview). It has been applied to a variety of tasks where global similarity of content is critical: scoring essays (as just mentioned), measuring textual coherence (Foltz, Kintsch & Landauer 1998), assessing student summaries (Foltz, Gilliam, & Kendall, 2000; Wade-Stein & Kintsch, 2003), and guiding an automated tutoring system (Lemaire, 1999; Wiemer-Hastings, P., Wiemer-Hastings, K., & Graesser, A. C., 1999a and b). In general, LSA and similar techniques are most useful when assessments must be made about the similarity of content of entire documents; because vector space methods do not take word order or document structure into account, they should be used with caution where the global content of documents is not the primary target of inference for task level scoring.

Feature-based methods and LSA have in common the fact that they largely discard the local linguistic structure of the text. This fact places important limitations on the sorts of inferences that can validly be derived from such techniques: they are, as a rule, most effectively used for evidence identification with respect to whole documents, or to form summary measures over other textual constructs, and are least useful where the precise phrasing and logical structure of a text is critical. There are a variety of techniques deriving from natural language processing that capture a larger portion of this local linguistic structure and thus support more fine-grained textual analysis. These range in complexity from methods that look only at local word sequences (typically word bigrams and trigrams, i.e., two- and three-word sequences) and information extraction techniques to methods that recapitulate a large portion of a full linguistic analysis. Such techniques can be used either to augment identification of linguistic features, such as by identifying vocabulary that supports a particular type of linguistic argumentation, or to support linguistic or structural analysis, such as identifying statements that match elements within an instructor rubric, or to identify constructs indirectly, as in vector space methods.

It is therefore worthwhile to outline the elements that must enter into a full, automated linguistic analysis of textual data, as these provide an additional dimension along which one may classify systems which use NLP techniques. Beginning at the level of individual words, and moving up to entire documents, analysis may focus on a variety of tasks.

At the word level, these include:

- *phonetic* and *phonemic* analysis—recognizing the sound structure of words and identifying words from acoustic signals;

- *tokenization* and *segmentation*—identifying individual word tokens and determining sentence and paragraph boundaries; this is not, in fact, a trivial problem as hyphenated words and abbreviations pose significant issues concerning the correct delimitation of boundaries in text;

- *lemmatization*—identifying the stem or root forms of individual words, such as *dog* for the plural *dogs*, or *sing* for the past tense *sang*;

- *finite-state analysis*—determining properties of words at a low level, where the focus is on the probability of token or lemma sequences without regard to linguistic structure, typically by considering statistical properties of word bigrams and trigrams. This is closely related to the next item,

- *term extraction*—identifying fixed phrases and collocations that should be treated as units for purpose of later processing; for instance, recognizing fixed phrases such as *social security* or typical phrase patterns such as might be found in the names of companies;

- *lexical semantic analysis*—identifying the relationship between the words that appear in the sentence and other words that could have been used in their place, including synonyms and antonyms.

At the next level, syntactic analysis, these tasks include:

- *phrasal chunking*—identifying the key phrases (noun phrases, prepositional phrases, verb phrases, etc.) that can rapidly be identified in a text;

- *clausal chunking*—identifying grammatical relationships such as subject and direct object within clauses that can be rapidly identified in a text;

- *parsing*—preparing a full analysis of the grammatical relationships within a sentence or other natural language expression, possibly including multiple alternative parses where appropriate.

At the third level, clause-level semantic analysis, these tasks include:

- *semantic role analysis*—identifying the semantic relationships that hold between a verb (or other linguistic predicate) and its arguments; role analysis is essential to understanding paraphrase because (for instance) a paraphrase may use different grammatical relationships to convey the same semantic relations; thus the person who dies is the subject of die but the direct object of kill;

- *word sense disambiguation*—identifying the intended meaning of a term where more than one meaning is possible.

At the fourth level, discourse analysis, these tasks include:

- *anaphora resolution*—identifying the intended antecedents of pronouns;

- *reference tracking*—more generally, identifying intended referents of noun phrases; this includes topic chain analysis, identifying chains of noun phrases referring to the same entity;

- *discourse chunking*—identifying sequences within a text or discourse that have a single rhetorical function, such as giving an example or providing a topic sentence; subtasks can include summarization, determining the coherence of a discourse sequence, and similar tasks;

- *discourse parsing*—building up a full representation of the discourse structure of a text; this may include a pragmatic analysis in which speech acts and other social communicative transactions are identified.

Where these tasks can be completed successfully, the result is a rich representation that captures a large amount of information not available in simple word-based methods. Such techniques appear to be particularly useful when analyzing short-answer questions and other texts not long enough for word-based statistical analysis to yield useful information.

The past few years have seen the emergence of commercial short-answer scoring systems performing at least partial automated linguistic analyses; these include the C-Rater scoring system developed by the Educational Testing Service (cf. Leacock & Chodorow, 2004) and the AutoMark system developed by Intelligent Assessment Technologies (cf. Mitchell, Russell, Broomhead, & Aldridge, 2002); both of these systems make use of a variety of NLP techniques to determine whether student answers match an instructor rubric. In addition to the fairly general architecture required for short-answer scoring, various of these techniques have been deployed for specific assessment purposes, such as identifying grammatical errors (Chodorow & Leacock, 2000).

It is therefore worthwhile to consider the full matrix of possibilities, particularly because the discussion will examine both *techniques* for analysis of textual response and actual *applications* which score textual responses. The same application may use multiple techniques, and the techniques can be classified both with respect to the level of linguistic analysis and to the analytic method deployed, which yields a fairly complex picture. The most important of these relationships are expressed in Table 9.1 for the applications to be discussed in the remainder of the chapter; the rows of the table correspond to the just listed hierarchy from word level to discourse analysis. Note that the full application of such linguistic techniques yields a characterization of a text not primarily as a vehicle for assessment, but as a linguistic product. Determining which aspects of the linguistic product matter most for a particular assessment purpose is essential from an ECD perspective.

TABLE 9.1.
Alignment of Analytical Method, Linguistic Level, and Application in
Modern Automatic Scoring Technologies

	Linguistic Feature Analysis	Vector Space Analysis	Linguistic Structure Analysis
Word-Level (Lexical Constructs)	Lexile Framework Project Essay Grade E-rater	LSA (Intelligent Essay Assessor, Summary Street, Autotutor, Select-A-Kibitzer) E-rater Larkey & Croft BETSY	C-rater Automark
Syntactic Analysis	Biber E-rater Project Essay Grade (modern version)	Biber	C-rater Automark
Clause-Level Semantic Analysis			C-rater Automark
Discourse Analysis	E-rater		

Summary of Applications
    Reading Level Analysis:
      Lexile Framework
    Automatic Essay Scoring:
      Project Essay Grade, E-rater, Intelligent Essay Assessor, Larkey & Croft, BETSY
    Short Answer Scoring:
      C-rater, Automark
    Genre Analysis:
      Biber
    Tutoring & Instructional Feedback:
      Summary Street, Select-A-Kibitzer, Autotutor

Given the complex relationship between the linguistic level of evidence used, the kind of student model being developed, and the analytic method deployed, it is impossible to discuss some applications (e.g., E-rater) under a single heading. The discussion that follows will be organized primarily in terms of the primary method of evidence identification (linguistic features, vector space analysis, linguistic structures) with specific applications being considered in due sequence under these larger headings.

FEATURE-BASED METHODS

One of the chief advantages of feature-based methods in text analysis is that they are generally well understood and computationally straightforward. Because they are designed to provide direct measurements of the appearance of construct categories in the text, their interpretation is relatively straightforward both in the development of evidence identification tools and in process of evidence accumulation. Indeed many of the methods for evidence accumulation highlighted elsewhere in this book, such as Bayesian networks, have been applied to texts characterized in terms of linguistic features (cf. Rudner & Liang, 2002).

In evidence identification based upon the extraction of linguistic features, there are fundamentally two issues that must be addressed from the point of view of evidence-centered design: first, the tightness of the inferential relationship between the features as measured by the scoring algorithm and the construct they are intended to measure, and second, strength of association between the identified features and the elements of the task and student model to which they are linked, and thus the feature's value in an evidence model. That is, if features are to be extracted and summarized at the level of task performances, they should be both conceptually and empirically relevant as evidence about the student proficiencies that are the target of the assessment. Both of these implicate the nature of the feature being extracted, as relatively surface features may have a weaker connection both conceptually and statistically to the underlying cognitive structures and processes. Thus the discussion that follows will start with relatively surface word-based features, moving step-by-step to more complex linguistic features and their use in automatic assessment. In particular, the sections that follow examine three examples of linguistic feature-based analysis: the use of features to assess reading levels, to perform genre classification, and to score essays.

Application I: Assessment of Text Readability

One of the oldest foci for text assessment lies in the area of readability (cf. Bashaw & Rentz, 1977; Bormuth, 1966; Davidson & Green, 1988; Davidson & Kantor, 1982; Klare, 1963; Zakuluk & Samuels, 1988). With some significant caveats, the reading difficulty of text can be measured by a few very simple variables; in the case of the Lexile framework (Stenner, 1996; Stenner & Wright, 2002) for instance, the readability of a text is measured as a function of average word frequency and average sentence length. Moving from a characterizations of the reading level of a text (the work product) to a characterization of a student model for verbal sophistication (judged by the reading level of the text they produce) or to a task model specifying what students must do to demonstrate mastery of the relevant linguistic constructs, is quite another matter. It goes without saying that neither average word frequency nor average sentence length provides direct access to reading comprehension: both are proxies, chosen because they can be easily measured, yet are strongly correlated with demand for important underlying abilities. Such proxies can be attractive due to the ease of implementation, but at the risk of threatening the construct representation embodied in scoring. The use of such proxies relies on their correlation with the true construct variable of interest. As a result, variation, and therefore uncertainty, is introduced in the construct representation of the scoring when proxies are used to measure related constructs of convenience rather than the primary construct of interest. When the outcomes of scoring are evaluated with respect to external variables, such as a student grade level, additional variation, and associated uncertainty, are introduced with respect to the nomothetic span of the scoring. In other words, attention must be directed at both the degree to which the variables computed and used for scoring represent the construct of interest rather than a construct of convenience *and* the degree to which resultant scores are true representations of the nomothetic span criteria. Mismatches in either area can undermine the utility of a particular approach for some uses.

In the case of the Lexile reading level framework, the proxies deployed to measure the "grade level" construct are justified by two hypotheses: (a) that the average corpus frequency of words is strongly correlated with the probability that a reader will have learned them, and thus with their ease of comprehension, and (b) that the average length of sentences is strongly correlated with the probability that the author has chosen to use complex syntactic structures highly correlated with sophisticated discourse strategies. But despite the correlations that can be obtained (Stenner, 1996, reported that they explain 85% of the variance in reading difficulty in Peabody Individual Achievement Test reading comprehension items, though see the following discussion), the indirect nature of the correlation raises serious issues of face validity, and the risk of misclassifying deviant texts where the usual correspondence does not hold; if similar variables are then interpreted as evidence about a student or task model, introducing an additional layer of analysis, the uncertainties grow quickly under an ECD perspective.

These evidentiary issues make the Lexile framework for the assessment of reading difficulty/reading comprehension an excellent example of both the power and very real limitations of a simple linguistic-feature-based approach. As described in Stenner (1996), Stenner and Burdick (1997), and Stenner and Wright (2002), the Lexile reading difficulty scores for a document entirely derive from two features, one based on word frequency, the other on sentence length. The argument for these two variables is fairly straightforward (Stenner & Wright, 2002):

> *The semantic axiom*: the more familiar the words, the easier the passage is to read; the more unfamiliar the words, the harder.

> *The syntactic axiom*: the shorter the sentences, the easier the passage is to read; the longer the sentences, the harder. (p. 11)

Neither of these "axioms" is truly an axiom when subjected to linguistic analysis. Familiarity—if reduced to simple frequency—is clearly not sufficient by itself to account for ease of use; other linguistic processes can affect ease of use rather seriously, such as morphology. The plural of a rare word may be vanishingly rare, yet it is not likely to be much harder to understand than the singular; similarly, a transparently derived word such as *antigovernmental* may be unattested yet instantly comprehensible. Nor is sentence length necessarily tied to comprehension difficulty. There are circumstances where breaking up a long sentence decreases readability by eliminating the cues that support readers' constructing coherent understandings of texts as wholes. Yet despite these issues there is a strong statistical value for word frequency (as measured by a large corpus) and for in-text sentence length when it comes to predicting readability. Stenner (1996) obtained the following formula by regression, which he then transformed into a scale of reading levels (Stenner, 1996):

$$(9.8227*LMSL) - (2.14634*MLWF) - \text{constant} = \text{Theoretical Logit}$$

$$\text{where: LMSL} = \text{Log of the Mean Sentence Length}$$

$$\text{MLWF} = \text{Mean of the Log Word Frequencies. (p. 12)}$$

A strong correlation is claimed between the Lexile reading levels so calculated and a whole series of measures of reading difficulty, including reading comprehension tests (Stenner, 1996, p.16), and basal readers (Stenner, 1996, p.17), with correlation values generally above 0.9. For instance, Stenner & Burdick (1997) present correlations for a series of reading comprehension tests, including NAEP and the Peabody Individual Achievement Test, in which they report quite high correlations (generally about 0.75 for the raw correlations and above 0.9 for most of the tests after theory based calibrations), between the Lexile framework and each of these tests.

In principle, a case such as this is fairly close to the ideal situation for a simple feature-based approach: there is a direct and easily explained connection between the measured variables (i.e., word frequency and sentence length) and the underlying construct (i.e., vocabulary familiarity and structural complexity), and agreement with other measures of the same construct may be high. (Note, however, that the criterion measure, difficulty of test items based on the passage, is restricted to what might be called basic comprehension.)

However, considerable caution must be exercised in interpreting results from feature-based analyses of this type, and the Lexile framework is a case in point. In particular, the use of features, given their abstraction from the underlying data, requires careful examination of what the features are providing evidence *about*. In this case, the features arguably directly provide evidence about *passage* difficulty—about the reading difficulty of texts—and not the actual difficulty of items on a test such as those listed in the table above—and it is important not to lose track of this distinction. For instance, in the case of the NAEP reading test, IRT item difficulty estimates were available for 189 passage-based reading items. Although these item difficulty estimates would have provided a useful test of the validity of the Lexile difficulty predictions, information relevant to the outcome of the test is not provided. Instead, the table lists the correlation coefficient obtained after first averaging over all the individual item difficulty estimates that referred to a common passage, then correlating those passage difficulty estimates with the difficulty predictions obtained from the Lexile Equation. The resulting correlation is .65, indicating that the Lexile equation is successful at explaining about 42% of the observed variation in passage difficulty ($.65^2 = .42$). Since the difficulty of items is only partly determined by the difficulty of source passages, considerable caution would have to be exercised in extending the passage reading difficulty predictions to predictions of item difficulty on an assessment. There are also other analytic issues that raise questions about these correlations. The report notes that for some texts (e.g., the Peabody Individual Achievement Test or PIAT), empirical item difficulty was not available but it was known that item order was determined by difficulty, so empirical item difficulties were approximated by the rank order of the items in the test booklets, raising the question of whether some of the correlations are theory-to-theory correlations rather than theory-to-data correlations. Also in this study, a significant number of items were excluded from the final analysis, raising issues about the extent to which excluded items differed from retained items, and thus, the extent to which misfitting data might have been excluded before the correlations were calculated.

Even assuming very strong correlations between identified features and test scores, however, there is clearly room for significant slippage between the linguistic features that are directly measured and the assessed construct (e.g., reading comprehension), for the observable variables are only indirectly associated with relevant underlying competencies required to read at high comprehension levels (i.e., possession of linguistic knowledge and the ability to hold complex linguistic structures in working memory). Where there is a mismatch between them (for instance, where use of connectives may increase apparent sentence length yet decrease the load on working memory), there is the potential for an assessment based on such features to yield misleading results. Although such misleading results are more likely with weaker correlations, caution must be exercised even with very strong correlations, as the correlation may be mediated through a number of intermediate variables. (See, e.g., Smith, 1988, for a more detailed discussion of factors that affect sentence complexity, and White & Clement, 2001, for more detailed assessment of the Lexile framework.)

In many ways, the Lexile framework is an example of a linguistic feature system cut to the bare bones. In its development the framework appears to have been focused on choosing features with the strongest connection to the underlying construct and the best correlation with task performance, without developing elaborate methods of integrating evidence over multiple features. This is arguably driven by the readability construct itself: given a construct such as reading comprehension that places students along a simple unidimensional scale, the critical issue for the student model is finding variables that will correlate well with differing levels of performance. However, if such features were to be used in a scoring model, perhaps to score the verbal sophistication of a student's writing, the evidential inference from simple linguistic features to evidence for a score level would be far from watertight. And that is, in general, the critical issue with respect to relatively simple feature analyses of this type:

the evidential argument for the feature as operationalized is critical, not merely the strength of the correlation.

Application II: Genre Detection

Use of a few relatively simple features can work where the correlations are particularly strong, but many properties of text do not reveal themselves so readily. Or, to phrase the matter somewhat differently, the student model variables one wishes to measure may not correlate strongly with simple, surface features of the text they write, and thus drive the development of evidence by forcing the analyst to identify measurable linguistic features that correspond to rather more abstract constructs. Thus more sophisticated analysis may require (a) use of more features in combination with multivariate methods; (b) use of features more closely tied to abstract linguistic structures in the text, such as the presence or absence of particular grammatical structures. In combination, these methods can tease out less easily recognized text properties, and thus provide an evidentiary basis for inference beyond the text for scoring purposes.

The work of Douglas Biber and his associates on genre categories (Biber, 1995, 1998; Biber, Conrad & Reppen, 1998; Biber, Conrad, Reppen, Byrd, Helt et al. 2004) serves as an excellent example of how this technique can be applied to analyze important attributes of texts. Although Biber et al.'s (2004) work is not directly applied to scoring, the techniques have obvious applications, as is discussed next. Here, as with simpler feature-based methods, the key issue is whether there is a clear evidentiary case that the features being abstracted are, in fact, directly relevant to the intended construct. It is critical to note, however, that features extracted from an analysis designed, like Biber's, to identify major differences between types of tests would not directly transfer to developing a scoring algorithm for items drawn from a much narrower range of text types. That is, the design of such features is not independent of the purpose to which they will be put.

Biber et al. (2004) reported on a study designed to capture the properties of academic English, whether spoken or written. They collected a corpus, the TOEFL 2000 Spoken and Written Academic Language (T2K-SWAL) Corpus, which contained the types of documents indicated in Table 9.2 (Biber et al., 2004, p. 4).

TABLE 9.2.
Composition of the T2K-SWAL Corpus

Register	# of texts	# of words
Spoken:		
Class sessions	176	1,248,811
Classroom management[*]	(40)	39,255
Labs/In-class groups	17	88,234
Office hours	11	50,412
Study groups	25	141,140
Service encounters	22	97,664
Total speech:	251 (+40)	1,665,516
Written		
Textbooks	87	760,619
Course packs	27	107,173
Course management	21	52,410
Other campus writing	37	151,450
Total writing:	172	1,071,652
TOTAL CORPUS:	423	2,737,168

Note. [*]Classroom management texts are extracted from the "class session" tapes, so they are not included in the total tape counts.

Biber et al. sought to extract a wide range of features that capture both syntactic and semantic text attributes; to support this effort, the corpus is tagged for grammatical part-of-speech categories, enhanced to support analysis of "the distribution of particular syntactic constructions in particular lexico-grammatical contexts" (Biber et al, 2004). Biber et al. extracted 159 features covering the following major headings:

1. Pronouns and pro-verbs

2. Reduced forms and dispreferred structures

3. Prepositional phrases

4. Coordination

5. Wh-questions

6. Lexical specificity

7. Nouns

7a.   Semantic categories of nouns

7b.   Frequency features for nouns

8.   Verbs

8a.   Tense and aspect markers

8b.   Passives

8c.   Modals

8d.   Semantic categories of verbs

8e.   Frequency features for verbs

8f.   Phrasal verbs

9.   Adjectives

9a.   Semantic categories of adjectives

9b.   Frequency features of adjectives

10.   Adverbs and adverbials

10a.   Adverb classes

10b.   Semantic categories of stance adverbs

10c.   Frequency features of adverbs

11.   Adverbial subordination

12.   Nominal post-modifying clauses

13.   That complement clauses

13a.   That clauses controlled by a verb

13b.   That clauses controlled by an adjective

13c.   That clauses controlled by a noun

14.   WH-clauses

15.   To-clauses

15a.   To-clauses controlled by a verb

15b.   To-clauses controlled by an adjective

15c.   To-clauses controlled by a noun

16.   Lexical bundles (i.e., idioms)

In this first stage of analysis Biber is essentially inventorying the syntactic resources of English at a certain level of abstraction—one much deeper than the word-token level employed in the Lexile framework, but still quite limited in its scope and easily measurable by automatic techniques. The result of this initial phase of evidence identification is the inventory of linguistic features just listed. These features in effect provide a detailed syntactic and fairly general semantic profile; while there is not necessarily a strong correlation between any particular feature and particular genres or text types, there are systematic differences in the overall profiles that can be uncovered by multivariate analysis. Biber et al. (2004), in particular, constructed a "Multidimensional" analysis of the genres of text covered in this corpus, using factor analysis to identify dimensions of text variation, and identified the following:

1. Involved vs. Informational Production

2. Narrative vs. Non-narrative Concerns

3. Situation-Dependent vs. Elaborated Reference

4. Overt Expression of Persuasion

5. Non-Impersonal vs. Impersonal Style

The poles of each of these dimensions correlate with specific features, as follows:

- *Involved Production*: Correlated with private verbs, that deletion, contractions, present-tense verbs, second person pronouns, DO as a pro-verb, analytic negation, demonstrative pronouns, general emphatics, first person pronouns, pronoun IT, BE as main verb, causative subordination, discourse particles, indefinite pronouns, general hedges, amplifiers, sentence relatives, WH-questions, possibility modals, non-phrasal coordination, WH-clauses, final prepositions.

- *Informational Production*: Correlated with above-average use of nouns, longer word length, above-average use of prepositions, a higher type-token ratio, and above-average use of attributive adjectives.

- *Narrative Discourse*: Correlated with past-tense verbs, third-person pronouns, perfect aspect verbs, public verbs, synthetic negation, present-participial clauses.

- *Situation-Dependent Reference*: Correlated with time and place adverbials and frequent use of adverbs.

- *Elaborated Reference*: Correlated with WH-relative clauses on object positions, pied piping constructions, WH-relative clauses on subject positions, phrasal coordination, and nominalizations.

- *Overt Expression of Persuasion or Argumentation*: Correlated with infinitives, prediction modals, suasive verbs, conditional subordination, necessity modals, split auxiliaries.

- *Impersonal Style:* Correlated with conjuncts, agentless passives, past participial adverbial clauses, by-passives, past-participial postnominal clauses, and adverbial subordinators.

Using these feature clusters, Biber et al. then examined where each spoken and text register or genre fits along each dimension, with the following results:

- Spoken university registers are strongly involved and situation-dependent; written university registers are strongly informational, impersonal and tend to use elaborated reference.

- All university registers avoid narrativity.

- Classroom management, office hours, and course management registers tend to be overtly persuasive; course packs and textbooks are not.

Although Biber et al.'s study is focused on characterizing particular genres or registers in terms of linguistic variables, the potential application to assessment is clear: given an analysis that identifies major factors in variation among documents, any given document can be assessed for its position on the dimensions identified, which can serve as the evidentiary basis for an assessment. To the extent that dimensions can validly be linked to appropriate constructs, certain of these linguistic features can provide the evidence for effective methods of automated scoring. The critical issue is the extent to which the features can be identified without manual intervention, as certain of these features require extensive checking and correction of tagger output. Although the precise set of features Biber used could not, therefore, be directly applied to automated assessment, the general style of analysis could readily be adapted.

In this example, the conjecture to be addressed with regard to automated scoring of students' work would be that successful productions in a given genre are distinguished from unsuccessful productions in terms of their status on the relevant dimensions. However, the best ECD design for such a study would examine a range of documents correlating with the actual construct to be measured—perhaps a series of documents of varying quality within the same genre—and would construct a multivariate analysis designed to predict differences in score level. Although heavy loading on the properties characteristic of a genre might correlate well with score levels, they might prove irrelevant to the task of differentiating documents within the same genre class, in which case, an analysis which correlated linguistic features with score levels would isolate an entirely different set of factors.

Another way to make the point is this: Biber's use of multivariate analysis could be interpreted in two quite different ways if it were applied to scoring. If Biber's features are used solely to classify texts along the dimensions identified in the study—that is, if the intention is simply to score student productions stylistically—then the second, multivariate step is essentially an evidence accumulation phase, with the identification of linguistic features constituting evidence identification. This would correspond to the use of automated scoring in the analysis of texts, rather than in the assessment of students. However, if the position of a document on Biber's dimensions is itself to be used as a construct, and the student model will be informed by the classification of a student's several productions' classifications on these dimensions, then the multivariate analysis becomes part of the evidence identification phase, and is in fact quite parallel from an ECD perspective to the use of Latent Semantic Analysis as a vector space technique to measure similarity among documents for the purpose of assessing students, as discussed later.

It remains important to consider the evidentiary basis for the features. It is no accident that the dimensions in Biber et al. are almost entirely concerned with what a writing handbook would call *style*. Most of the dimensions Biber et al. isolate have to do with choices about the use of specific syntactic constructions: passives versus actives, pronouns versus definite descriptions, and so forth. Where writers and speakers have a choice of syntactic pattern to express the same conceptual content, the choices are driven by essentially rhetorical and pragmatic considerations, so that analysis and/or scoring in terms of (mostly syntactic) linguistic features is most appropriate where the assessment is concerned with stylistic and grammatical choices rather than content. That is, automated task-level scoring of students' texts via the features and then dimensions in Biber's analysis is more likely to produce useful evidence for inferences about students' use of stylistic and pragmatic knowledge than about their knowledge of the substance of the text. At the same time, because Biber's analysis is based on linguistic features (the presence or absence of certain grammatical categories), the features identified in such an analysis would not be well suited for drawing inferences about such things as the nature of argumentation in a text, which would depend on the identification of relations among topics and arguments, and would not depend only on detecting that certain categories are used more frequently than others In other words, one would be driven to using evidence of the sort that Biber's methods identify just in case the student model implicated constructs best identified in terms of the stylistic properties of documents.

Application III: Essay Scoring

Project Essay Grade, or PEG, is the oldest automated scoring system for text, developing from Ellis Page's pioneering work in the 1960s (Page, 1966a, b, 1967; Page, Fisher, & Fisher, 1968; Page & Paulus, 1968). PEG represents a pure linguistic feature approach to essay scoring, and in its early versions the features were entirely based on word tokens. Quite strikingly, despite this limitation, even the earliest versions of PEG returned excellent correlations with human graders. More recent versions of PEG have employed parsers and other natural language processing tools to enhance performance by extracting more abstract syntactic or stylistic features.

Page's approach focused from the beginning on the distinction between the intrinsic variables one wished so measure (or *trins*), such as fluency, spelling accuracy, level of diction, syntactic complexity, and so forth, and the approximations to such variables (or *proxes*) that could be measured by computer. The proxes employed in Page's work in the 1960s had to be fairly simple, reflecting the limitations of computer technology at the time. They included such measurements as:

- length of the essay in words

- average sentence length

- counts of commas, periods, and other punctuation marks

- counts of prepositions, subordinating conjunctions, and other grammatical formative types

- number of spelling errors

- number of common words

- average word length

Even using features as simple and approximate as these, Page was able to achieve correlations with human graders comparable to the agreement among graders (though early results ranging from correlations of 0.5 to 0.7 are far lower than the current state of the art.)

In later work Page (1994, 1995) made use of emerging technologies to recognize more linguistically sophisticated features, mining spell-checkers, taggers, and parsers to extract useful information about document features, and reported continued improvements in computer scoring. Applied to a large set of NAEP (National Assessment of Educational Progress) writing samples, PEG obtained 0.87 agreement with human scorers; in a blind test conducted by the

Educational Testing Service, PEG predicted scores better than did three human judges (Page, 1995).

Despite the strong correlations PEG returned, there has been significant resistance to scoring essays using linguistic features alone. A number of issues should be noted, though since the features used in PEG have been varied continuously through different incarnations of the system, the criticisms will apply more to some versions of PEG than to others:

1. *Face validity*. The single most important variable in PEG regression analyses is essay length (in much of the reported work, Page uses the fourth root of length, as what is typically important is that essays achieve a minimum length.) Although essay length and other obviously-surface variables can be interpreted as proxies for valid essay-production abilities, the lack of a direct connection between quality and the measured variable raises serious issues, some of which are discussed below.

2. *Coachability*. To the extent that the features can be reduced to easily recognized, surface properties of text, they are potentially coachable. In particular, what PEG values can almost completely be reduced to stylistic features: if students write longer essays, preferring long words in longer sentences with a variety of punctuation marks and remembering to throw in certain grammatical function words, then PEG will value their essays more highly than if they express the same content more concisely in relatively simple language. It is possible, of course, that this tendency rather accurately reflects biases of human graders, as the classic student recipe for creating a bad faith essay prescribes exactly this course of action: expressing as little content as possible while throwing in as many long words relevant to the topic as one can in as elaborate a style as one can manage. This is of course the classic example of the criterion problem: to what standard should automated scoring be held for validation? To hold it to human scores is to explicitly include all the problems of human scoring as an implicit goal of automated scoring, yet to rest entirely on the construct representation suggests the lack of substantial empirical evidence of the appropriateness of the scores until some track record of usage can be established. However, from an ECD perspective, the critical point to note is that PEG is vulnerable to this criticism because the evidence being used to support inferences about writing quality (essentially, linguistic features that measure stylistic properties of text) is at best a partial measure for one aspect of the construct we actually wish to measure (quality of student writing, which involves measurements of quality and appropriateness of content, among other things, and not sophistication of style divorced from any actual content.)

3. *Content versus Style*. The preceding points indicate one of the most critical issues. PEG is arguably quite general in its applicability, precisely because the variables it uses can be measured on any text, regardless of content. But that general applicability means that (barring introduction of features measuring domain-specific content), PEG grades essays on style. To the extent that an appropriate score depends on content coverage, linguistic feature analysis must be supplemented by content analysis, which implicates rather different techniques.

4. *The Discounting of Structure.* One of the problems with linguistic features, at least of the sort that have generally been deployed thus far, is that by their very nature they discount structure in favor of global frequencies. Using a long word is all well and good, but unless the word is used appropriately in its sentence context, one risks awarding points for malapropism. Preferring sentences joined with grammatical connectives is excellent, but if the connectives suggest the wrong logical relationship, one may be rewarding students for incoherence. An approach that extracts feature counts, discarding structural information, must by its very nature take such risks.

None of these considerations invalidates the use of linguistic features for scoring, but they clearly indicate the strengths and weaknesses of feature-based approaches. If what is being scored is closely related to stylistic issues, it can be measured effectively with linguistic features alone; if, on the other hand, content is implicated, or if there is a significant evidential distance between measurable feature and underlying construct, then the use of linguistic features may not be indicated for scoring.

VECTOR SPACE METHODS

A second family of methods for text analysis derives from work in text classification and information retrieval: this is the *vector space* approach to text analysis. In a vector space model, the fundamental datum is co-occurrence: two words (or other measurable features) occur in the same document, the same paragraph, the same sentence, or within a window of 1, 2, 3, or n words. This co-occurrence may be treated as a binary presence or absence, or weighted by frequency or some other measure of importance; it may be used directly, or subjected to further processing. But ultimately, all information derives from patterns of co-occurrence within text. Unlike linguistic feature-based systems, where particular linguistic categories are abstracted and given special status, vector space systems can draw their data from every word in the document, and are thus particularly well suited to classification and assessment tasks where content rather than style is the primary consideration. As elsewhere in this chapter, the technique we are considering is not specific to scoring; it is a general method for analyzing text, and can be used as a scoring methodology as long as there is a clear evidentiary relationship between the method and the construct to be measured.

From an ECD perspective, it is important to note that vector space methods are not fundamentally construct-centered. In linguistic feature approaches, considerable effort is expended to guarantee that individual features are *transparent*—that they correspond reasonably directly to elements of the student model that one wishes to measure. Vector space approaches, by contrast, accept much weaker evidence in much larger quantities, and rely on mathematical techniques which extract correlations from the mass of evidence thus assembled. In other words, the primary evidence is evidence of proximity of usage, without any direct mapping from individual sources of evidence to particular constructs.

In essence, vector space models are equivalent to the *bag-of-words* model commonly used in text classification (cf. Lewis, 1992), where each document is represented by a set of binary attributes corresponding to the presence or absence of particular words. Classifiers can then be trained to recognize probable instances of a category by the extent to which they match combinations of attributes characteristic of the training set.

Slightly more information can be brought in using so-called *content vector* approaches based on information retrieval techniques (cf. Salton, Wong, & Yang, 1975), where documents are represented by a vector representing (some function of) the relative frequency of component terms. In this case, documents can be classified by their cosine similarity to the vectors associated with documents in the training set, as it has been found that the cosine of the angle between two vectors is a relatively robust and accurate measurement of agreement in these vector space analyses.

Perhaps the most sophisticated of the context-space methods is Latent Semantic Analysis (LSA), which uses information from a corpus to produce a vector representation that captures far more of the underlying semantics of a text than a mere word count can express. The particular technique employed (Singular Value Decomposition) can be very effective at capturing similarities between words that appear in the training set and words that do not, yielding a more robust classification technique. See Landauer, Laham, and Foltz (1998), Landauer, Foltz, and Laham (1998), and Landauer and Dumais, (1997) for general overviews of the subject.

All of these techniques share certain common liabilities: unless *stemming*—reduction of related words to a common form—is performed, they treat word-forms as unanalyzed units, ignoring important connections among morphologically related forms; they completely ignore word order and syntax and (unless otherwise augmented) topical subdivisions within the text. In short, they rely entirely on information about word-choices; information about the order and relationships among the words—that is, linguistic analysis of any sort—is excluded. Landauer (2002) argued that there are strong *a priori* reasons to believe that the choice of words is a much more significant factor than word order, essentially because the amount of information conveyed by word choice is in principle much larger than the amount of information that can be conveyed by word order alone.

This argument appears to have some merit, particularly given the performance of context-space systems, which often perform well above correlations of 0.8 in comparison to human judgments. However, the lack of linguistic analysis entails clear limits on what one can reasonably expect of a vector space approach to textual scoring: in short-answer scoring, for example, one would not wish to count a sentence like "Einstein's career promoted the theory of relativity" as equivalent to a sentence like "The theory of relativity promoted Einstein's career." In short, the failure to consider linguistic structure is an exclusion of information, and does limit the types of analysis that can be effectively performed using content vector techniques alone.

From an ECD perspective, the most important attribute of vector space methods is that they depend for their efficacy on combining many sources of evidence to get as strong a set of correlations as possible, limited only by their failure to take structural and positional information into account. This makes them particularly effective when the constructs being measured can be treated as attributes of entire texts, as in essay scoring. They are least effective for shorter texts (clause-length or less) and for measuring constructs where the exact order and arrangement of textual material is critical (such as measuring the quality of argumentation) or for providing diagnostic information on performance.

The sections that follow discuss several applications of vector space methods, including three essay scoring approaches (the Larkey system's use of standard text classification techniques, the E-rater system's use of content vector analysis, and the Intelligent Text Assessor's use of Latent Semantic Analysis), followed by a number of other applications of Latent Semantic Analysis, including assigning reading levels, assessing textual coherence, providing summary feedback, and enabling tutorial feedback in an automated system.

Application I: Essay Scoring Via the Larkey System

There are a number of systems that apply standard text classification techniques to the task of essay scoring, including the system discussed in Larkey (1998) and Larkey and Croft (2003), and the BETSY system discussed in Rudner and Liang (2002).

Larkey's system used a standard bag-of-words model in which stopwords were removed (a total of 418 common words), the remaining words were stemmed, and a subset of these were selected as features using an algorithm that ranked them by expected mutual information (EMIM, cf. van Rijsbergen, 1979).

Two types of classifiers were trained: Bayesian independence classifiers (cf. Lewis, Shapire, Callan, & Papka, 1996), and K-nearest-neighbors classifiers, using *tf-idf* [term frequency/inverse document frequency][3] weighting for the similarity metric (cf. Salton 1990). The Bayesian classifiers were binary classifiers, and several were trained to recognize the difference between various score points (e.g., essays were scored from 1–4, and the classifiers were trained to recognize 1 vs. 2, 3, 4; 1, 2 vs. 3, 4; 1, 2, 3 vs. 4). The K-nearest-neighbor method assigned each essay a score based on the average score of its K nearest neighbors in the training set, with the value of K set during training. The training set consisted of 5 sets of manually scored essays, two of which covered general subjects; the remaining three covered specific subjects (in the fields of social studies, physics, and law).

Larkey's experiments also calculated a number of general textual features essentially parallel to the kinds of features used in PEG and included these in a regression analysis. Larkey and Croft (2003) concluded that:

> It is striking that a certain fairly consistent level of performance was achieved using the Bayesian classifiers, and that adding text-complexity features and k-nearest-neighbor scores did not appear to produce much better performance. The additional variables improved performance on the training data, which is why they were included, but the improvement did not always hold on the independent test data. These different variables seem to measure the same underlying properties of the data, so beyond a certain minimal coverage, addition of new variables added only redundant information. (p. 63)

The performance of the system was in the same general range as other modern essay scoring systems, as the correlation with human scores ranged in the high .70s and .80s, and with exact accuracy (the percentage of essays assigned exactly the same grade as by the human scorers) ranging between 0.5 and 0.65.

Larkey's system is in its essentials a simple bag-of-words model. It uses for evidence little more than the presence or absence of certain keywords, and accumulates the evidence with Bayesian classifiers. Despite its simplicity, it performed well, but it is important to note its limitations. This approach depends on the availability of significant quantities of labeled data with which to train each Bayesian classifier, and the number of texts in the training set must be

---

[3] TF-IDF weighting is a method for assigning the greatest value to those words that are relatively infrequent in a document collection as a whole, but are relatively frequent in some subset of documents within the collection, as these words tend to be strongly correlated with the topical content on which such documents are focused.

large enough to avoid spurious associations in which words are chosen as classifiers because they happen to co-occur frequently with particular categories in the training set. In general, text categorization systems of this type must be trained on sets containing thousands of examples of each category, and where such data is lacking, other techniques are likely to be preferable.

A second text classification approach is reported in Rudner and Liang (2002), which used Bayesian networks for essay scoring[4]. Rudner and Liang's approach was essentially parallel to Larkey and Croft (2003), except that Larkey and Croft experimented with the use of features other than single words, that is, *key phrases* (two-word phrases with a high value using the *tf-idf* [term frequency-inverse document frequency] metric) and *arguments* (any bigram or two-word phrase that appeared in at least 2% of the calibrated essays). The use of arguments appeared to improve accuracy significantly over baseline levels; with optimal performance exceeding 80% accuracy.

Both Larkey and Rudner and Liang were able to achieve reasonable performance with relatively small training sets (as low as 40 documents per set in Rudner and Liang, between 200 and 600 per set in Larkey.) However, one must underscore the importance of the training set in these approaches. The training set defines what features will be used and how important they will be, and since all features are derived from the presence or absence of specific words in training set documents, there is no recovery from accidental gaps: if a word does not appear in the training set, it cannot affect scoring. This is one point where use of linguistic knowledge could improve results; one technique that has been used in the information retrieval literature (i.e., *thesaurus expansion*) is to introduce manually compiled information about close synonyms (cf. Qiu & Frei, 1993; Voorhees, 1993).

Statistically, the major issue with standard text classification techniques is that there is no established methodology for determining the training set size needed to guarantee accurate results, though in the text classification literature the usual approach is to use training sets containing thousands of documents per category. Viewed in this light, the size of the training set is potentially an issue, as it is not clear what number of sample essays will adequately sample the realm of possibilities for any given prompt, and the number of manually scored essays will often be in the hundreds or even thousands, and not the 10s or 20s.

---

[4] Note Rudner and Liang use Bayes nets for evidence identification, in contrast to the use of Bayes nets for evidence accumulation discussed in Williamson, Mislevy, Almond, and Levy (chap. 7, this volume).

Despite these limitations, text classification techniques of this type have the advantage that they are very easy to implement and require very little explicit linguistic or construct information to be supplied in advance. From an ECD perspective, the major drawback is that once a classifier has been trained using these techniques, it will be very difficult to interpret the classifier to explain in construct-centric terms why the method works, as its success depends upon exploitation of correlations over many weak sources of evidence.

Application II: E-Rater–Content Vectors as a Component in a Hybrid Essay-Scoring System

Content vector analysis is essentially parallel to the text classification methods discussed previously, differing primarily in the fact that it uses cosine distance (calculated over word frequencies) as a metric for identifying similar documents instead of the simpler tf-idf metric employed in standard text categorization methods. This technique is an important part of the E-rater scoring system discussed in Burstein (2003), Burstein et al. (1998a, 1998b, 1998c), and Powers et al. (2001). The E-rater system is reported to show agreement with human rater scores ranging from 87% to 94% on earlier versions, and 97% on a more recent version (Burstein, 2003, p. 114), which is significantly above the values reported by many other automatic essay scoring systems. This level of performance may be due to E-rater's hybrid, modular design and its relatively heavy use of natural language processing (NLP) techniques. It has been in use for operational scoring of the GMAT Analytical Writing Assessment since February 1999. The discussion that follows is specifically a discussion of the first version of E-rater, deployed in 1999. A more recent version has been developed, which operates on somewhat different principles, including significant use of a more highly elaborated discourse analysis module (cf. Burstein, Marcu, & Knight, 2003).

The E-rater scoring system has three main modules: one designed to capture information about *syntactic variety*, another that focuses on the *organization of ideas*, and a third that measures *vocabulary usage*. To support these modules a number of NLP modules are applied:

- a part of speech tagger (Ratnaparkhi, 1996) to assign part-of-speech labels to all words in an essay;

- a syntactic "chunker" (Abney, 1996) to identify phrases and assemble them into clauses, combined with COMLEX, a program that assembles chunks into clauses, providing a shallow parse;

- a discourse parser that identifies discourse markers that signal the boundaries of discourse units (or "arguments") and uses them to divide the essays into coherent discourse chunks.

The part-of-speech tagger and the chunker are primarily used to identify linguistic features, such as the presence of infinitive, complement, and subordinate clauses and thus to measure syntactic variety. The discourse parser is put to two uses: first, to extract linguistic features reflecting the extent to which appropriate discourse organization is signaled; second, to divide the essay into argument segments for use in the analysis of content and vocabulary usage. There are two separate content analyses:

- a global analysis, which provides a measure of how well the total vocabulary in each essay matches essays in the reference set;

- an analysis by argument segment, which determines how well each rhetorical chunk of the essay matches essays at one of the six score points to which essays can be assigned.

As discussed in Burstein et al. (1998a, 1998b, 1998c), the first of the two content vector components is a simple k-nearest-neighbors method using cosine similarity. Each training document is converted to a vector, where content words correspond to features whose weights derive from document word frequency. A similar vector is constructed for an essay to be graded, and the essay score suggested by the module is the mean of the scores associated with the six nearest neighbors in the training set. Then the second content vector component merges all essays associated with each score point into a single "super-vector". The six super-vectors are compared with the vector for each individual argument segment to produce a set of scores that indicate which essay score point typically contains a section with comparable content.

The contribution made by content, syntactic features, and discourse features is not permanently fixed; that is, it depends on the specific prompt. A regression is performed during training to assign appropriate feature weights for each essay prompt. Thus E-rater's performance can be fine-tuned to maximize accuracy by prompt.

A number of notes are in order about the E-rater system. First, note that the primary use of the NLP resources within E-rater is to enable the accurate identification of relatively abstract linguistic features. The structural relationships identified by the sentence-level linguistic analysis plays no independent role in the scoring. Second, note that the two content vector analyses clearly have an important role to play, since the primary difference among different prompts for the same test is likely to derive from differences in verbal content. The E-rater system is designed to extract a very wide range of features, many of which may be at least partially redundant, but by exploiting the redundancy, it is capable of maximizing performance.

However, some of the issues that arise with text categorization also arise here. How large a training set is needed for statistical reliability? How much information is lost by the non-use of word order in the content analysis? To what extent are the linguistic features extracted by E-rater subject to the critiques directed at feature-based systems like PEG? (See Powers et al., 2001, for a discussion of some of these issues.) Ultimately, E-rater can be viewed as a hybrid model, exploiting both vector space analysis and linguistic features, and thus many of the issues that arise with these models in isolation are worth considering with respect to E-rater. (It should be noted that the second version of E-rater, partially documented in Burstein (2003) and Burstein, Chodorow, and Leacock (2003), in fact addresses many of these concerns, with particular attention being paid to such issues as the size of the training set and need for discourse-level analysis to avoid some of the issues that arise with a pure feature-based system.)

Application III: Essay Scoring Via Latent Semantic Analysis

Latent Semantic Analysis (LSA) is the most powerful of the vector space methods, for two reasons: (1) unlike simpler text categorization methods it uses a corpus to acquire information about how words are related in general, information that makes it easier to generalize from training sets for specific prompts; (2) moreover, it uses a powerful mathematical technique, Singular Value Decomposition (SVD), to generalize the data that it extracts from the corpus. It has been applied in particular to the task of essay scoring, and a wide variety of other applications have also been developed, some of which are discussed next. The most important application in this context is essay scoring, though other applications, including the assessment of textual coherence, will be discussed in future sections.

An Overview of LSA as an Analytical Technique. Before examining the details of essay scoring with LSA, it is useful to review the essence of the method and some of the theoretical issues with which it is associated. Latent Semantic Analysis begins with a corpus of texts, preferably one that represents fairly evenly the major concepts and conceptual distinctions with which users will be concerned. To be useful, the corpus must be sufficiently large—in the millions of words; for instance, useful results have been obtained with encyclopedias running to about 10 or 11 million words of text.

The first step in an LSA analysis is the preparation of a word-by-document frequency matrix that indicates for each document the number of occurrences of every word that the document contains. Untransformed, such matrices have been used for a variety of purposes within information retrieval and natural language processing; for instance, HAL, a semantic retrieval system quite similar in application to LSA, but using a much larger corpus (cf. Burgess, Livesay, & Lund, in press; Lund & Burgess, 1996). In LSA, the log of word frequency is used.

The next step in an LSA analysis is the application of the linear algebra technique of singular value decomposition (SVD). SVD is formally defined as a mathematical operation in which a matrix A is decomposed into three component matrices in the following manner:

$$A = U D V^T,$$

where D is a diagonal matrix which identifies a set of dimensions, and two additional square matrices (U and V) characterize the original rows and columns in terms of the dimensions in the diagonal matrix. Conceptually, SVD can be viewed as a mathematical generalization of principal component analysis (a relative of factor analysis), with a diagonal matrix corresponding to the ideal factorization, such that each cell in the diagonal indicates how important that factor is in the overall composition of the original word-by-document data matrix.

The third step is the critical step. The less heavily weighted dimensions in the diagonal matrix are set to zero, reducing the total number of dimensions to some predetermined number. (In Landauer's work, that number is usually around 300, as he has found that that generally works well with natural language data.) When the three matrices are multiplied together again, the elimination of minor dimensions induces generalizations based on the properties of the major dimensions. For instance, it may be that *festive* never appears in combination with *wedding*; but if *joyous* does, and there is a strong association between *joyous* and *festive*, the final matrix will indicate the presence of an association between *festive* and *wedding*. (For an overview of the mathematics of LSA, see Golub and Loan (1996); an implementation of SVD is described in Berry (1992), and is available at http://www.netlib.org/svdpack/index.html.)

The following illustration may help to elucidate how LSA actually works. The core data for LSA is a matrix *A* containing the rows in which are the words that appear in a corpus, or collection of texts, and the columns are discrete documents within the corpus. The individual cells contain a weighted (log normalized) transform of the raw frequency with which words appear in each document. That is, the raw data *A* that goes into the determination of *A* takes the form in Table 9.3.

TABLE 9.3.
Raw Data Used in a Latent Semantic Analysis (*A*)

Word	Document #1	Document #2	Document #3	Document #4	Document ...
the	35	12	40	75	
house	5	23	1	7	
analyse	22	1	3	5	
Total number of words in document	546	600	250	180	

Application of weighting followed by singular value decomposition to this raw data results in an analysis in which each word and document is assigned a vector in a factor space of dimensionality *N*, where *N* is the number of factors maintained from the singular value decomposition. The two matrices *U* and *V* would take the forms shown as Tables 9.4 and 9.5. The product of these two matrices and the third (reduced) weight matrix D^* approximates the original matrix *A* on which the singular value decomposition was performed.

TABLE 9.4.
Latent Semantic Analysis Word/Factor Matrix (*U*)

Word	Factor #1	Factor #2	Factor #3	Factor #4	Factor N
the	.05	.22	.11	.0001	
house	.002	.003	.01	.10	
analyse	.05	−.09	.45	−.04	

TABLE 9.5.
Latent Semantic Analysis Document/Factor Matrix (V)[5]

Document	Factor #1	Factor #2	Factor #3	Factor #4	Factor N
#1	.50	.02	.15	.0006	
#2	.023	.34	.002	−.20	
#3	.01	.008	.15	−.001	

---

[5] The data in these tables is purely illustrative.

LSA then allows three operations: (1) a comparison of words to words, to see how similar two words are with respect to the factors identified by the singular value decomposition; (2) a comparison of documents to documents, to see how similar two documents are with respect to the same factors; (3) a comparison of words to documents, to see how strongly associated any given word is with any given document.

There are two important points to note about this form of analysis. First, and critically, no construct claims are made for the base data (the word/document frequency tabulations) or for the factors in and of themselves. In most applications of LSA it is only the similarity induced by the factor analysis that is treated as corresponding to independently specifiable constructs, such as intuitions about word meaning or similarity of document content. Second, the LSA analysis induces a considerable amount of generalization, since the extraction of factors induces inferences about how probable words will be in all contexts, not merely those contexts observed in the original matrix.

The Construct Status of LSA Representations.   It is important to note that although proponents of LSA do not make any construct claims for the raw data or the factors that enter into the analysis, they do argue that the outcome of the analysis—the space of semantic similarities induced by LSA—does have construct status, and going beyond that, that it corresponds fairly closely to actual processes of human learning. They argue that it provides a coherent account of a variety of psychological facts and results (cf. Laham, 1997; Landauer, 2002; Landauer & Dumais, 1994, 1996, 1997; Landauer, Laham, & Foltz, 1998; Landauer, Laham, Rehder, & Schreiner, 1997). The structure of their argument is worth examining from an ECD perspective, as in effect they argue for a method of inducing variables in the student model by finding empirical relationships (a strong nomothetic span) between a structure induced in the evidence identification process and external criteria such as human scores and other psychological and psycholinguistic data. This form of indirect inference is quite different from the feature-based approach, which depends on prior theory about the construct domain. There is much to be said for such an approach, which involves adoption of an evidence identification method that induces a structure based upon analysis of large amounts of raw data, followed by studies that establish a correlation between the structure thus induced and external variables, though care must be taken to avoid oversimplifying the structure of the phenomenon under study.

In the present case, the data on which LSA operates clearly places limits on what portions of a model of students' knowledge and skill it can be fairly used to infer. Like other vector space techniques, LSA is a bag-of-words method that ignores word order and adjacency and morphology and other known elements of linguistic structure. Landauer (2002) comes close to endorsing a position that rejects any significant role not just for word order but for syntax in the analysis of meaning, and that reduces the role of syntax to little more than an error-correction mechanism and a culturally transmitted set of styles. There is a danger here: given the success of a technique like LSA, it can be tempting to minimize the significance of the aspects of the construct that the technique cannot successfully address. But LSA in its essence only covers generalizations at the level of lexical constructs, and does not extend to cover syntactic, logical or discourse structure. In effect, if viewed as a model of meaning, an LSA space appears to be roughly equivalent to a propositional calculus in which each word is an independent proposition, despite efforts such as Kintsch (2001) to extend it. Detailed applications of LSA are reviewed in the following section, but it is best to remember that LSA is, strictly speaking, a model of the statistical probabilities with which words will occur in the same documents, and thus is most directly relevant to such constructs as topical coherence within or among documents.

Statistical Issues.   As LSA is currently implemented, there are known statistical problems, which can be summarized as follows (Shelby Haberman, personal communication, August, 2002).

First, LSA uses log word frequency for its input data. Using logarithms in this fashion has a number of undesirable properties. The mean frequency of words is lower than desired for modeling the probabilities of discrete events, which (all other things being equal) would cause a bias toward lower probability estimates. As LSA is currently implemented, this possibility must be weighed against the tendency for unsmoothed maximum likelihood estimates to overestimate the probability of words that actually appear in the corpus. While LSA could be modified by adopting smoothing techniques such as those suggested in Good (1953) or Baayen (2001), given the unreliability of maximum likelihood estimation with infrequent words, there is the added problem that the logarithms will be rather variable when word frequencies are low.

Second, Singular Value Decomposition is only stable when the elements of the decomposition are well-separated; in other words, the generalizations induced by SVD can change significantly with minor changes in input data unless the data supporting the generalizations are very strong. (See, e.g., Wilkinson, 1965, for mathematical analysis.) Use of log word frequency input, with its sampling bias, is likely to produce significant perturbations of the resulting SVD analyses of unknown magnitude and significance; these effects are particularly likely with less-frequent words.

Latent semantic analysis has been applied rather widely to a variety of scoring tasks. Most of these tasks involve direct matching of content against a standard, including:

- holistic essay scoring (Foltz, Laham & Landauer, 1999; Dessus, Lemaire & Vernier, 2000; Lemaire & Dessus, 2001; Miller, 2003);

- readability assessment (Wolfe, Schreiner, Rehder, Laham, Foltz et al., 1998);

- measuring coherence within a text (Foltz, Kintsch, & Landauer, 1998);

- evaluating summaries for content coverage (Foltz, Gilliam, & Kendall, 2000; Kintsch, Steinhart, Stahl, Mathews, Lamb et al., 2000);

- assessing student answers to guide the responses of an automatic tutoring system (Lemaire, 1999; Graesser Person & Harter, 2001; Wiemer-Hastings & Graesser, 2000; Wiemer-Hastings, Wiemer-Hastings, & Graesser, 1999a and b)

Essay Scoring.   Application of LSA to automated essay scoring begins with Foltz, Britt, & Perfetti (1994) and Foltz (1996). Foltz' approach was to obtain a body of instructional materials covering a particular subject and to build an LSA model based on that corpus. Student essays on the same subject were scored sentence by sentence for similarity to sentences in the instructional materials, and the results were compared to human raters' judgments about the likely source for information contained by the sentences in each student essay. On this task the agreement between human raters was 0.63, somewhat higher than the LSA performance, with 0.59 agreement with human raters. Having established that LSA performed reasonably well at matching by semantic content, Foltz examined the performance of LSA as a measure of essay quality. Two methods were assessed. In the first method, essays were scored by the extent to which they matched the content for the entire collection of source materials. In the second method, essays were scored for how well they matched a list of 10 sentences that expert graders classified as the most important in the instructional materials. Excluding one of the four graders whose grades did not correlate well with the other three, the correlations for the first method ranged from .317 to .552, and for the second method, from .384 to .626.

These methods, based on a sentence-by-sentence comparison, arguably do not use LSA to full advantage, as content-vector methods generally work best when applied to large amounts of text, and perform less and less reliably as the amount of text is reduced. The information that LSA ignores—for example, syntactic relationships and other structural sources of information—are most salient at the sentence level, and least salient at the level of entire documents. Thus, it is not surprising that later work on essay scoring focuses on more holistic methods. Landauer, Laham, Rehder, and Schreiner (1997) use a k-nearest-neighbor method similar to that employed by E-rater, and report a correlation with human graders of 0.77, agreeing with human raters about as often as human raters agreed with one another. Foltz, Laham, and Landauer (1999b) report another test in which holistic LSA scoring was applied to a set of essays for the GMAT provided by the Educational Testing Service. On this test, which employed a significantly larger training set than Landauer, Laham, Rehder, and Schreiner (1997), the automated system's correlation with human graders was at or just above 0.86, exactly matching inter-grader agreement.

The Intelligent Essay Assessor is a product based on Foltz, Laham, and Landauer's approach. Assessments of its performance also show correlations with human graders above 0.8 (Landauer, Laham, & Foltz, 2003). This system incorporates some additional measurement of linguistic features to handle such issues as plagiarism and errors in mechanics such as misspelling, and supports internal analysis of a set of essays on a single topic. Landauer, Laham, and Foltz (2003) show that this internal analysis can also be used for essay scoring, as student essays that cover a topic well will combine information that appears separately in more poorly written essays.

Another essay scoring system based on LSA is Apex (Dessus, Lemaire, & Vernier 2000; Lemaire & Dessus, 2001). Apex is designed to support instructor-designed essay prompts, and so its methods are somewhat different. At the core of the system is an instructor-supported markup of the instructional materials which identifies a series of "notions" (paragraphs or sections) that divide up the instructional content. The instructor is allowed to specify for an essay prompt which notions are to be matched by the student essays, and essay scores are assigned by their LSA cosine similarity to the selected notions. Dessus, Lemaire, and Vernier (2000) report correlations to human graders between 0.59 and 0.68; Lemaire and Dessus (2001; table 2) also report somewhat lower correlations ranging between 0.38 and 0.46.

The optimal performance of LSA, a purely content-based method, as a method for automatic essay scoring appears to be about as strong as a pure linguistic feature system such as PEG; as noted earlier, both achieved correlations with human graders just above 0.85 in blind tests. It is possible, given the published results, that both fall short of the best results for the hybrid E-rater system, which uses both linguistic features and content. However, there have been no direct head-to-head comparisons of the three systems to determine their relative efficacy. Note that the results for LSA in particular span a wide range, with holistic essay scoring performing most effectively; the human-grader correlations for LSA when applied to smaller text units than an entire essay can be quite low.

There are a number of questions that are raised by these validity studies. One of the most interesting is the extent to which different constructs may be correlated with one another in the student model, yielding high correlations for a variety of methods. LSA-based studies yield correlations with human graders in the same general range as the correlations yielded by purely feature-based approaches to automatic essay scoring such as Project Essay Grade. When one approach (based on similarity of content between essays) yields results quite comparable to another approach (based on similarity of style among essays), there are several issues that must be confronted.

First, one must ask whether the data that goes into Latent Semantic Analysis is in fact truly homogeneous, yielding evidence about a single construct, or whether it represents a statistical model that combines evidence about multiple constructs. Significant in this regard is the large proportion of information which appears to be carried by very frequent function words in an LSA analysis (Peter Folz, personal communication, October 22, 2003.) The relative frequencies with which such words appear in a document has little direct connection to content per se, but certainly reflects the stylistic and grammatical choices made in each document.

Second, one must ask whether the evidence provided by the method is sufficiently direct to yield confidence that one is actually measuring the student model variables one intends to measure. In the language of validity theory, when evidence of construct representation is lacking, we must rely on studies of nomothetic span or correlations with other measures of students' proficiencies. It is common enough for various student abilities to be strongly correlated with one another, particularly in a core competence like language. The usefulness of any given scoring method then should be measured not just by whether it yields a strong correlation with human graders, but whether it makes sense of statistical outliers, yielding results as good for them as it does for the main statistical trend where many different student model variables are strongly correlated. Few of the validity studies for LSA (or indeed for any of the automatic scoring systems) have examined this question in depth, yet it is crucial. By way of illustration, observe (as noted as early as Page's early work on essay scoring) that as simple a measure as essay length may be strongly correlated with human scores. It does not follow that it is measuring the student model variable of essay quality; rather, that there is a strong correlation between one student model variable (fluency of writing in a test situation) and another (quality of the resulting essay.) However, this correlation will break down at the margins, in cases where outstanding writers are capable of writing with extraordinary clarity and succinctness, or in the case of writers who are capable of producing large quantities of text swiftly with very little actual content or quality of argumentation. And it is precisely these outliers that measure the true value of one automatic scoring method over another, given the strong correlations among a variety of writing skills. These considerations should be kept in mind when examining the wide range of tasks to which LSA has been applied, as the argument from evidence identification to student model varies considerably from one application to the next.

Application IV: Readability and Learnability

Standard readability measures as discussed previously are based on a few general linguistic features and can, at best, determine whether a text is roughly at the right grade level for a student's reading ability. One of the more interesting potential applications for LSA lies in the area of matching texts to students' level of knowledge of a particular subject. Since LSA is content-based, it should in principle be possible to determine whether an instructional text is "too easy" or "too hard" for particular students' current level of knowledge. Initial results from Wolfe et al. (1998) suggested that this application is possible: they demonstrated strong correlations between LSA scoring of student essays and other evaluations of student knowledge, and demonstrated a differential effect of essay difficulty (as measured by LSA) and student learning depending on students' initial knowledge state. If these results are corroborated, LSA potentially could be applied to provide subject-specific readability/learnability estimates, helping match readers to appropriate texts given their current knowledge state.

Since this application of LSA is directly tied to content—to whether the choice of vocabulary is appropriate to the skills of the reader—the argument from evidence identification to student model variables is fairly direct, and thus from an ECD perspective, this application of LSA could provide fairly direct evidence about readability or, at least, that component of readability that is tied to level of vocabulary rather than style.

Application V: Textual Coherence

An important concept within discourse analysis is the concept of *coherence*. Essentially, the more a sequence of sentences "hangs together" as being about the same subject and following a logical sequence of thoughts, the more coherent it will be perceived as being. Foltz, Kintsch, and Landauer (1998) argue that LSA is particularly well-suited to measurement of textual coherence. They present a number of studies in which LSA cosines among sentences correlate strongly with independent measures of textual coherence, and thus argue that textual coherence can be measured simply by observing the degree to which sentences overlap in content as measured by LSA.

This claim raises a number of interesting questions. To begin with, early work on coherence (e.g., Halliday & Hassan, 1976) identified a number of distinct factors that contributed to textual cohesion. These included (a) pronoun–antecedent relationships across sentences, (b) clausal connectives that indicate the logical relationships among clauses, (c) lexical chains (i.e., sequences where the same or closely related words are repeated within a text segment), and (d) more general sorts of lexical coherence having to do with related concepts appearing in adjacent portions of the text. Foltz, Kintsch, and Landauer's argument that LSA can measure textual coherence clearly has to do with items (c) and (d); the other sorts of coherence, even if strongly correlated with lexical coherence patterns, depend upon syntactic information to which LSA is insensitive. But the claim that LSA measures lexical coherence comes very close to being a tautology.

Latent semantic analysis is not a direct measure of word-word similarity of meaning. What it is is a direct measure of how likely two words are to appear in the same or statistically similar text chunks, where that text chunk is defined in various ways—in Foltz, Kintsch, and Landauer, as a 2000-character window. When the corpus is large enough, probability of co-occurrence within a discourse window will approximate semantic similarity, simply because non-synonyms cannot be used together coherently in all possible contexts; but in a smaller corpus, all that LSA similarity can strictly be said to measure is (an estimate of) the magnitude of the conditional probability that two words will appear or co-occur within statistically comparable text segments. By definition, authors seek to produce text segments that are coherent, which means they are likely to choose words that produce coherent text when used together. Thus there is a stronger case in principle that LSA measures textual coherence than there is that it measures semantic similarity.

This is particularly true when, as is the case in a number of educational applications of LSA, the training corpus consists of a relatively small body of instructional materials. Given that the corpus does consist of instructional materials, one can expect that particular care will have been taken to make each section coherent in terms of the course content covered, and thus one can have reasonable confidence that LSA, by measuring probability of lexical co-occurrence, will also be providing a reasonably accurate measure of lexical coherence. But it is questionable whether a corpus of a (say) few hundred thousand words will provide reliable statistical inference beyond a minimum measure of likelihood of appearing in the same text paragraphs.

In addition, certain of the issues that Foltz, Kintsch, and Landauer encounter are symptomatic of issues that must always be addressed to determine the relative effectiveness of LSA as a technique. They observe that simple lexical overlap—the repetition of exactly the same word—accounts almost as well for textual coherence as does LSA. They are able to show that LSA does better than literal word repetition in a head-to-head comparison, but it is important to note that literal word repetition is always a factor when the LSA similarity between two texts is calculated. Very few applications of LSA provide a head-to-head comparison with simple keyword-based content-vectors, yet that is the baseline against which LSA must be measured.

From an ECD perspective, the inference from Latent Semantic Analysis to judgments of topical coherence is very direct; that is, one can make a strong case that the construct to which LSA is most directly applicable is, in fact, a propensity to produce text with topical coherence as expressed by its direct reflex, the probability that words will co-occur in the same document.

Application VI: Summary Feedback

One of the most instructionally valuable uses of writing is as a method for consolidating student learning. If students summarize what they have read in texts, the active thought needed to produce the summarized text usually improves both comprehension and recall of the target concepts. One of the standard instructional cycles is for a teacher to assign a writing assignment to students, to evaluate their content knowledge based on their writing, and then to intervene to improve their writing either through additional assignments or by requiring revisions to the original text. (See, e.g., Bean & Steenwyk, 1984; Brown & Day, 1983; Brown, Day, & Jones, 1983; Casazza, 1992; Gajria & Salvia, 1992; McNeil & Donant, 1982; and Winograd, 1984, for studies of the importance of this skill for student learning.) This instructional cycle is highly time-intensive, however, as its use requires extensive interaction between the teacher and each student. Automation of the feedback cycle could potentially allow teachers to assign a much larger number of writing assignments and thus to obtain more benefit from the fact that students learn more when they have to express their knowledge in written form. Foltz, Gilliam, and Kendall (2000) and Kintsch et al. (2000) describe attempts to use LSA for automated scoring to support an interactive process in which students write essays summarizing course content and revise them in response to feedback.

Foltz, Gilliam, and Kendall provide a study in which an LSA essay scorer was used to provide feedback to students about essays summarizing a topic from a class in psycholinguistics. The LSA space was based on the textbook used for the course; a web-based scoring system was developed that allowed students to submit an essay based upon a specific prompt, and that provided them with differential feedback based on how closely their answer matched a rubric for the prompt. Essays were scored by human scorers both for form and content, and the resulting scores were correlated with the performance of the LSA system. The correlation between human graders and the automatic scoring system was 0.89; however, the study did not examine whether use of the automated scoring system improved student performance on other tasks reflecting comprehension of the text, and it did not provide a comparison with a baseline keyword system.

Kintsch et al. (2000) described an automated scoring system, *Summary Street*, explicitly designed to provide interactive computer support for writing. Summary Street is a web-based system allowing both automated scoring of student essays and interactive revision of the essays by students in response to the feedback provided by the automatic scoring system. LSA is used for this purpose; it is trained on a general-purpose corpus of 11 million words. The LSA scoring system is created by dividing a source text into sentences, and determining the most typical sentence in each section of the document (as determined by mutual LSA similarity among all sentences in the same section.) Students' essays are scored by the coverage they provide for each section of the text. Comparison to blind human grading indicated that the feedback provided by Summary Street did improve student summaries; once again, however, the study did not examine the effects on student comprehension outside the writing task, nor did it examine how well students would have done if a keyword system had been substituted, though in this case, with the use of a fairly large corpus, the odds that the LSA system would outperform a keyword system were significantly higher.

The results of these two studies suggest that LSA could be useful to support implementation of an essay feedback system, without clear demonstration that it would effectively increase student comprehension of course material; hopefully evidence in this regard will be forthcoming from future work.

It is important to note, however, that there is rather more room for slippage in the evidentiary chain in this application. Summarization is rather more than producing a text with a high occurrence of words likely to appear in documents like the source document. A good summary replicates the logical and rhetorical relationships among the most important concepts in the source document, whereas LSA would yield the same score for a document even if all the words in the document were scrambled. Applications like Summary Street have the advantage of being relatively easy to implement, but it would be a mistake to assume that students will get equally good feedback about all aspects of their summary. The strength of such systems is that they provide a fairly strong evidentiary argument about a purported summary's content coverage, but that is all that they do.

Application VII: Tutoring Systems

Latent Semantic Analysis has been applied by a number of researchers to the task of building an intelligent tutoring system. These include a number of systems reported on in Lemaire (1999) and Zampa and Lemaire (2002) and the Autotutor and Select-a-Kibitzer systems developed by Wiemer-Hastings and Graesser (Wiemer-Hastings, Wiemer-Hastings & Graesser, 1999a, 1999b; Wiemer-Hastings, 1999).

Lemaire (1999) and Zampa and Lemaire (2002) focus on three potential applications where LSA could provide a useful model. The first is a model of lexeme misunderstanding, where student responses are used to judge whether their use of particular novel words is in accord with an internal LSA model; the second is a game-playing tutor which develops a model of students' abilities by observing the sequences of moves they make and matching them to an internal database; the third is a system which seeks to provide texts neither too hard nor too difficult for student learners of a foreign language. Since these papers take the form of initial reports, without detailed evidence of system performance, it is difficult to determine whether these models will lead to a successful tutoring system or are purely exploratory. Rather more developed is the work on the Autotutor system developed by Graesser and Wiemer-Hastings, where LSA is but one part of a sophisticated natural language tutoring engine.

Autotutor, as described in Graesser, Person, and Harter (2001), has a number of components: a rich tutoring database containing questions, preferred answers, and alternative moves for a tutor to take depending on the student response; graphics and animation to make the tutorial responses seem more naturalistic; linguistic analysis (speech act classification) to determine what sort of response is in order after a student enters a response; and a dialog management system that maps possible dialog moves in a finite state network, to name some of the most important. Latent semantic analysis is used primarily to determine how well student responses match desired responses stored in the tutoring database.

Wiemer-Hastings (1999) reported on the performance of LSA in comparison to keyword and content vector techniques. His results indicate that LSA provides a significant but not very large(less than 20%) improvement in performance over techniques that do not make use of singular value decomposition. These results were with a fairly small corpus (2.3 MB of text consisting entirely of instructional materials plus the curricular script). Wiemer-Hastings, Wiemer-Hastings, and Graesser (1999b) examined the effect of corpus size on performance, and found that performance degraded relatively little when only the curriculum script was included, though the difference was significant (the performance of the system with the full corpus exceeded the curriculum-script-only system by a value which generally ranged between .05 to .15 at various threshold settings).

These results are not particularly surprising given some of the concerns raised earlier: given a relatively small corpus to work with, the advantages of LSA are minimized, and simple keyword-based systems are potentially competitive if not quite as accurate. However, within the limitations thus imposed, the correlation with human raters was, as usual, fairly good: the correlation between LSA and the average human rater was 0.47, virtually identical to the correlation between human raters (Wiemer-Hastings, Wiemer-Hastings, & Graesser 1999a). It is, however, an open question as to how much of the correlation is due to the quality of the tutorial scripts and their relative richness (i.e., in containing the vocabulary patterns most likely to occur in tutoring sessions on particular subjects.) There is only a weak evidentiary argument that LSA has contributed significant evidence with which to apply the student models used in this application.

The Select-a-Kibitzer system reported in Wiemer-Hastings and Graesser, 1999, represents a different strategy, in which specialized LSA systems identify different aspects of good writing as part of a feedback system where students are exposed to the sometimes-conflicting advice of a series of agents specialized for particular aspects of essay analysis. One agent asks questions encouraging more coherent text, using LSA to assess the coherence of sentence sequences; another focuses on whether essays develop the material in standard ways; another addresses whether they stick to the assigned topic; and another produces automatic summaries by selecting sentences which reflect the most important material in each paragraph. This approach appears to represent a more focused application of LSA, in that LSA is being used to assess specific student model variables, such as content coverage and coherence of topic development, where the evidentiary basis for using LSA is fairly strong.

Except for Autotutor, the tutoring systems seem to be in early stages of development, and information about their overall performance is fairly limited. What is also not clear is how well a system that used manually compiled lexical systems (e.g., online thesauruses and lexical databases) might have performed where such systems are available. One of the advantages of LSA is precisely its trainability: since it can operate purely on corpus data, it can be applied to relatively domain-specific text without significant degradation of performance.

Discussion. From a technical point of view, LSA is one of a family of vector space techniques with well-known strengths and weaknesses. LSA is a relatively simple member of the family, as it does not make use, for example of some of the smoothing techniques and clustering methods used in statistical natural language processing (see Manning & Schütze, 1999, for an overview.) It appears to give better performance than pure keyword/vector space systems, though generally not orders of magnitude better when trained on small corpora. Its performance is strongly influenced by the size and content of the corpus used to train it, with best results when the corpus is large and the texts it contains are highly coherent. It appears to provide good results in essay scoring, particularly when the texts contain hundreds of words, and to perform less well when applied to smaller text units, such as phrase- or sentence-size chunks.

From an ECD perspective, LSA essentially provides evidence regarding topical coherence when applied to words (e.g., it is a measure of the likelihood that words will co-occur within the same documents and hence be relevant to the same topics.) When applied to documents, LSA is essentially a measure of content overlap, rendered more robust by the underlying dimensionality reduction which allows it to detect similarity of content even when different words are used to express the same information. Because LSA does not take textual structure into account (e.g., morphology, syntax, or logical and rhetorical relationships) it should not be viewed as a panacea covering all aspects of language structure and use, but rather as an important and powerful tool which has the potential to provide access to important aspects of a student model.

LINGUISTIC STRUCTURE ANALYSIS

Earlier in this chapter, it was pointed out that a full linguistic system for text analysis includes at least the following components:

- tokenization and segmentation

- lemmatization

- finite-state analysis

- term extraction

- lexical semantic analysis

- phrasal chunking

- clausal chunking

- parsing

- semantic role analysis

- word sense disambiguation

- anaphora resolution

- reference tracking

- discourse chunking

- discourse parsing

Many of these methods, used in isolation, are extremely effective for the extraction of linguistic features; the more accurate the computational linguistic foundations, the more likely the methods applied are to provide useful and accurate classificatory features. However, there is another way in which these methods could be applied for scoring. For certain purposes, there is no substitute for constructing as accurate a model of the full linguistic structure of a text as possible, with the full text model serving as the input to an automatic scoring system.

Certain caveats should be noted here. Construction of a linguistically-based system offers the opportunity for an in-depth analysis not otherwise available, and for a degree of precision not otherwise possible, but there are limits to what can currently be achieved due to limits on the size and accuracy of language resources, the accuracy of parsers, and so forth. Detailed linguistic analysis can only be justified if the benefits from an in-depth linguistic analysis outweigh the costs and risks in the current stage of development of natural language processing technologies.

Currently, the major area where full linguistic scoring systems are justified is automatic scoring of short free-text responses—the type of item where a fairly precise question demands a precise answer in less than a paragraph of text generated by the test subject. Short-answer scoring is ill-suited to the other scoring techniques reviewed in this chapter because its demands for coverage and accuracy are too high for methods like LSA to work well. Often, a correct answer cannot be specified by a list of words, however appropriate. A correct answer must cover specific points, and it must say specific things about each point. Short-answer questions of this type are a knowledge-elicitation technique, and nothing short of a complete linguistic analysis can determine whether the answer actually contains the requisite knowledge or merely skates around it throwing out appropriate words in more-or-less appropriate ways. An automated short-answer scoring system has to deal with these facts:

1.   that the same words can be the right, or the wrong, answer, depending on how they are put together;

2.   that different words can be the same answer if they paraphrase the same information.

In short, there is no escaping from a syntactic and semantic analysis that seeks to extract propositional knowledge from the student answer; and the scoring algorithm must determine whether the student answer matches the rubric closely enough to get full or partial credit.

There are presently two systems that provide linguistically-based scoring of short answer responses: the C-rater system developed by the Educational Testing Service, and the Automark system developed by Intelligent Assessment Technologies. Both appear to function fairly similarly, as they implement morphological, syntactic, and semantic analyses of student answers in order to extract a propositional structure which can be matched against an instructor rubric.

Application I: Scoring Constructed Response Items Via C-Rater

C-rater is a technology developed by the Educational Testing Service for the purpose of automatically scoring constructed-response short-answer verbal items where the scoring rubric is based upon an evaluation of content (Leacock, 2004; Leacock & Chodorow, 2003, 2004). It is appropriate for any constructed-response verbal item that has the following characteristics:

•   Answers are in verbal form and range between one sentence and a few paragraphs in length.

•   The rubric can be stated as a series of points (each about a sentence long) specifying the content that must be contained in a correct answer.

•   Scoring is entirely based upon content, without penalties for grammatical errors, misspellings and the like as long as the intended meaning is clear.

C-rater has been tried successfully in a number of large-scale assessments, including the NAEP Math Online project, where it was used to score student explanations of mathematical reasoning, and the State of Indiana's English 11 End-of-Course Assessment, where it scored in excess of 100,000 student responses per year for 2002, 2003, and 2004. C-rater exploits several natural language processing (NLP) technologies, including the following:

- *spelling correction* (identifying the intended spelling when words are misspelled)

- *morphological analysis* (identifying the correct stem or root form of a word)

- *chunking* to specify key word-to-word relationships and identify paraphrases, with a predicate-argument structure extracted from the chunks to identify propositional content

- *pronominal reference resolution* (automatically determining the antecedents of pronouns)

- *synonymy and semantic similarity* (using corpus data to identify semantically related words)

In combination, these technologies support C-rater's capacity to identify when student responses match clauses in the scoring rubric even if they use entirely different words and grammatical structures.

C-rater is essentially a paraphrase recognizer; however, in internal structure, C-rater is roughly similar to certain NLP-based question-answering and information retrieval systems, insofar as it makes use of similar arrays of linguistic analysis techniques. Such systems feature detailed sentence-level analysis with a series of algorithms intended to arrive at a representation of sentence meaning; instances include the InFact information retrieval engine (http://www.insightful.com/products/infact/default.asp), the MeaningMaster (formerly Inquizit) search engine (http://www.meaningmaster.com), and the Cyc NL system (http://www.cyc.com/nl.html), among others (cf. Pradhan, Krugler, Ward, Jurafsky, & Martin, 2002). C-rater differs from these systems in being configured and optimized to identify paraphrases to support scoring of short verbal responses, rather than deploying the linguistic structure analysis it creates for one of the many other potential applications to which analysis of linguistic structure can be put. Like these systems, it performs a partial NLP analysis; unlike them, it is optimized to extract information needed to score short-answer free response text. In ECD terms, it provides a first pass at evidence identification, providing input to a second pass whose nature and success will depend on the project at hand.

In essence, what C-rater does is create a template from the points specified in the instructor rubric; this template specifies configurations of meanings in grammatical relations which must appear in the student answer if it is to receive full credit. The syntactic and semantic analysis C-rater performs is abstract enough to detect synonyms and paraphrases, enabling it to identify very different responses as providing the same conceptual content without giving credit to inaccurate replies.

Results from tests of C-rater indicate that it obtains about 84–85% agreement with human raters, whereas human raters agreed about 92% of the time (Leacock, 2004; Leacock & Chodorow, 2003). It thus performed well enough to enable automated scoring of short answer responses for the very large test volumes involved in the Indiana assessment.

Application II: Scoring Constructed Response Items Via Automark

The Automark short answer scoring system is described in Mitchell, Russell, Broomhead, and Aldridge (2002). In general structure it is very similar to C-rater: student responses are scored by subjecting the text they produce to NLP analysis. Automark performs syntactic preprocessing and sentence analysis to standardize spelling and punctuation, identify the main syntactic constituents, and determine their grammatical relationships. The output of the sentence analysis is passed through a pattern matching component which determines which of one or more *mark schemes* matches the answer. Mark schemes are simply syntactico-semantic patterns; Mitchel et al.'s example is presented here as Figure 9.1 (Mitchell, Russell, Broomhead, & Aldridge, 2002: p. 236).

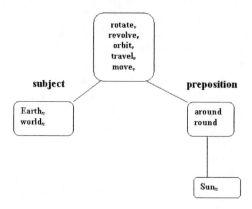

FIG. 9 1. An Automark mark scheme.

Development of mark schemes is an offline process: instructor rubrics and possibly sample student answers are analyzed to develop a set of mark schemes that will correctly classify student responses; when the system is run, the pattern matching subsystem matches student answers against the available mark schemes and assigns a score according to rules associated with the available schemes.

Mitchell et. al's discussion does not make some details clear; it is not clear, for instance, whether the creation of synonym lists within a mark scheme has an automated component or is entirely created by hand; neither is it clear whether the handling of syntactic paraphrases is handled automatically, or manually by increasing the number of mark schemes. But the essential nature of the system is clear: analyze the patterns in student answers, and match against a mark scheme devised to match the instructor rubric

Mitchell et al. reported a number of studies that illuminate the strengths and weaknesses of the system. On a series of blind tests, they found that the Automark scheme worked well for short answers ranging in length from single words to single sentences. On a more complex question requiring multiple clauses, it performed less well, with a significant number of false negatives: the mark scheme simply did not anticipate all the possibilities for alternative phrases inherent in the relatively complex answer required by the rubric

In general, the errors Mitchell et al. reported fall into two classes:

1.   errors in the linguistic coverage of the system, e.g., spelling errors, synonyms and grammatical patterns not recognized or not covered by the mark scheme;

2.   errors that reflect fundamental issues with how the system operates.

Coverage issues will, in principle, be eliminated as the linguistic resources used in a system like Automark are extended, but it would be a mistake to ignore their importance. In general, when NLP systems are developed, the largest errors can be eliminated quickly, but a large residue of issues remains that cannot be resolved easily or quickly. However, for a system like Automark, this issue is counterbalanced by the fact that human scorers can be inconsistent when dealing with relatively open-ended constructed-response texts; certainly the performance levels Mitchell et al. reported are clearly well above the level that would make automatic short-answer scoring an attractive option, though the published studies thus far seem to be fairly preliminary.

It should be noted that Automark appears to focus on relatively specific patterns (e.g., words and sentence fragments), whereas C-rater is being used for 11th grade reading comprehension prompts, but as there has been no head-to-head comparison of the two systems, a full evaluation of their relative performance is not yet available.

Some General Considerations

With short answer scoring systems like C-rater and Automark, it is important to be aware of what information they are using and what information they are ignoring in their analysis, and thus what evidence they can reasonably be expected to respond to. Both Leacock (2004) and Mitchell et al. (2002) provided an analysis of error patterns.

Some of the errors are simply due to the limitations of a partial paraphrase analysis engine: where the engine allows too much leeway in paraphrase, false positive results; where it fails to identify paraphrases correctly, correct answers are missed. Such errors can be reduced as the underlying paraphrase identification engine is improved, but is unlikely to be eliminated completely in the foreseeable future; indeed, even human scorers disagree, in part because it is not always clear whether a particular phrasing correctly paraphrases the desired answer.

Perhaps even more interestingly, many of the ways in which these systems can go wrong are directly linked to the fact that they are focused on sentence level analysis, with relatively little higher level discourse or conceptual analysis of content. For instance, the Automark system gave full marks where an instructor took off when an answer contained both correct and incorrect information. That is, if the scoring system expected a single word answer such as "melting", and the student answered "melting—condensation", the instructor did not give credit, and the system did. This illustrates a general problem that requires an analysis beyond the level of individual phrases and clauses: the problem of distinguishing between relevant additions that display an elaboration of the required answer, and irrelevant additions that suggest a buckshot approach to getting (at least partial) credit. In short, scoring algorithms for short answer questions cannot be reduced to a simple checklist approach to content; some measure of the overall appropriateness and relevance of "unnecessary" added text is also necessary. Leacock (2004) reported similar limitations for C-rater; when a response contains a correct answer, the presence of information that makes the overall answer incorrect is not taken into account.

In general, these systems do worst when answer scoring requires analysis above the sentence level; the systems do not conclude a discourse parser that can identify how the pieces of a longer answer fit together, and so the current limit of short answer scoring arises with questions which require complex (multiclause) answers with specific relations among the pieces. Both Automark and C-rater appear likely to work well with multisentence answers if the instructor scoring guide can be reduced to a series of bulleted points that are combined using a scoring algorithm based on the number and distribution of points covered. More complex logical and rhetorical relations among clauses appear to be beyond the capacities of either system.

However, within the constraints just identified, systems like C-rater and Automark have considerable promise, making it possible for the first time for short-answer free-text response items to be scored automatically. The existence of these systems underscores the importance of being aware of the different methods that exist for automatic scoring of text. What they are able to do that none of the other systems do is provide for scoring that is very sensitive to the precise structure and content of text, rather than focusing on general trends in the data or characterizing content without regard to structure. They do this by simulating certain aspects of the process of human comprehension of text (e.g., parsing and text interpretation) without constructing a full model of text understanding. Thus, the evidentiary argument from scoring rubric to automatically scored short answer text is very direct and very strong, based as it is on an explicit reconstruction of the underlying construct.

CONCLUSIONS

The purpose of this chapter has been to provide an overview of methods for automatic scoring of linguistic (primarily textual as opposed to verbal) materials, with an evaluation of each method from the point of view of Evidence-Centered Design. Now that this overview is complete, it is worthwhile to step back and examine the current state of automatic text scoring.

The field is in the midst of a major series of advances, fueled by the influx of methods developed in information retrieval, text categorization, and natural language processing. Simple statistical analysis of surface linguistic features, which dominated the field from early work on readability theory and essay scoring, are being replaced by approaches which extract more sophisticated linguistic features using NLP techniques, by content vector approaches such as Latent Semantic Analysis, which leverage text corpora for statistical knowledge of language, and by more advanced NLP systems that have made possible accurate automatic scoring of short free-response verbal items for the first time. There is every reason to think that this ferment in automatic scoring will continue as more sophisticated natural language processing systems allow more and more accurate automatic analysis of textual materials.

At the same time, the new methods are not panaceas, and adoption of new techniques should be accompanied by thoughtful evaluation of the evidence they use and how they use it. If systems like C-rater or Automark are used where discourse analysis is critical, they can hardly be expected to perform well; if LSA is used where syntactic structure is critical, or without an adequate corpus, results will hardly be better. And so forth. In general, the new methods for automatic scoring offer powerful new tools, but their efficacy depends as ever on a careful matching of assessment methods to the evidence needed to design an appropriate instrument.

From an ECD perspective, these methods illustrate a number of different strategies for achieving the necessary linkage between the construct representation in the student model, the nomothetic span connecting the model to task performance, and the engineering decisions needed to achieve feasible automatic scoring.

In linguistic feature-based approaches, the design process achieves engineering feasibility by narrowing focus to cover only a selected range of textual attributes, with the selection of features being driven jointly by engineering feasibility and the plausibility of each feature as a direct reflex of desired construct categories. The quality of the nomothetic span that links student model to task performances is evaluated separately from the engineering solution to the problem of evidence identification; however, the engineering solution does not rely on a detailed theory of the student model, only on the identification of features that are likely to provide evidence about the aspects of knowledge and skill intended to be represented by student model variables.

Vector space approaches illustrate a less theoretically "heavy" approach to building a student model, one in which textual data is analyzed without preexisting theory, and the resulting analysis is correlated directly with task attributes. The value of the student model thus inferred is entirely driven by the strength of the correlations thus obtained. Engineering feasibility is guaranteed by selecting methods (such as singular value decomposition) with known computational and inferential value. The major weakness of this approach is that it can be something of a black box, as weaknesses in the inferential process can be obscured by the uniform application of a known technique without regard for known complexities of the underlying construct.

The linguistic structure approaches have the advantage because they directly simulate the process of text comprehension, of being completely explicit about the student model variables being postulated, and enjoy the additional advantage of providing far more detail about the structural aspects of language which are necessary for fine-grained textual analysis. In effect, the inferential step from evidence to student model is as strong as possible to get, and because these models are typically applied to short answer scoring, where precise matching of text content and structure is the scoring criterion, the relation to task performance is equally direct. The chief drawback of linguistic structure-based approaches is the heavy demand they place on the engineering implementation for accuracy and the risk that truly important data will be lost in the variety of linguistic and structural details such applications make available.

This tradeoff between the ease with which an automatic scoring system can be devised, the directness and accuracy with which the student model variables can be inferred from the evidence identification process, and the directness with which the variables are correlated with task performance, is typical of text-based applications due to the extreme complexity of human language and the high-level cognitive capacities deployed in human communication. It is, however, likely to feature in many other ECD design decisions when automatic scoring issues come into play. The ECD perspective facilitates achieving a clearer perspective when many different techniques are applicable to a single complex domain, since it forces the analyst to pay careful attention to the role of student model variables in the evidence identification process.

REFERENCES

Abney, S. (1996). Partial parsing via finite-state cascades. *Journal of Natural Language Engineering, 2*(4), 337-344.

Baayen, R. H. (2001). *Word frequency distributions*. Dordrecht, The Netherlands: Kluwer.

Bashaw, W. L., & Rentz, R. R. (1977). The National Reference Scale for Reading: An application of the Rasch model. *Journal of Educational Measurement 14*, 161-179.

Bean, T. W., & Steenwyk, F. L. (1984). The effect of three forms of summarization instruction on sixth-graders' summary writing and comprehension. *Journal of Reading Behavior 16*, 287-306.

Bejar, I. I., (1988). A sentence-based automated approach to the assessment of writing: A feasibility study. *Machine Mediated Learning, 2*, 321-332.

Berry, M. (1992). Large scale singular value computations. *International Journal of Supercomputer Applications 6*(1), 13-49.

Biber, D. (1998). *Variation across speech and writing*. Cambridge, UK: Cambridge University Press.

Biber, D. (1995). *Dimensions of register variation: A cross-linguistic comparison*. Cambridge, UK: Cambridge University Press.

Biber, D., Conrad, S., & Reppen, R. (1998). *Corpus linguistics: Investigating language structure and use*. Cambridge, UK: Cambridge University Press.

Biber, D., Reppen, R., Clark, V., & Walter, J. (2001). Representing spoken language in university settings: The design and construction of the spoken component of the T2K-SWAL corpus. In

R. Simpson and J. Swales (Eds.), *Corpus linguistics in North America*, (pp. 48-57). Ann Arbor, MI: University of Michigan Press.

Biber, D, Conrad, S., Reppen, R., Byrd, P., Helt, M., Clark, V., Cortes, V., Csomay, E., & Urzua, A. (2004). *Representing language use in the university: Analysis of the TOEFL 2000 spoken and written academic language corpus*. Princeton, NJ: Educational Testing Service.

Bormuth, J. R. (1966). Readability: New approach. *Reading Research Quarterly 7*, 79–132.

Brown, A. L., & Day, J. D. (1983). Macrorules for summarizing texts: The development of expertise. *Journal of Verbal Learning and Verbal Behavior, 22*, 1–14.

Brown, A. L., Day, J. D., & Jones, R. S. (1983). The development of plans for summarizing texts. *Child Development, 54*(4), 968–979.

Burgess, C., Livesay, K., & Lund, K. (1998). Explorations in context space: Words, sentences, discourse. *Discourse Processes, 25*, 211–257.

Burstein, J. (2003). The E-rater scoring engine: Automated essay scoring with natural language processing. In M. D. Shermis and J. C. Burstein (Eds.), *Automated Essay Scoring: A Cross-Disciplinary Perspective* (pp. 113–122). Mahwah, NJ: Lawrence Erlbaum Associates.

Burstein, J., Chodorow, M., & Leacock, C. (2003, August). Criterion: Online essay evaluation: An application for automated evaluation of student essays. *Proceedings of the Fifteenth Annual Conference on Innovative Applications of Artificial Intelligence*, Acapulco, Mexico.

Burstein, J., Marcu, D., Andreyev, S., & Chodorow, M. (2001). Towards automatic classification of discourse elements in essays. Proceedings of the 39th Annual Meeting of the Association of Computational Linguistics, Toulouse, France, July 2001.

Burstein, J., Marcu, D., & Knight, K. (2003). Finding the WRITE Stuff: Automatic identification of discourse structure in student essays. In S. Harabagiu & F. Ciravegna (Eds.), *Special Issue on Advances in Natural Language Processing, IEEE Intelligent Systems, 18*(3), 32–39.

Burstein, J. and Marcu, D. (2000, October). *Toward using text summarization for essay-based feedback*. Paper presented at Le 7e Conference Annuelle sur Le Traitement Automatique des Langues Naturelles TALN'2000, Lausanne, Switzerland.

Burstein, J. & Marcu, D. (2000). Benefits of modularity in an automated essay scoring system. Proceeding of the Workshop on Using Toolsets and Architectures to Build NLP Systems, 18th International Conference on Computational Linguistics, Luxembourg.

Burstein, J. & Chodorow, M. (1999, June). Automated essay scoring for nonnative English speakers. In *Proceedings of the ACL99 Workshop on Computer-Mediated Language Assessment and Evaluation of Natural Language Processing,* College Park, MD.

Burstein, J., Kukich, K., Wolff, S., Lu, C., Chodorow, M., Braden-Harder, L., & Harris, M. D. (1998a, August). Automated scoring using a hybrid feature identification technique. *Proceedings of the Annual Meeting of the Association of Computational Linguistics,* pp. 206-210, Montreal, Canada.

Burstein, J., Kukich, K., Wolff, S., Lu, C., & Chodorow, M. (1998b, August). Enriching automated essay scoring using discourse marking. *Proceedings of the Workshop on Discourse Marking and Discourse Relations, Annual Meeting of the Association of Computational Linguistics, Montreal, Canada.*

Burstein, J., Kukich, K., Wolff, S., Lu, C., & Chodorow, M. (1998c, April). Computer Analysis of Essays. Paper presented at the NCME Symposium on Automated Scoring, San Diego, CA.

Casazza, M. E. (1992). Teaching summary writing to enhance comprehension. *Reading Today, 9*(4), 26.

Chodorow, M., & Leacock, C. (2000). An unsupervised method for detecting grammatical errors. *1st Meeting of the North American Chapter of the Association for Computational Linguistics* (pp. 140–147). Seattle, WA.

Davison, A., & Green, G. M. (Eds.) (1988). *Linguistic complexity and text comprehension: Readability issues reconsidered.* Hillsdale, NJ: Lawrence Erlbaum Associates.

Davison, A., & Kantor, R. (1982). On the failure of readability formulas to define readable text: a case study from adaptations. *Reading Research Quarterly, 17,* 187–209.

Dessus, P., Lemaire, B., & Vernier, A. (2000). Free-text assessment in a virtual campus. In K. Zreik (Ed.), *Proceedings of the Third International Conference on Human System Learning* (CAPS'3; pp. 61–76)). Paris: Europia.

Embretson, S. (1983). Construct validity: Construct representation versus nomothetic span. *Psychological Bulletin, 93,* 179–197.

Foltz, P. W. (1996). Latent semantic analysis for text-based research. *Behavior Research Methods, Instruments and Computers, 28*(2), 197-202.

Foltz, P. W. (2003). Personal Communication–October.

Foltz, P. W., Britt, M. A., & Perfetti, C. A. (1994, July). *Where did you learn that? Matching student essays to the texts they have read.* Paper presented at the Fourth Annual Conference of the Society for Text and Discourse, Washington, DC.

Foltz, P. W., Gilliam, S., & Kendall, S. (2000). Supporting content-based feedback in online writing evaluation with LSA. *Interactive Learning Environments 8*(2), 111–129.

Foltz, P. W., Kintsch, W., & Landauer, T. K. (1998). The measurement of textual coherence with Latent Semantic Analysis. *Discourse Processes 25*(2–3), 285–307.

Foltz, P. W., Laham, D., & Landauer, T. K. (1999a). The intelligent essay assessor: Applications to educational technology. *Interactive Multimedia Electronic Journal of Computer-Enhanced Learning, 1*(2).

Foltz, P.W., Laham, D., & Landauer, T. K. (1999b). Automated essay scoring: Applications to educational technology. In Proceedings of the ED-MEDIA Conference, pp. 939-944, Chesapeake, VA:AACE.

Gajria, M., & Salvia, J. (1992). The effects of summarization instruction on text comprehension of students with learning disabilities. *Exceptional Children 58,* 508–516,

Golub, G. H., & Loan, C. F. V. (1996). *Matrix computations.* Baltimore, MD: Johns Hopkins University Press.

Good, I. J. (1953). The population frequencies of species and the estimation of population parameters. *Biometrika 40,* 237–264.

Graesser, A. C., Wiemer-Hastings, K., Wiemer-Hastings, P., Kreuz, R., & Tutoring Research Group, University of Memphis. (1999). AutoTutor: A simulation of a human tutor. *Cognitive Systems Research, 1,* 35–51.

Graesser, A. C., Person, N., & Harter, D. (2001). Teaching Tactics and Dialog in Autotutor. *International Journal of Artificial Intelligence in Education, 12,* 257-279.

Haberman, S. (2002). Personal Communication–August.

Halliday, M. A. K., & Hasan, R. (1976). *Cohesion in English*. London: Longman.

Kintsch, W. (2001). Predication. *Cognitive Science, 25* (2), 173–202.

Kintsch, E., Steinhart, D., Stahl, G., Matthews, C., Lamb, R., & the LSA Group (2000). Developing summarization skills through the use of LSA-based feedback. *Interactive Learning Environments, 8*(2), 87–109.

Klare, G. R. (1963). *The measurement of readability*. Ames, IA: Iowa State University Press.

Klare, G. R. (1974). Assessing readability. *Reading Research Quarterly, 1*, 63–102.

Laham, D. (1997). Latent semantic analysis approaches to categorization. In M. G. Shafto & P. Langley (Eds.), *Proceedings of the 19th Annual Conference of the Cognitive Science Society* (p. 979). Mahwah, NJ: Lawrence Erlbaum Associates.

Landauer, T. K. (2002). On the computational basis of learning and cognition: Arguments from LSA. *The Psychology of Learning and Motivation, 41*, 43–84.

Landauer, T. K. & Dumais, S. T. (1994). Latent semantic analysis and the measurement of knowledge. In R. M. Kaplan and J. C. Burstein (Eds.), *Educational Testing Service Conference on Natural Language Processing Techniques and Technology in Assessment and Education* (pp. 127–147). Princeton: Educational Testing Service.

Landauer, T. K., & Dumais, S. T. (1996). How come you know so much? From practical problems to new memory theory. In D. J. Hermann, C. McEvoy, C. Hertzog, P. Hertel, & M. K. Johnson (Eds.), *Basic and applied memory research: Vol. 1: Theory in context* (pp. 105–126). Mahwah, NJ: Lawrence Erlbaum Associates.

Landauer, T. K., & Dumais, S. T. (1997). A solution to Plato's problem: The Latent Semantic Analysis theory of the acquisition, induction, and representation of knowledge. *Psychological Review 104*, 211–240.

Landauer, T. K., Laham, D., & Foltz, P. W. (1998). Learning human-like knowledge by Singular Value Decomposition: A progress report. In M. I. Jordan, M. J. Kearns, & S. A. Solla (Eds.), *Advances in Neural Information Processing Systems 10*(pp. 45–51). Cambridge, MA: MIT Press.

Landauer, T. K., Laham, D., & Foltz, P. W. (2003). Automated scoring and annotation of essays with the Intelligence Essay Assessor. In M. D. Shermis & J. C. Burstein (Eds.), *Automated essay scoring: A cross-disciplinary perspective* (pp. 87–112). Mahwah, NJ: Lawrence Erlbaum Associates.

Landauer, T. K., Laham, D., Rehder, B., & Schreiner, M.E. (1997). How well can passage meaning be derived without using word order? A comparison of Latent Semantic Analysis and humans. In M. G. Shafto & P. Langley (Eds.), *Proceedings of the 19th annual meeting of the Cognitive Science Society* (pp. 412–417). Mahwah, NJ: Lawrence Erlbaum Associates.

Larkey, L. S. (1998). Automatic essay grading using text categorization techniques. In *Proceedings of the 21st Annual international ACM SIGIR Conference on Research and Development in information Retrieval* (pp. 90-95). New York, NY: ACM Press.

Larkey, L. S., & Croft, W. B. (2003). A text categorization approach to automated essay grading. In M. D. Shermis and J. C. Burstein (Eds.), *Automated essay scoring: A cross-disciplinary perspective* (pp. 55–70). Mahwah, NJ: Lawrence Erlbaum Associates.

Leacock, C. (2004). Automatisch beoordelen van antwoorden op open vragen; een taalkundige benadering. [Scoring free-responses automatically: A case study of a large-scale assessment]. *Examens, 1*(3) (in press). Available online at http://www.ets.org/research/crater.html.

Leacock, C., & Chodorow, M. (2003). C-rater: Automated scoring of short answer questions. *Computers and the Humanities, 37*(4), 389–405.

Leacock, C., & Chodorow, M. (2004, June). *A pilot study of automated scoring of constructed responses*. Paper presented at the 30th Annual International Association of Educational Assessment Conference, Philadelphia, PA.

Lemaire B. (1999). Tutoring systems based on Latent Semantic Analysis. In S. P. Lajoie & M. Vivet (Eds.), *Artificial intelligence in education; frontiers in artificial intelligence and applications, 50*, 527–534.

Lemaire, B & Dessus, P. (2001). A system to assess the semantic content of student essays. *Journal of Educational Computing Research, 24*(3), 305–320.

Lewis, D. D. (1992). Representation and learning in information retrieval. (Doctoral dissertation, University of Massachusetts at Amherst, 1992). Technical Report 91–93.

Lewis, D. D., Shapire, R. E., Callan, J. P., & Papka, R. (1996). Training algorithms for linear text classifiers. In *Proceedings of the 19th Annual International ACM SIGIR Conference on Research and Development in Information Retrieval* (pp. 298–306). New York: ACM Press.

Lund, K., & Burgess, C. (1996). Producing high-dimensional semantic spaces from lexical co-occurrence. *Behavior Research Methods, Instruments & Computers 28*(2), 203–208.

Manning, C. D., & Schütze, H. S. 1999. *Foundations of statistical natural language processing*. Cambridge, MA: MIT Press.

McNeill, J., & Donant, L. (1982). Summarization strategy for improving reading comprehension. In J. A. Niles & L. A. Harris (Eds.), *New inquiries in reading research and instruction* (pp. 215–219). Rochester, NY: National Reading Conference.

Miller T. (2003). Essay assessment with latent semantic analysis. *Journal of Educational Computing Research, 29*(4), 495-512.

Mitchell, T., Russell, T., Broomhead, P., & Aldridge, N. (2002). Towards robust computerized marking of free-text responses. Paper presented at the Sixth Conference on Computer Assisted Assessment, Loughborough University, UK, June 2002. Available online at http://www.lboro.ac.uk/service/ltd/flicaa/conf2002/pdfs/Mitchell_t1.pdf.

Page, E. B. (1966a). The imminence of grading essays by computer. *Phi Delta Kappan, 47*, 238–243.

Page, E. B. (1966b). Grading essays by computer: A progress report. Invitational Conference on Testing Problems. Princeton, NJ: Educational Testing Service.

Page, E. B. (1967). Statistical and linguistic strategies in the computer grading of essays. In *Proceedings of the 1967 Conference on Computational Linguistics* (August 23 - 25, 1967). International Conference on Computational Linguistics. Association for Computational Linguistics, pp. 1-13, Morristown, NJ.

Page, E. B. (1994). Computer grading of student prose: Using modern concepts and software. *Journal of Experimental Education 62*(2), 127–142.

Page, E. B. (1995, August). Computer grading of essays: A different kind of testing? Paper presented at APA Annual Meeting, New York.

Page, E. B. (1996, April). Grading essays by computer: Why the controversy? Paper presented at NCME Invited Symposium, New York.

Page, E. B. (2003). Project Essay Grade: PEG. In M. D. Shermis and J. Burstein (eds.), *Automated Essay Scoring: A Cross-Disciplinary Perspective* (pp. 43–54). Hillsdale, NJ: Lawrence Erlbaum Associates.

Page, E. B., Fisher, G. A., & Fisher, M. A. (1968). Project essay grade: A FORTRAN program for statistical analysis of prose. *British Journal of Mathematical and Statistical Psychology, 21*, 139.

Page, E. B., & Paulus, D.H. (1968). The analysis of essays by computer. Final Report to the U.S. Department of Health, Education and Welfare. Washington, DC: Office of Education, Bureau of Research.

Powers, D. E., Burstein, J. C., Chodorow, M. S, Fowles, M. E., & Kukich, K. (2001). Stumping *E-Rater*: Challenging the validity of automated essay scoring. GRE Board Professional Report No. 98-08bP; ETS Research Report 01-03. Princeton, NJ: Educational Testing Service.

Pradhan, S., Krugler, V., Ward, W., Jurafsky, D., & Martin, J. H. (2002, December). Using semantic representations in question answering. Paper presented at the *International Conference on Natural Language Processing (ICON-2002), Bombay, India.* Available online at http://oak.colorado.edu/~spradhan/publications/cuaq.pdf.

Qiu, Y., & Frei, H. (1993). Concept based query expansion. In R. Korfhage, E. Rasmussen, and P. Willett, (Eds.), *Proceedings of the 16th Annual international ACM SIGIR Conference on Research and Development in information Retrieval* (pp. 160-169). New York: ACM Press.

Ratnaparkhi, A. (1996, May). Maximum entropy part-of-speech tagger. In *Proceedings of the Empirical Methods in Natural Language Processing Conference* (pp. 133-142). Somerset, NJ: Association for Computational Linguistics.

Rudner, L. M., & Liang, T. (2002). Automated essay scoring using Bayes' Theorem. *Journal of Technology, Learning and Assessment 1*(2).

Salton, G. (1990). Developments in automatic text retrieval. *Science, (253)*, 974–980.

Salton, G., Wong, A., & Yang, C. S. (1975). A vector space model for automatic indexing. *Communications of the ACM, 18*(11), 613–620.

Shermis, M. D. & Burstein, J. (Eds.). (2003). *Automated essay scoring: A cross-disciplinary perspective.* Mahwah, NJ: Lawrence Erlbaum Associates.

Smith, C. (1988). Factors of linguistic complexity and performance. In A. Davison & G. Green (Eds.), *Linguistic complexity and text comprehension readability issues reconsidered* (pp. 247–278). Hillsdale, NJ: Lawrence Erlbaum Associates.

Stenner, A. J. (1996, February). Measuring reading comprehension with the lexile framework. Paper presented at the Fourth North American Conference on Adolescent/Adult Literacy, Washington, DC.

Stenner, A. J., & Burdick, D. S. (1997). The objective measurement of reading comprehension—In response to technical questions raised by the California Department of Education Technical Study Group. Retrieved from http://www.lexile.com/about_lex/tech-papers/documents/ObjectveMS.pdf.

Stenner, A. J., & Wright, B. D. (2002, February). Readability, reading ability, and comprehension. Paper presented at the Association of Test Publishers Presentation, San Diego, California.

van Rijsbergen, C. J. (1979). *Information retrieval* (2nd Ed.). London: Butterworths.

Voorhees, E. M. (1993). Using Wordnet to disambiguate word senses for text retrieval. In R. Korfhage, E. Rasmussen, and P. Willett, (Eds.), *Proceedings of the 16th Annual International ACM SIGR Conference on Research and Development in Information Retrieval* (pp. 171–180). New York, NY: ACM Press.

Wade-Stein, D., & Kintsch, E. (2003). Summary street: Interactive computer support for writing. University of Colorado, Boulder Institute of Cognitive Science Technical Report 03-01.

White, S., & Clement, J. C. (2001). Assessing the lexile framework: Results of a panel meeting. National Center for Education Statistics Working Paper Series, Working Paper No. 2001-08, August 2001.

Wiemer-Hastings, P. (1999). How latent is latent semantic analysis? In T. Dean (Ed.), *Proceedings of the 16th International Joint Conference on Artificial Intelligence* (pp. 932-937). San Francisco, CA: Morgan Kaufmann.

Wiemer-Hastings, P. & Graesser, A. C. (2000). Select-a-Kibitzer: A computer tool that gives meaningful feedback on student compositions. *Interactive Learning Environments. 8*(2), 149–169.

Wiemer-Hastings, P., Wiemer-Hastings, K., & Graesser, A. C (1999a). Improving an intelligent tutor's comprehension of students with Latent Semantic Analysis. In S.P. Lajoie and M. Vivet (Eds), *AI in Education–Proceedings of the AIED'99 Conference* (pp. 535–542). Amsterdam: IOS Press.

Wiemer-Hastings, P., Wiemer-Hastings, K., & Graesser, A. C (1999b). Approximate natural language understanding for an intelligent tutor. In A. N. Kumar and I. Russell, (Eds.), *Proceedings of the 12th International Florida Artificial Intelligence Research Symposium* (pp. 192–196). Menlo Park, CA: AAAI Press.

Wilkinson, D. H. (1965). *The algebraic eigenvalue problem.* Oxford, UK: Oxford University Press. Reprinted in 1988.

Williams, J. (1982). Non-linguistic linguistics and the teaching of style. In H. B. Allen and M. D. Linn, (Eds.), *Readings in applied English linguistics, 3rd Edition* (pp. 417–427). New York: Knopf.

Winograd, P. M. (1984). Strategic difficulties in summarizing texts. *Reading Research Quarterly, 19,* 404–425.

Wolfe, M. B. W., Schreiner, M. E., Rehder, B., Laham, D., Foltz, P. W., Kintsch, W., & Landauer, T. K. (1998). Learning from text: Matching readers and text by latent semantic analysis. *Discourse Processes, 25,* 309–336

Zakulak, B. L., & Samuels, S. J. (Eds.). (1988). *Readability: Its past, present and future.* Newark, DE: International Reading Association.

Zampa V., & Lemaire B. (2002). Latent semantic analysis for user modeling, *Journal of Intelligent Information Systems, 18*(1), 15–30.

10

Analysis and Comparison of Automated Scoring Approaches: Addressing Evidence-Based Assessment Principles

Kathleen Scalise
University of Oregon

Mark Wilson
University of California, Berkeley

> *The only man who behaved sensibly was my tailor; he took my measurements anew every time he saw me, while all the rest went on with their old measurements and expected them to fit me.*—George Bernard Shaw (1903, Man and Superman, Act 1).

This book presents a variety of approaches to automated scoring for computer-based assessments. In this chapter, our task is to try and compare among the various approaches, giving our consideration to strengths and weaknesses. In order to do so, we need to adopt a common perspective on how assessments function. For this purpose, we will use the principles of the Berkeley Assessment and Evaluation Research (BEAR) Assessment System (Wilson & Sloane, 2000). These principles place evidence-centered ideas in a practitioner's context, and consider what the role and range of assessment evidence can and should be.

Before introducing BEAR principles, we should first consider what we mean by "technology" when we speak of automated scoring. Commonly when considering how technology may help in assessment, developers often tend to focus on what we might call *information processing* technology, such as the technology used to distribute assessments to respondents, record responses, score responses and generate reports.

Interestingly, however, the traditional technology associated with assessment, and the one that has been around much longer in educational measurement, has to do with technology for the *statistical interpretation of scores*, or in other words, measurement technology. This means that once a student has completed an assessment and has been assigned scores on *items* (questions and tasks), using whatever approach whether online or offline, s*tatistical technology* helps us understand measurement issues such as (a) how likely would we be to get the same result if we measured again, and (b) are certain items or tasks biased (i.e., show a tendency to unfairly favor certain individuals over others) and so forth.

A third type of technology involved in assessment has to do with the content-based underpinnings of test development and interpretation, addressing questions such as (a) what is the fundamental construct we are measuring; (b) what are the interpretable levels of the construct that can be defined; and (c) question and task creation. This might be called the *construct technology*.

Together, these three types of technology considerations—information processing technology, statistical technology and construct technology—comprise what we might call, "the technologies of assessment" (Wilson, 2003). All three must be considered together in any comprehensive discussion of automated scoring.

This volume on automated scoring covers an interesting blend of these assessment technologies. Chapter authors combine both statistical and information processing technology innovations to explore what might be most useful for automatic scoring of online assessments. Throughout the discussion in this review chapter, we should keep in mind that although automated scoring can be an important consideration in large-scale testing such as accreditation and achievement examinations, it is also a key consideration in the rapidly growing field of computer-based testing (CBT) more broadly, such as in e-learning products and in classroom-based assessments. This emerging CBT market emphasizes formative assessments, individualized learning materials, dynamic feedback, cognitive diagnosis, course placement considerations, and assessment as metacognitive intervention for students and teachers, especially in higher education and adult education where the digital divide is much less of a limitation than in K–12.

In order to analyze the many technology innovations explored in this book, we will next introduce the four BEAR principles for assessment, which should be addressed to support the premise of evidence-centered design:

1.   Developmental perspective;

2.   Match between instruction and assessment;

3.   Generation of quality evidence; and

4.   Management by instructors or other targeted users of assessment data, to allow appropriate score reporting, feedback, feed forward, and follow-up, as the case may be depending on the purpose of the assessment.

BEAR Assessment Principle 1, having a developmental perspective of student learning, most directly means building a system with the potential to interpret the development of student understanding of particular concepts and skills over time, as opposed to, for instance, making a single measurement at some final or supposedly significant time point. Of course, should the needs of the assessment tool be a one-time summary score, a developmental perspective might be considered to be less important—but in this case we argue that it is crucial to be able to consider how the distribution of students represents a range of development of student understanding, and to be able to map this distribution back to a meaningful interpretation of the construct. This is usually done by having some type of criteria describing what is being measured, and the ranges of performance that might be expected. We look at how each chapter addresses this concept of development perspective. BEAR Assessment Principle 1 sets up the purpose of the assessment.

BEAR Assessment Principle 2, the match between instruction and assessment, implies not that the needs of assessment must drive instruction, nor that the description of instruction will entirely determine the assessment, but rather that the two, assessment and instruction, must be in step—they must both be designed to accomplish the same thing, the aims of learning, whatever those aims are determined to be. Many large-scale assessment developers claim that a virtue of their assessment instruments is that they are not closely tied to a curriculum or instructional approach, but in this case the match between instruction and assessment comes down to a match between learning goals (for instance, "standards") and what is measured by the test. BEAR Assessment Principle 2 establishes important constraints on the test that allow for meaningful interpretation.

BEAR Assessment Principle 3, quality evidence, gets to the technical heart of evidence-centered design. Technical problems with reliability, validity, fairness, consistency or bias can quickly sink any attempt to measure students, scored automatically or otherwise. To ensure comparability of results across time and context, procedures are needed to (a) examine the coherence of information gathered using different formats; (b) map student performances onto meaningful constructs to address validity concerns; (c) describe the structural elements of the accountability system—for instance, tasks and raters—in terms that can consider their effects; and (d) establish uniform levels of system functioning, especially quality control indices such as reliability. Although this type of discussion can become very technical to consider, it is sufficient to keep in mind that the traditional elements of assessment standardization, such as validity and reliability studies and bias and equity studies, must be considered in evidence-centered assessment design. It is not enough to have evidence: procedures must be in place to ensure the evidence satisfies the usual quality control rules and expectations.

BEAR Assessment Principle 4, management by instructors or other relevant audiences (including the students themselves), suggests that if information from the assessment tasks is to be useful, it must be couched in terms directly related to the instructional goals and must reach the audiences who are intended to have the information. In large-scale testing, this suggests score reports need to be meaningful and to reach points in the educational system where the data can be used for intervention, for instance at the student, teacher, school, district, state or other level, depending on the purpose of the assessment. Furthermore, open-ended and other complex tasks, if used, must be quickly, readily, and reliably scorable. Here, of course, automated scoring and computer-based systems, as this book points out, can offer advantages that are hard to match offline. Note, however, that especially for class-room based assessments, BEAR Assessment Principle 4 suggests there should be a balance between the time constraints and needs of instructors for automatic machine scoring against the metacognitive needs of students to have their instructors understand, engage and react to information about student levels of performance. An example where a failure to consider the broader context can be problematic is where automated scoring derails the feed-forward loop of student progress to instructors, which can weaken rather than enhance the educational goals.

As we consider each scoring approach in the prior chapters, and as in the future one might assess approaches that come on the scene in the emerging arena of online assessment, we encourage attention to how all four of these principles are addressed. Take away any one principle and the whole threatens to topple—without knowing what you want to measure, how can you design what to measure it with or how to interpret the scores obtained? Conversely, without quality observations and sound interpretation that pays attention to validity and reliability, there is less basis for believing that what you wanted to measure really has been measured.

As a quick review of the chapter contents to be reviewed here, chapter 2 describes evidence-centered design. Chapter 3 provides an overview of human scoring, but much of the chapter addresses issues of construct development, specifically the problems of consistent scoring and rater reliability in the absence of well-developed ideas about what is being measured. Chapter 4 explores the power of assessments when the construct is modeled through the extraction of rules for scoring from work products that satisfy clearly defined performance standards. This is a scoring approach that uses complex "rules" encoded into programming algorithms, by which computers score according to a usually fine-grained and codified understanding of what is being measured. Chapters 5 through 9 focus primarily on a variety of statistical approaches to scoring, score adjustment, or score accumulation. They base their innovations mostly on unique approaches to measurement methods, and therefore the authors mainly are discussing innovations in statistical technology rather than information processing technology as a basis for automated scoring in their examples.

Most of the examples in these later chapters explore how data that computers are good at collecting, such as frequency counts for how often a certain behavior is performed, can be manipulated with statistical models to say something meaningful about what a student can do. In Chapter 5, a regression-based transformation is applied to certain frequency measures based on the assumption that regression analysis can show how to "weight" evidence from such observations to statistically identify high performing and lower performing students. Chapter 6—Testlet Response Theory—suggests what to do when assessment questions share common material, thus violating statistical assumptions of independence between items in measurement models. Chapter 7 discusses how surface features of writing as well as vector methods such as latent semantics—the most commonly known versions of latent semantics are concept maps—can be converted into proxy measures for linguistic assessment and interpreted with measurement models. This chapter raises the challenge of how relevant proxy measures are to measurement. Chapter 8 uses neural networks for another type of exploratory measurement analysis, also employing a regression-based transformation but capitalizing on the fact that neural nets are able to use nonlinear and hierarchical approaches to identify patterns in a collection of data. Finally, chapter 9 explores Bayesian networks, which use some observed measures, combined with conditional probabilities on other related measures, to infer the probability of unobserved outcomes. Each chapter is explored in the following sections.

We noticed that one area where much of the emerging work in automated scoring is now taking place is not discussed in this book, so we will mention it briefly here. It involves the *design* of assessment tasks and responses, or in other words part of what we previously included in the category of *construct technology*. An especially fertile area here for automated scoring involves assessment questions and tasks constructed such that responses fall somewhere *between* fully constrained responses—such as the traditional multiple-choice question that is sometimes far too limiting to tap much of the potential of new information technologies—and fully constructed responses, such as the traditional essay, which remains a formidable challenge for computers to meaningfully analyze, even with sophisticated statistical tools such as those just discussed. We call these "intermediate-constraint" items. Intermediate-constraint item and task designs are beginning to be used in CBT, with response outcomes that are promising for computers to readily and reliably score, while at the same time offering more freedom for the improvement of assessment design and the utilization of computer-mediated functionality. In another publication, we have described a 16-class taxonomy of iconic intermediate-constraint item types that may be useful for automated scoring (Scalise, 2003). Intermediate-constraint tasks can be used alone for complex assessments or readily composited together, bundled and treated with bundle (testlet) measurement models to form a nearly endless variety of complex task designs (Scalise & Wilson, 2005), that are often readily scorable by machine.

It should be noted that some of the most successful examples of automated scoring in this book also utilize intermediate-constraint item designs, although this is not in most cases explicitly discussed by the chapter authors. For instance, in the case of the Bayesian nets NetPASS example, the authors have interesting work in "point-and-click" item development, in which data is selected and assembled from tables, and used by students in response to items (Mislevy, 2001). Such an example falls within the iconic intermediate-constraint types we have identified. It is readily computer scored, as the computer can record which elements are selected and how they are assembled, and experts can decide in advance how the various permutations of elements and assembly would be scored. Possible combinations of response are numerous enough to generate data that can discriminate among different types of respondent thinking and strategy. For instance, the response possibilities can be in the range of tens to hundreds of patterns compared to five or less for standard multiple-choice, but still arguably well within reasonable quantities for experts in advance to group and score meaningfully.

We now return to reviewing the chapters, and start again at chapter 2. In the National Research Council report, "Knowing What Students Know: The Science and Design of Educational Assessment" (Pellegrino, Chudowsky, & Glaser, 2001), the authors state that whether formative or summative, every assessment involves three elements: a model of student cognition and learning, observations of the student, and an interpretation of what the observations mean in order to relate them back to student cognition and learning. This is directly related to the assessment needs as outlined in chapter 2 of this volume, "Evidence-Centered Design."

In ECD:

1. The model of cognition is represented as the "student model" in the terminology of evidence-centered design. This is the concept of a construct in Bear Principle 1 and can, for instance be a framework for what components are to be measured, such as based on sets of standards, or the specification of variables that show a theoretical view of developing knowledge in a field, among other approaches.

2. The observation component of assessment, which represents the questions and activities by which the respondent will be observed, is called the "task model" in chapter 2.

3. The interpretation component of assessment, which maps to the "evidence model" in chapter 2, represents both the outcome space, or scores generated from the responses, and any transformations of scores such as may occur when measurement models are applied.

Throughout this volume, the chapter authors use the terminology of evidence-centered design to explore how each chapter example addresses these assuredly key assessment concepts. These concepts are very important in measurement and chapter 2 does an excellent job of exploring why they are important. Thus chapter 2 is a key chapter for this volume and additionally an excellent resource for anyone wishing to better understand the purposes of assessment. One caveat, however, is that the terminology and representations employed in chapter 2, and generally throughout the conceptualization of evidence-centered design, may confuse some readers, especially if they do not come to assessment with the information processing background from which terms such as *student model* and *task model* are derived.

That said, whatever the terminology and representations employed to discuss these core assessment concepts, take away any one leg of the assessment process that the concepts represent and the whole threatens to topple—for example, without knowing what you want to measure, how can you design what to measure it with or how to interpret the scores obtained? Conversely, without quality observations and sound interpretation that pays attention to validity and reliability, there is less basis for believing that what you wanted to measure has been measured. Chapter 2 thus describes extremely important assessment considerations that directly bear directly on automated scoring approaches.

Of course, for online assessment settings, these core ideas of assessment can be placed within a larger framework that represents augmentations provided by the technology or that are necessary to implement the technology. The Conceptual Assessment Framework (CAF) introduces this larger framework, including: considerations for the computer environment and interface specifications; the delivery mechanism, for instance via Internet, CD, server or other mechanism; and specifications for the order in which items are delivered.

As described in chapter 2, these various components of online assessment can take on many different manifestations and suit many different assessment approaches, with the caveat that each must be adequately addressed for the assessment purpose of the instrument.

Chapter 3, "Human Scoring", describes an important element in human scoring as "the variability introduced by raters into the scores," citing subjectivity on scoring more open-ended tasks and questions as a long-standing problem going back a century or more in assessment. The authors review some of the literature in clinical judgment and educational assessment, and conclude that modeling of raters to see how they perform on scoring is necessary to assess reliability. G-theory approaches, item-response facets models and hierarchical rater models are briefly discussed as methods of evaluating and responding to concerns of rater variability.

The crux of the chapter argument is that although automated scoring can come up short if computer approaches to evaluating the evidence are inadequate, so too human scorers have weaknesses, especially if raters must generate scores so quickly that it precludes reflective work or if there is inconsistency in interpreting and executing rubrics across raters. In addition, the cost of employing raters and the infrastructure that may be required to support them, especially under secure conditions for large-scale assessments, can be high.

The rest of the chapter explores case studies of raters and "the unique set of features" individual raters see or look for in a work product. It points out that in "naturalistic and undirected efforts," subject matter experts (SMEs) can bring very different perspectives to scoring. However, this caveat about undirected efforts is very important in interpretation of these case studies. The case studies of human scoring purposely use extremely open-ended scoring designs in which raters intentionally receive little or no instruction or standardization on how to score, or what to look for and value in their judgments. Rubrics and exemplars, standards of good measurement, are *not* provided to raters in order that the case studies can explore a native condition of naive scoring. These conditions, although interesting to explore the concept of what raters natively value, are very different from current assessment practices for human scoring, which call for evidence-centered construct modeling and good practices of rubrics, work product exemplars, scoring moderation, and other mechanisms to bring human scorers into agreement and to model the cognitive construct the instruments are intended to measure (Wilson & Case, 2000). Thus the large inter-rater differences cited in these case studies seem more strongly related to the intentional lack of direction for the raters than to the issues involved in contemporary good practices in human scoring. From another perspective, open-ended informant scoring such as in these case studies can be especially good for rubric generation.

These case studies point out the importance of BEAR Assessment Principle 1, a developmental perspective that allows a clear description of how developing student understanding is to be described within the construct. If we don't know what we intend to measure, how can human raters be expected to measure it consistently? This can be artificially simulated in automated scoring algorithms by implicitly assuming that whatever the algorithm measures, which can be expected to be consistent, is what we intended to measure. But this is a duck-and-cover approach to specifying a construct—duck the difficult specification and let the computer cover for you—and isn't consistent with evidence-centered design. The measurement construct must be well-specified, and also should reflect BEAR Assessment Principle 2, a match between instruction and assessment, or learning goals and assessment, whether the scoring is automated or not.

Other good practices in human scoring that respond to BEAR Assessment Principle 3, good quality evidence, can include spiral rather than nested scoring designs. In spiral designs, one rater scores all cases for a given set of items; in nested designs, one rater scores all items for a given set of cases. Spiral designs help ensure the individuality of a given rater more equally affects all cases. Rater training and timeliness in intervening with inconsistent raters during the scoring process also can be important in protecting against threats to the evidence of the scores. Processes that involve re-rating of selected student responses, in particular rater overlap patterns, such as when two raters score the same work product and discrepancies in scores are referred to a third rater, provide a high standard for good quality evidence on complex assessments and are often implemented for scoring complex assessments.

While the limitations of human scoring may seem oversold in chapter 3, it helps to make the point that good construct modeling is needed in the construct aspect of assessment. Automated scoring may be especially useful when near real-time results are needed or where resource constraints make human scoring problematic or limiting, but there are many situations in which human rating with proper attention to construct modeling has proven a reasonable approach, especially when combined with a variety of overlap rater patterns, for instance in the Graduate Management Admissions Test, where automated scoring also involved one human rater (Enbar, 1999). Certainly for most, if not all, cases of automated scoring within evidence-centered design, human ratings are needed in at least the assessment design process to help specify how the automated scoring should be valued and assigned.

When considering whether to employ automatic scoring, it is furthermore critically important, especially as e-learning approaches move ever more into the area of classroom-based assessment, to consider not only what may be lost or gained in the quality of the inferences made for students, but also what may change for the raters themselves if machine scoring is substituted. This gets to the heart of BEAR Assessment Principle 4, that teachers and other users of the data must be able to interact effectively with the assessment approach. Chapter 3 says the primary goal of selecting the scoring approach "is to maximize construct representation in the least costly fashion." Yet especially in formative assessment situations where many e-learning products with automatic scoring systems are rapidly being deployed, they may be replacing teachers who currently are performing as raters. This can profoundly affect (a) the feed-forward loop by which teachers monitor student understanding, and also (b) the role of human scoring as a powerful professional development tool for teacher instructional practice. Teacher scoring is an intervention targeted at the metacognitive functioning of teachers, with the practice of evaluating assignments not only offering teachers the opportunity to give direct feedback to students, but also providing a feed-forward loop by which teachers can monitor their instructional practice and the resulting student understanding. It should be noted that although chapter 3 says that human scoring occurs most frequently "as part of large-scale assessment," the scoring that teachers do in classrooms everyday probably far exceeds anything done in large-scale assessments.

Furthermore, even in the context of large-scale assessments, as described in Bennett's chapter on future directions for automated scoring, human experts may be preferable in a variety of scoring contexts if they are more readily "justified to disciplinary communities (e.g., writing instructors)" and this may need to be a consideration in the choice of scoring method.

The assertion in chapter 3 that the assessment literature shows the "persistent superiority" of statistical scoring over human scoring also needs some contextualizing. As other chapters in this book indicate, sometimes automated computer scoring approaches can match or beat human reliability, in other cases not. This usually depends on how well the tasks lend themselves to interpretation by the computer, and what supports and models are in place for human scoring. However, what is discussed as "statistical scoring" throughout the chapters of this book often means an actuarial approach that refers not to computer automated scoring of *individual* items, but to statistical interpretation of *combined or accumulated* scores over an instrument or instruments. Just as in all tests for statistical significance, computers can be very good at comparing complex patterns of data and aggregating and summarizing results according to specified statistical transformations. Human raters of course would be challenged to match machine results for such statistical patterns of scoring in the evidence accumulation phase, just as people would have a hard time generating an accurate regression equation by glancing at a dataset—but this does not suggest that scoring of individual items requires or necessarily lends itself to the same computational burdens or that computers always offer the clear advantage for evidence identification. Indeed, the chapter describes human scoring in the evidence identification stage as a strength of humans. Thus, it is important to consider whether the computer is being used for actual scoring of complex tasks and items, or for informative statistical ways of combining the scores to obtain consistent results once item-level scores, frequency counts, or other data minings have already taken place.

One caveat for statistical models that aggregate human scores and can estimate rater parameters is what to do with the information they provide.

Should the performance estimates of individual students actually be adjusted when they involve scores from raters who overall are found to be "lenient" or "harsh" relative to other raters? This raises fairness concerns. In actual practice, it is more likely that these models are used to, for instance, confirm that raters are scoring consistently or to identify raters who need more training or need scoring intervention (Wilson & Case, 2000).

The authors of chapter 4, rule-based methods and mental modeling, discuss traditional elements of human scoring—such as the establishment of detailed scoring rubrics, calibration of grading practices against a set of work products, and the representation of known performance standards—as foundational building blocks for rule-based methods. Here, rule-based methods are defined as groups of "if–then logical analyses," written into programming code, that represent "a consensus of the best evaluative practices of human expert graders." Scores identified at this grain size are then combined, or accumulated, according to further hierarchical rules, here called *mental modeling*. Thus scoring in a rule-based approach primarily is evidence identification, built on mining the processes of human scoring to define logical and reproducible scoring algorithms for items and tasks.

In many rule-based systems, much attention is paid to BEAR Assessment Principle 1, developmental perspective, and BEAR Assessment Principle 2, the match of assessment with instruction or with learning goals. Constructs are extensively described by area experts in order to codify scoring rules. Scoring rules are machine-tested and iteratively improved by content experts with item construction, critique, and revision, incorporating such details as exceptions to scoring rules identified by new work products.

For strongly codified domains with direct and well-understood relationships, such as troubleshooting flow-charts used to train on or fix mechanical systems, these rule-based expert systems have been in use for some time. The authors state that for "relatively open-ended assessment tasks," presumably such as would allow multiple pathways for solution and could result in original solutions, this approach is still in its early stages.

The chapter example shows rule-based methods and mental modeling for scoring the Architectural Registration Examination, a national test battery for licensure, which according to the chapter authors was the first fully computerized licensure test to operationally incorporate complex automated scoring. The exam consists of multiple-choice items combined with several graphic design tasks that require the examinee to draft architectural structures and layouts on the computer.

In this example, no examinee ability estimate is ever explicitly estimated. The "evidentiary requirement" for the exam is to determine whether or not the examinee can achieve a minimum cut score for competency. This is key in this example because the rule-based methods and subsequent mental modeling of this example do not need to "support making fine distinctions between different levels of competent practice," or to show growth in competency over time, both of which would put much more pressure on fine-tuning the automated scoring approaches and rule-based accumulation. Instead in the development of scoring algorithms, an acceptable or unacceptable mark was specified such that by expert opinion it was highly likely the examinee possessed or did not possess the ability measured by the feature being assessed. Indeterminate marks on a feature were awarded by the rule-based system if actions taken were not highly probable to be acceptable or unacceptable, and more measurement proceeded.

Because rule-based systems often require fairly elaborate models of human scoring based for instance on extensive think-aloud protocols, cognitive task analysis and committee/expert decisions to determine relevant factors to be extracted from the candidate's solution, the grain size of the analysis needed can become a limiting factor. Also, although the chapter authors do not emphasize it, the scored tasks cited here use item designs that lend themselves to computer data collection—for instance, in the drawing of structures that do or do not exceed architectural setback limits, the computer can readily capture and store x–y coordinates drawn on screen by the examinee and compare these against the tolerance of allowed targets. This type of item design is an intermediate-constraint type, as discussed earlier in this review chapter, and allows a readily scorable constructed response in which the variable measured would be considered a "direct assessment" of the targeted knowledge—if the goal is to assess understanding of setback limits, then the examinee is directly constructing diagrams that do or do not meet setback limit specifications.

Weaknesses of rule-based systems of course include the challenges of constructing appropriate rules. BEAR Assessment Principle 3, high-quality evidence, can sometimes be jeopardized from a psychometric standpoint in rule-based systems. Possible threats to validity, the chapter authors argue, include the rejecting of certain assessment tasks because constructing rule-based automated scoring would be too difficult, possibly introducing a selectivity of tasks that underrepresents the construct. Threats to reliability evidence in many rule-based systems include the absence of a probabilistic ability estimate, and therefore possibly more limited information on the certainty and standard errors surrounding the awarding of scores. The chapter authors point out that rule-based logic without an uncertainty mechanism "implies that for each profile of performance the corresponding inference is known with certainty," which is a strong assumption often without sufficient evidence for it to be tested. Sometimes fuzzy logic and other comparison approaches are combined with rule-based methods to address such concerns, but not often. Also, often equating of items is less feasible in rule-based systems than with standard psychometric methods, making securing the item pool of extreme importance, and item leaks possibly difficult to detect, because parameter drift tests and other such standard evidence are not necessarily available to this method.

However, rule-based systems, when they are well designed and appropriate to a given domain, seem promising regarding BEAR Assessment Principle 4, the management of systems by instructors and others who need to employ the evidence. Because the scoring approach so closely matches human scoring, scores on items and tasks are often readily understood and their relationship to the construct more transparent to instructors than in statistical scoring methods such as are the topic of later chapters of this book. Furthermore, assessment blueprints and score reports can lean on the well-explicated constructs to explain the assessment design and to make examinee scores meaningful for the appropriate audiences.

By contrast, chapter 7[1], "Strategies for Evidence Identification through Linguistic Assessment of Textual Responses," has both a finer grain target— accurate essay scoring over the range of possible scoring rather than a dichotomous cut score decision—and measures that are more indirect than the architectural example of chapter 4. In chapter 7, essay scoring examples range from correlations with "simple, surface features of the text," such as average sentence length and counts of commas, to more sophisticated linguistic analysis, such as how often past-tense verbs and third-person pronouns are used within an essay, combined with factor analysis to identify dimensions of text variation. An example applied to a large set of NAEP writing samples uses simple surface features of writing style combined with spell checkers and other emerging automated technologies to obtain a .87 agreement with human scorers. The authors note considerable resistance to this indirect approach, however, citing criticisms ranging from face validity about grading essays on "style" rather than on content to coachability on the indirect variables.

The authors continue their explorations of automatic linguistic analysis by next considering vector space methods, or how closely together words occur in the essay, for instance "the same paragraph, the same sentence, or within a window of 1, 2, 3, or n words." All such information "derives from patterns of co-occurrence within text."

The vector space methods scoring approach moves radically away from the expert-based and rule-based construct modeling employed in chapters 3 and 4. In these earlier chapters, the rules of scoring were "construct-centered" and drew

---

[1] For the sake of a contrast we wish to make at this point, we will skip reviewing chapters 5 and 6 for the moment and return to them later in this chapter.

on a performance construct and expert analysis to specify the preferred performance characteristics. According to the chapter 7 authors, vector-space methods, perhaps most commonly known in latent semantics through concept map designs, "accept much weaker evidence in much larger quantities," and rely on statistical techniques to extract meaningful correlations that might not be apparent to a human rater. Thus, the evidence accumulation validity may be less interpretable from a human perspective than in some other automated scoring approaches.

In the simplest "bag-of-words" form, vector space methods simply categorize the presence or absence of particular words tracked to generate a score. In more sophisticated latent semantic analysis, the distance between words is considered, but usually not word order. The authors present compelling information that such statistical word location scoring models can correlate well with human scorers. However, as the authors say, there is always the concern that even with high correlations between the proxy and construct measures, caution must be exercised as the correlation may be mediated through a number of intermediate "noise" variables.

From the point of view of BEAR Assessment Principle 1, obfuscation of why measures and scoring are related to the construct can be problematic. When primarily statistical measures make the score identification or interpretation link to the construct, addressing this principle calls for building a theoretical case for the high correlation of proxy variables, and implies a responsibility for investigating intervening lurking variables that may throw off construct measurement.

Just as important, however, is BEAR Assessment Principle 2, the match between instruction and assessment, and BEAR Assessment Principle 4, instructor management. When scoring models fail to take structural and positional information of words and phrases into account, and are not capable of delving into actual "mean-making" in essay construction, this may not meet key goals of instruction in this area. This would seem to leave vector space methods with some of the same face validity and coachability concerns as previously cited for the more primitive surface feature models, with teachers perhaps instructing students to write essays that throw in the right words in certain patterns, but paying less attention to meaningful arguments and supportive evidence in writing development. In other words, "what gets measured gets taught" and whether the measure is indirect by statistical analysis or indirect by surface analysis, indirect proxy measures can tweak instruction toward the proxy rather than the intended construct. Should this happen, it would be a case of assessment driving instruction rather than finding an appropriate balance with learning goals.

However, as a caveat to this, often a current practice in complex assessment scoring when automated scoring is employed, such as for the Graduate Management Admission Test discussed in chapter 11, is to have each work product rated by a person as well as a computerized approach, which is seen as a persuasive compromise that reduces the scoring burden while maintaining strong construct validity. A direct assessment of quality is applied by human scorers and an indirect assessment by the statistical models, which have been previously validated for good reliability with human scoring. Of course, as is usual in dual-rater patterns, scores that differ substantially between the two scoring approaches, by some set target, should be flagged and re-evaluated in some way.

For more examples of where the field is moving with textual analysis, readers may be interested in learning more about the ETS E-rater and C-rater products. E-rater provides a holistic score for an essay, with a companion product, Critique, that provides near real-time feedback about grammar, mechanics and style as well as essay organization and development. E-rater employs a combination of feature analysis, vector space methods and linguistic analysis. E-rater 2.0 was reviewed in a 2004 study (Attali & Burstein, 2004) that looked at scoring results from 6th to 12th grade users of Criterion as well as GMAT and TOEFL (Test of English as a Foreign Language) essay data. It reviewed students who completed two essays and compared the scores as test-retest scores. E-rater had a reliability of .6 as compared to .58 when human raters scored. Although the raw score correlation was not reported in the review paper, the "true-score" correlation, or correlations after scores were corrected for unreliability, between E-rater and human scoring was reported as very high (.93).

C-rater by comparison is intended to automatically analyze short-answer open-ended response items. C-rater is designed to recognize responses that "paraphrase" correct responses, looking for syntactic variations, substitution of synonyms and the use of pronouns, as well as misspelling. It was reviewed in a 2004 study (Leacock, 2004) of a large-scale assessment of 11th graders in Indiana that scored 19 reading comprehension and five algebra questions. Over a sample of 170,000 short-answer responses in this study, C-rater was found to obtain 85% agreement with human raters.

Of course, as chapter 11 points out, and relevant to BEAR Assessment Principle 3 of standards for high quality evidence, reliability matching human scoring and high machine-human agreement are only *some* relevant pieces of evidence in a validity/reliability argument. As evidence-centered design strategies suggest, building a case for why the automated scoring approach effectively measures the construct, and bringing forward external validity and other evidence is also needed for the scoring criterion comparisons.

The remaining chapters to be reviewed continue and extend the use of advanced statistical models for automated scoring, with methods varying on the degree to which statistical rather than substantive criteria are used to select variables and weight them in the process of scoring an examinee's performance.

In chapter 5, case management results from a regression-based procedure for automated scoring of a complex medical licensure assessment are evaluated. The statistical method used to generate scores—regression—was found to successfully compare with human inter-rater reliability. Here, in regard to BEAR Assessment Principle 1, observables in this example that are scored by the computer directly reflect important performance characteristics for the construct measured, such as frequency counts of inappropriate and appropriate medical tests specified for the hypothetical patient in the case study. As compared to an example such as the latent semantics statistical approach previously discussed, the regression approach of chapter 5 is thus a much more direct measure, and less fraught with the complexities of using indirect or proxy measures.

Because scores in this example are meaningful relative to the construct, a good match between instruction and/or learning goals and assessment (BEAR Assessment Principle 2) seems possible, depending on the selection of variables and how much careful attention is paid to the articulation process. However, because weightings of the score variables are automatic in this statistical process, it would be important to select cases in which the *weight* of assessment variables for the scores properly reflected their relative importance in learning goals.

Here, with direct measures and reasonable reliability in the norming sample as compared to human scoring, the utility of automated scoring seems to rest, in part, on how well the empirical data can be expected to satisfy the statistical models employed and how well the statistical models capture the variance in the data. These are issues in regard to BEAR Assessment Principle 3, the quality of evidence. A good deal of unexplained variance in the modeled data could of course be problematic. As is the case whenever statistical methods are employed, relevant assumptions should be satisfied within the robustness of the statistical test to the assumptions, for instance as in the case of linearity and normality assumptions. The regression model must also capture performance of the respondent population, accounting for unspecified variables that might affect the score assignments. If hierarchical data is employed to generate model parameters, such as students within schools, it may be important that the model reflects the nested nature and within-class or within-school dependency of the data, for instance employing multilevel modeling in which some parameters are specified as variable over schools rather than fixed. Of course, such considerations could introduce considerable scoring complexity and may not be easy or straightforward to implement.

In the simplest form in this example, seven independent variables were included in the regression equation. Three variables represented counts of good actions taken by examinees in simulated case studies, three represented counts of bad actions taken by examinees, and the last variable represented how quickly the examinee worked by recording when the last of the essential actions was taken. Other treatments included, for instance, adding variables on the ordering of actions, because the order in which actions were taken could make a difference in treatment outcomes. In general, each simulated case study was scored with its own regression equation.

Generalizability analyses were used to examine the comparison generalizability of human ratings, regression-based scores and rule-based scores. Findings included that regression-based procedures were more generalizable than the rule-based approach used in this example and as generalizable as scoring based on using a single human rater, but less generalizable than scoring based on using an overlap pattern of four human raters per each work product. Of course four raters would be a very high evidence standard.

In regard to BEAR Assessment Principle 4, whether or not regression-based scoring procedures could be well-managed by instructors and/or the relevant users of the data, this would seem to depend on how well the regression-based scoring could translate transparently into understandable score reports and, in formative settings, whether or not instructors could generate or tailor their own assessment items and still employ a regression-based scoring algorithm. This last concern impinges on usability for all the more elaborate scoring approaches discussed in this volume: Is there a way for instructors to develop and integrate items into these assessments or are these closed-scoring systems that can only be employed by advanced test developers? It would appear that in most of the examples discussed in this book, with the exception of human scoring, the expertise required to implement the scoring systems precludes instructor development of assessments, unless special tools are developed and made available for this purpose. This last might be a good future direction of research for the field.

Chapter 6 introduces a testlet approach to handling local dependence within groups of items. This chapter is somewhat different than the other chapters in the volume because it does not include an automated scoring example but instead suggests approaches for dealing with dependency in complex items, whether online or off line. Testlets generally are a set of assessment items or tasks that share some common stimulus material, common context, or other common element. Often in measurement language they also are called "item bundles" (Rosenbaum, 1988). Bundles of items that share common elements violate conditional independence assumptions in many measurement models. Therefore the simpler models may overestimate the precision of estimate, thus overestimating the reliability of the overall instrument. They also may jeopardize the evidence accumulation process and throw off parameter estimation, for instance.

However, as an item type, testlets are a promising format in computer-based assessment. By allowing numerous assessment items within a single context, a richer exploration of an assessment can take place, for instance with simulations, case studies, new media inclusion, and other items designs that build a body of shared content and take advantage of the powerful representations of the electronic platform.

Polytomous IRT approaches have often been used to handle the modeling of dependency in testlets, although chapter 6 authors argue that this discounts the available information too much and is an overly conservative model for handling testlets, although they do not discuss IRT-type approaches that make full use of the vector of item information in each bundle (Wilson & Adams, 1995). Chapter 6 proposes an alternative model, where a within-testlet effect is used to correct for local dependence within each testlet or item bundle.

Presumably, a variety of testlet effect models could be anticipated in the family described by the authors, for instance in which there is a standard testlet effect estimated for certain types of bundles, or in which each testlet is modeled with a unique effect parameter. Authors here add a testlet effect parameter to a 3PL IRT model for dichotomous items and to an ordinal response model for polytomous items. MCMC estimation is used. The example in this chapter involves applying the new testlet model to human ratings of clinical skills in a medical certification exam. The 8-hour assessment consists of 10 simulated encounters with patients.

As the chapter authors describe, the testlet effect parameters can be thought of as student ability estimates that apply to a given testlet only. In other words, the parameters project how much a given student is helped or hurt by the fact that the entire set of items for one particular testlet is in that particular context, or shares those common elements. If for instance an entire simulated encounter on a general skills instrument regarded diagnosis and treatment of pneumonia and a particular examinee had, by chance, specialized in this area but other examinees had not, the pneumonia specialist could be expected to score higher on that particular testlet than his or her general proficiency score might otherwise suggest. The testlet effect parameters would estimate and attribute this difference not to the examinee proficiency but to the presence of the testlet.

The authors describe how they obtained more accurate estimates of uncertainty by properly accounting for local dependence, how ease of equating was improved and how their model more closely mirrored the structure of the test.

From the perspective of the BEAR Assessment Principles, the testlet models as discussed in this example mostly address BEAR Assessment Principle 3, the quality of evidence. The proposed testlet models help us do a better job of handling issues such of dependency that threaten to undermine reliability estimates in complex assessments with common elements.

Testlets can be a nice unit for item design, especially on a computer platform. They allow a powerful approach to construct modeling, since the testlet can be a question or task and series of subsequent probes that adaptively move up and down a construct. Testlets can closely align instruction and assessment, so the entire assessment can become a learning activity. Testlets can allow for automated scoring using a wide array of intermediate-constraint item types. These attributes allow testlets to be highly authentic to the classroom experience and still easily constructed and used by instructors. Bundled items can act like any other assessment item, and so are amenable to many current approaches for collection and accumulation of assessment evidence, and can offer such indices as reliability estimates, standard errors, and fit statistics.

Our own work has shown that testlet approaches for item design, teamed with multifacet bundle models to control for dependency, can be effective both for creating rich assessments that can be automatically scored and for generating high quality assessment evidence (Scalise & Wilson, 2005). We developed a computer-adaptive automated scoring approach with testlets for dynamically delivered content, in which homework sets adjusted for individual students depending on embedded assessment information and using IRT models for evidence accumulation. This was a first implementation of BEAR CAT: "Berkeley Evaluation & Assessment Research Computer Adaptive Tools." We found reasonably high reliability for the BEAR CAT instrument with 15 testlet item bundles—an EAP/PV reliability of .82 as compared to a slightly lower reliability of .80 for a non-adaptive paper-and-pencil comparison post-test instrument with constructed response answers. Also, students were able on average to generate this slightly more reliable score on the adaptive BEAR CAT testlet instrument in about 35 minutes in observational studies as compared to about 50 minutes as reported by teachers for the paper-and-pencil post-test instruments. Three different testlet designs were developed and successfully alpha- and beta- tested with adaptivity in Berkeley's Distributed Learning Workshop *Learning Conductor* Homework Tool (Gifford, 2001). All three bundle designs showed good item discrimination, with a mean of .53 (SD .06), and incorporated automated scoring.

To us the question about testlets includes how this potentially powerful item design can be used most effectively. It may be quite straightforward to estimate a "testlet effect," in which, for instance, the total amount of information from a set of items is in effect "discounted" for the dependency, and in which aggregate scores are adjusted with a variety of transformations that are specified by testlet, or by testlet type. But how is this useful in improving the meaningfulness of scores? If the testlet effect is used only to better represent that the total amount of data available is somewhat less than the number of total items would suggest, because of the dependency, then this is good in terms of score interpretation and is most likely a well-warranted adjustment when dependency is present.

But to reflect back on evidence-centered design and the BEAR Assessment principles, a more powerful use of testlet theory would be to understand how augmenting the measurement model with testlet parameters contributes to the meaningfulness in terms of the construct modeling and task development components of the assessment process. In other words, what does it mean to have a testlet effect? Is one effect over an entire bundle sufficient? Are there meaningful pathways to shared scores in hierarchical and nonhierarchical bundles? Can we anticipate why certain testlets behave in certain ways? What is a meaningful way to describe the within and between reliability of testlets, and what is a meaningful testlet analog for instance to point biserial? What other testlet models might be useful and why?

The caveat here, even truer in the next two chapters we review, is that we may be able to estimate new models before we have a reasonable way to fully utilize the power of what they offer, and to reflect on the meaning of what they tell us. But, as was suggested earlier in our chapter, new items designs, of which intermediate-constraint types and testlets are good examples, may be among the most effective ways to achieve automated scoring of complex online assessments. Thus, the hard work of developing interpretation frameworks must accompany the technical side of model development (De Boeck & Wilson, 2004).

The IMMEX project at UCLA and an artificial neural net exploratory scoring approach provides the example of chapter 8. IMMEX has been involved in innovative approaches to instructional and assessment design in science education for some time, and in a number of areas. Although the project has important goals in modifying task design and developing teaching and learning theory for science classrooms, the primary focus of the chapter in this volume is on IMMEX's approach to accumulation and aggregation of evidence in assessments using artificial neural net statistical models and simulation task designs.

Artificial neural networks are models that attempt to loosely "mimic the massive parallel processing that occurs in the brain" (Harvey, 2003). Real neurons can be thought of as collecting data from their environment and passing information along, or transmitting it, to other neurons. This allows signals to be sent within the body. Although such biological control systems can be complex, the basic idea of the signal is simple. A neuron can for instance receive a signal of 0, not firing, or 1, firing, from other neurons around it. The receiving neuron accumulates the signals—adds them up—over some period of time until a threshold is met. Then the neuron fires and itself delivers a signal.[2]

There are numerous topographies and approaches to the specification of artificial neural network models. The 1PL and 2PL item response models—as well as presumably many other IRT models—are mathematically analogous to semilinear neural net models (Scalise, 2004). Indeed, most IRT and neural-net models, except the neural-net linear function (NNLF), are nonlinear regression models, and can be considered part of the larger class of generalized linear models (De Boeck & Wilson, 2004; McCullagh & Nelder, 1989) which also encompasses the NNLF. To quote Russell and Norvig, authors of a leading textbook in Artificial Intelligence, learning in a nonlinear neural net "just becomes a process of tuning the parameters to fit the data in the training set—a process that statisticians call nonlinear regression" (Russell & Norvig, 1995).

Based on the example in chapter 8, here IMMEX appears to be primarily exploring unsupervised neural networks, which rely on statistical methods alone to extract dominant features of a dataset during "training," or the period in which the model tunes parameters to fit the data. A key issue for such *unsupervised* neural networks in the context of assessment, and reflective of the BEAR Assessment Principle 1 (concern about an appropriate developmental perspective), is that unsupervised neural nets do not incorporate expert opinion, or in other words do not start from a model of a construct. Neither can they be iteratively improved by expert analysis. Results are generated entirely statistically. This gets at the heart of how much automated scoring should rely on substantive as compared to statistical evidence.

The IMMEX "work product" in this example is a trace of all the problem-solving actions a student takes in the course of solving a "case," or complex task (in this example in the area of genetics). IMMEX uses neural networks to cluster, or find meaningful patterns, in the "paths" that students take while

---

[2] Signals can for instance be excitatory—"adding to" the accumulating threshold value of neighboring neurons—or inhibitory, "subtracting from" them. Many different properties of artificial neural networks have been studied, for instance signals that propagate outward or that feedback in loops.

attempting to solve complex assessment items. Paths here for instance include the pattern of computer "library" resources and data sets that students draw on while solving a particular set of problems. The chapter authors state that they believe the path patterns might reveal student thinking about the sequence of steps necessary to reach a logical conclusion, and to eliminate other possible conclusions, but that the performance data might be noisy or rich with outliers.

The IMMEX example employed a 6 x 6 Kohonen neural network grid trained in a diamond configuration.[3] Results included that the predictive power of the model was weak at the grain of the individual node (a 36-node map), but that in grouping over nodes to classify students and their pathway traces into four "states," a prediction accuracy of more than 80% was achieved. The four states were:

- Limited/guessing pathways, which showed evidence of students answering the problem before collecting enough information to make a logical choice.

- Prolific pathways, categorized by the student's access of many resources and a thorough trial-and-error search of nearly the entire problem space.

- Redundant pathways, for which students also participated in a fairly comprehensive search of the data domain, but made the search somewhat more parsimonious by eliminating some redundant resources.

- Efficient pathways, which mostly accessed information relevant to the problem solution.

Students often employed prolific strategies in the first assessment tasks (cases) they attempted, and they tended to switch to Efficient strategies over time, as more tasks (cases) were presented. Also a sample of University students in a study presented in the chapter switched to Efficient strategies sooner than a sample of Community College students, showing some validity evidence of difference in strategy pathway by criterion group (although it is not clear from the information presented in the chapter that the University students in the sample should be expected to be higher performing, or to transition sooner to more effective strategies, than the Community College students).

It is not clear whether a four-state model such as this requires the modeling complexity described in this chapter, or that similar results could not have been achieved with simpler approaches. But it was an interesting exploration and for these chapter authors and the IMMEX project, this is only one exploratory approach among many methods they have employed.

It is also unclear how an unsupervised neural net approach would be reconciled with BEAR Assessment Principle 2, the match between instruction

---

[3] See chapter for a description of this network topography.

and assessment, and BEAR Assessment Principle 4, management by teachers or other intended users of the data, since the statistical process is selecting the dominant features to extract.

In regard to BEAR Assessment Principle 3, high-quality evidence, it is true that neural networks sometimes can be promising in identifying traceable components of patterns in empirical data. However it is not always clear what specific criteria are being iteratively optimized. The greatest successes to date of neural network architectures have been in areas such as natural language processing and image visual processing where the outcome variables are *manifest*. For instance, an artificial neural network might be used in an online search engine to identify the presence of images that include, say, tigers in a particular image bank. The training set might include digitized information on pixel ranges in each photo and the neural network algorithm would also be told which images did and did not include tigers. Even unsupervised, the neural network might be able to identify pixel ranges with an orange frequency, for instance, as one good classification strategy for finding tigers in photos, and might combine this with other patterns discovered, for instance the presence of black stripes in the orange pixel pattern, to come up with a useful algorithm for tiger-finding generally. However, tigers are manifest variables. Given a tiger of sufficient size, it is readily obvious to humans whether or not one is present in a given photo. Thus not only can this information be supplied to the training algorithm with nearly 100% confidence but also once a neural net is "trained" and comes up with its algorithm, the algorithm can readily be tested to see how well it picks out the tigers in another dataset.

Neural networks that attempt to use latent variables as the outcome, as is the case in chapter 8, are much more challenging, because it is not possible to describe with absolute clarity what the proper final classification of the data should be, or what final groups it should be organized into. Although tigers/not tigers can be readily decided on, the relative proficiency of students is harder to specify. So besides the usual difficulties of selecting a useful nodal architecture, which is a challenge for both manifest and latent constructs, concerns of this method for latent spaces often are in interpretability of results for the patterns identified—similar in some senses to the well-known problems of meaningful interpretation of exploratory factor analysis (Loehlin, 1998). IMMEX's interesting solution to validating neural net results for a latent space is to closely tie neural net analysis with construct modeling through the student and task models, allowing theory to provide an explanatory basis for neural net findings, and validating results with other criteria. In this way, IMMEX suggests a similar approach to construct validation and evidence-centered design as introduced in Wilson's BEAR Assessment approach (Wilson, 2005), but with an unsupervised neural network architecture rather than a dimensionally specified item-response model.

It is also unclear how reliability evidence might play out in this neural net context. Note that most neural network architectures to date are calibrated with a step function rather than a sigmoidal or semilinear function, which is what would be called an item characteristic curve (ICC) in IRT. Sigmoidal models in neural net architectures are not considered to be well developed (Russell & Norvig, 1995), although may be rapidly developing. By contrast, the more prevalent step functions are cruder approximations than ICCs and assume zero probability of a respondent exhibiting a correct response until a certain level of student proficiency is reached and then a 100% probability that the item will be achieved. They introduce an absolute certainty assumption that cannot expect to necessarily be well-satisfied by most assessment data. Substituting a sigmoidal function, such as in item response models, would, of course, overcome this concern but estimation complications increase substantially, especially for more elaborate and cyclic neural net architectures.

Chapter 9 introduces Bayesian networks. This approach represents beliefs about student proficiencies as a joint probability distribution over the proficiency variables. The Bayesian network diagram, which is constructed by the developer of the assessment, embodies these beliefs, representing variables in the model as nodes in the network. As for path diagrams in some other statistical models, a key assumption is that any two nodes not directly connected by an arrow are conditionally independent, and can only act on each other through mediating variables.

Note that Bayesian nets should not be conflated with Bayesian estimation, a common confusion among those with limited experience with the Bayes net model. While both rely on Bayes theorem, Bayesian networks adds some strong assumptions not present generally for Bayesian estimation. As Bayesian estimation has secured a strong foothold in the measurement community, this confidence in the use of the method is sometimes inadvertently conferred to Bayes nets as well. Whether or not the additional Bayes net assumptions are warranted for a given situation should be the basic test of use for the Bayes net method.

These assumptions include that building the model requires not only the specification of which variables are conditionally independent, but also (a) the order of how they act on each other as parents and children,[4] and (b) the specification of the full joint distribution of the set of proficiency variables. The

---

[4] Based on assumptions of the method, Bayesian networks are acyclic directed graphs, where the direction of influence points from parent to child nodes, which must be specified. No cycles back to the originating variables are allowed as the network of relationships must be traversed by forward arrows only.

full joint distribution can be specified with starting values (predictions) and updated with empirical data from trials. But as in other path diagram approaches with conditional independence, it is often harder to know how to update assumptions on how the path model itself is specified. A strong theoretical basis usually is required for specifying conditional independence and parent/child node relationships in Bayes nets. Theoretically, many path diagrams could fit the data (Loehlin, 1998), especially as the networks become complex and include more than a few nodes (variables). Yet, results are entirely dependent on the specification of these path assumptions.

This concern about when the conditional independence assumption is justified might suggest simply connecting many nodes in the network. But as for other path models, parsimony is also important. The more relationships specified the more calculations that must be performed to propagate data through the model and achieve an estimate. Nodes with many connections dominate the cost of working with Bayesian network models.

Bayesian networks can be an attractive structure for evidence accumulation as they seem to combine the best of several worlds: the ability to capitalize on the expertise of content experts in the form of the structure of the network, and the advantage of being able to update priors with extensive empirical data. Furthermore, network structures can be highly complex and unconstrained, allowing architectures that seem to better fit real world data (be more authentic) than more constrained linear dimensional or categorical methods. This flexibility argues well for BEAR Assessment Principle 2, the match between instruction or learning goals and assessment. As for artificial neural nets, Bayesian networks are highly flexible and don't face the hard coding limitations of defining scoring rules needed in fine-grained rule-based systems.

However, as an author in this book at one point mentioned, there is "no such thing as a single-edged sword" and the double edge of the Bayesian net is that we have limited tools to "falsify" the network, or in other words to understand whether it is a sound representation of the true structure of constructs measured. Furthermore, varying the network structure and independence assumptions can vastly change assessment results (Russell & Norvig, 1995).

For Bayesian networks to offer a widely useful approach, ways to help content experts express their knowledge through the network specifications need much development and would need to be adapted to a wide range of different possible applications. It is not clear what these ways might be, and how they might be developed.

The example in this chapter is NetPASS, a Cisco Learning Institute assessment of computer networking skills. It is a performance-based instrument and uses simulations and live interactions as tasks in computer network design, implementation, and troubleshooting.

As with neural nets, Bayesian nets have achieved some great success in manifest constructs, such as in medical applications where a disease is clearly present or not present. Use in latent constructs presents formidable challenges to validity and reliability, with arguments analogous to the neural net chapter discussion. However, unlike unsupervised neural networks, in which the variables themselves and the relationships among them are entirely extracted statistically and expert opinion cannot be used to inform and iteratively improve the model, Bayesian network model specifications are often strongly dependent on expert opinion. Indeed, path structure and model fit is often validated primarily by whether the posterior distribution for the variable of interest is similar to the expectations of SMEs. But knowing what this posterior distribution should look like for latent variables is often a huge challenge, and in many cases for latent variables expert opinion can vary vastly. It often depends how strongly the construct and developmental perspective, BEAR Assessment Principle 1, are understood. In summary, although the challenges are formidable, this method's potential power suggests that further exploration is highly warranted.

A few words should be said about the discussion of reliability in the Bayes net chapter. This directly concerns both BEAR Assessment Principle 3, the quality of evidence, and BEAR Assessment Principle 4, management by instructors and, in this case, students. As for other approaches, reliability for a Bayesian network depends mostly on having enough data, usually in the form of enough items, to make a reliable estimate of student proficiency on the variables of interest. The authors of the Bayes net chapter state that for large-scale assessments involving high stakes, this usually means pushing the Bayes net model toward including few variables, since only a few parts of the domain can be well measured. This might imply to the reader that in formative or classroom-based assessment, it is okay to include more variables and achieve low reliability in instruments. This is often the case in Bayesian network approaches, which are so highly flexible that it is tempting to include many variables and perhaps also because many Bayes nets instruments have been developed by technologists rather than measurement professionals. However, the acceptance of low reliability in instruments is a violation of BEAR Assessment Principle 3, which calls for high quality evidence in assessments. Especially when espousing an evidence-centered design to assessments and promoting instruments as representing sound evidence, the consequences of low reliability, whether in summative or formative settings, can be particularly troubling. Speaking generally and not in relation to this chapter example, if Bayes net or any other systems award students with credit for "achieving" proficiencies in certain areas based on an observation in one session and then promptly take the credit away from students in the next session, due to low reliability, this can create problems. Students can be left anxious and concerned about what this means, for instance, how they could have "forgotten" what they "knew." But, in fact, if the instruments have low reliability, developers can easily see that the mastery inference was questionable in the first place. For students, lack of control in being able to effectively monitor their own learning, especially if supposedly sophisticated measurement systems are providing unreliable results that students use to monitor their performance, might have serious consequences. These might include moving some students from mastery learning patterns to helpless learning patterns (Dweck & Leggett, 1988). Questions of fairness, metacognition and effective teaching and learning strategies argue against endorsing instruments with known low reliability. This would be true when employing Bayes nets or other methods.

SUMMARY

In summary, the chapters in this volume provide much food for thought in the rapidly developing field of computer-based assessment and automated scoring. With the surge in availability of assessment software, this is a key time to consider the topics in this volume. For example a paper at the latest General Teaching Council Conference in London, England, on Teaching, Learning and Accountability described assessment for personalized learning through e-learning products as a "quiet revolution" taking place in education (Hopkins, 2004). Automated scoring is an important part of this "revolution." Principles of assessment design that draw on evidence to support inferences clearly need to be a standard in CBT, no matter the method of scoring. These chapters present some thought provoking examples for how such evidence can be accumulated and interpreted—to which we have added a few more ideas, including the BEAR Assessment principles.

In addition to innovations of evidence identification and accumulation as shown in these chapters, we strongly encourage investigation of what can be done with new task designs, for instance with intermediate-constraint types offering many relatively simple solutions for scoring, well suited to the strengths of online environments.

Finally, in weighing the strengths and weaknesses of various automated scoring approaches, we hope the advantages of retaining a bedrock in human scoring also are well appreciated. It is essential that human rating and expertise remain an important component in the development of assessment designs and scoring formats. These may be subsequently automated partially or fully for various degrees of efficiency, timeliness of feedback and so forth, which are very worthy goals. But especially in classroom-based assessments, it is imperative for teachers to have effective feedback, feed-forward and professional development loops in their instructional practice. It would indeed be a technical marvel if we could somehow capture all pertinent assessment knowledge for scoring and store it neatly in a computer—but it would be a terrible shame if in the process we undermined the practice of teachers constructing and informing their own knowledge base to effectively teach students.

REFERENCES

Attali, Y., & Burstein, J. (2004). *Automated essay scoring with e-rater V.2.0.* Paper presented at the Annual Meeting of the International Association for Educational Assessment, Philadelphia, PA.

De Boeck, P., & Wilson, M. (2004). *Explanatory item response models: A generalized linear and nonlinear approach.* New York: Springer.

Dweck, C. S., & Leggett, E. L. (1988). A social-cognitive approach to motivation and personality. *Psychological Review, 95,* 256–273.

Enbar, N. (1999). *This is E-Rater. It'll be scoring your essay today.* Business Week Online, 2003. Retrieved from http://www.businessweek.com/bwdaily/dnflah/jan1999/nf90121d.htm.

Gifford, B. R. (2001). Transformational instructional materials, settings and economics. In *The Case for the Distributed Learning Workshop* (pp. 1–71). Minneapolis, MN: The Distributed Learning Workshop.

Harvey, C. R. (2003). *Campbell R. Harvey's Hypertextual Finance Glossary.* Retrieved from http://www.duke.edu/~charvey/Classes/wpg/bfglosn.htm.

Hopkins, D. (2004 November). *Assessment for personalised learning: The quiet revolution.* Paper presented at the Perspectives on Pupil Assessment, New Relationships: Teaching, Learning and Accountability, General Teaching Council Conference, London, England.

Leacock, C. (2004). Scoring free-responses automatically: A case study of a large-scale assessment. *Examens, 1*(3).

Loehlin, J. C. (1998). *Latent variable models* (3rd ed.). Mahwah, NJ: Lawrence Erlbaum Associates.

McCullagh, P., & Nelder, J. A. (1989). *Generalized Linear Models* (2nd ed.). New York: Chapman & Hall.

Mislevy, R. J. (2001, August). *Modeling conditional probabilities in a complex assessment: An application of Bayesian modeling in a computer-based performance assessment.* Presented at the conference Cognition and Assessment: Theory to Practice, University of Maryland.

Pellegrino, J., Chudowsky, N., & Glaser, R. (Eds.). (2001). *Knowing what students know: The science and design of educational assessment.* Washington, DC: National Academy Press.

Rosenbaum, P. R. (1988). Item bundles. *Psychometrika, 53,* 349–359.

Russell, S., & Norvig, P. (1995). *Artificial intelligence, A modern approach.* Upper Saddle River: Prentice Hall.

Scalise, K. (2003). *Innovative item types and outcome spaces in computer-adaptive assessment: A literature survey.* Berkeley, CA: UC Berkeley Evaluation and Assessment Research (BEAR) Report.

Scalise, K. (2004). *BEAR CAT: Toward a theoretical basis for dynamically driven content in computer-mediated environments.* Berkeley, CA: University of California, Berkeley.

Scalise, K., & Wilson, M. (2005, April). *Bundle models for data driven content in E-learning and CBT: The BEAR CAT approach.* Paper presented at the National Council on Measurement in Education and UC Berkeley Evaluation and Assessment Research (BEAR) Report, Montreal, Canada.

Wilson, M. (2003, April). *The technologies of assessment.* Invited Presentation at the AEL National Research Symposium, Toward a National Research Agenda for Improving the Intelligence of Assessment Through Technology, Chicago, IL.

Wilson, M. (2005). *Constructing measures: An item response modeling approach.* Mahwah, NJ: Lawrence Erlbaum Associates.

Wilson, M., & Adams, R. J. (1995). Rasch models for item bundles. *Psychometrika, 60*(2), 181–198.

Wilson, M., & Case, H. (2000). An examination of variation of rater severity over time: A study of rater drift. In M. Wilson & G. Engelhard (Eds.), *Objective Measurement: Theory into Practice* (Vol. 5; pp. 113–134). Stamford, CT: Ablex.

Wilson, M., & Sloane, K. (2000). From principles to practice: An embedded assessment system. *Applied Measurement in Education, 13*(2), 181–208.

11

Moving the Field Forward: Some Thoughts on Validity and Automated Scoring

Randy Elliot Bennett
Educational Testing Service

> *Where principle is involved, be deaf to expediency.*—James Webb; retrieved February 4, 2006, from www.jameswebb.com/speeches/navalinstaddress.htm

What do we need to do to move the field of automated scoring forward? Before answering that question, we might first consider what factors motivated automated scoring in the first place. The primary factor has, without question, been efficiency. Scoring by human judges is costly and slow. The advent of web-based online scoring—that is, where judges read scanned or typed responses via the Internet—appears to have reduced the cost and increased the speed with which results can be returned to users. There is no costly and time-consuming movement of paper, and no gathering, feeding, or housing of judges. Several major testing companies now commonly use web-based online scoring as a routine component in response processing because they believe it to be an efficiency improvement ("ePEN Electronic Performance Evaluation Network," 2003; "ETS Online Scoring Network," 2003).

Automated scoring can make similar efficiency claims. For the Graduate Management Admission Test, for example, the use of automated scoring allows the program to employ one human rater instead of the two it formerly utilized (Enbar, 1999). For other programs, like the National Council of Architectural Registration Boards' Architect Registration Examination, no human judge is employed (except for quality control), so scoring could, in principle, be immediate.

The claim that automated scoring has achieved efficiency improvements can be most reasonably made under two conditions.[1] The first condition is that

---

[1] This analysis presumes that the test is already electronically delivered and that the question of interest revolves around the incremental cost of automated vs. traditional scoring and *not* around the incremental cost of computer vs. paper delivery.

the process required for preparing the automated system to score responses to new test items is rapid and inexpensive to implement. The second condition is that the examinee volume is large. The greater the examinee volume and the more efficient the scoring preparation for new items, the more competitive that scoring will be vis-à-vis human raters.

Although automated scoring may have achieved, at least in some cases, the efficiency goals of its progenitors, it has yet to achieve fully a potentially more important goal. This goal was, in the beginning, a secondary, almost incidental one. Automated scoring, as Bennett and Bejar (1998) pointed out, allows for relatively fine construct control. That is, the assessment designer can implement through the scoring program the particular set of response features, and a feature weighting, thought to best elucidate the construct of interest. The construct can be tuned by removing features, or reweighting them, at will. Once the best set of features and weights has been selected, it will be implemented consistently. Human scoring, in contrast, affords only gross control because it is more difficult for humans to deal with multiple features simultaneously, to weight them appropriately, and to apply scoring rules consistently (Bejar, chap. 3, this volume; Dawes, 1979).

As noted, we haven't yet achieved that fine construct control to the same extent as our original efficiency goal. Here are some thoughts about how we might approach the former goal more effectively.

AUTOMATED SCORING NEEDS TO BE DESIGNED AS PART OF A CONSTRUCT-DRIVEN, INTEGRATED SYSTEM

In an article titled, "Validity and Automated Scoring: It's Not Only the Scoring," Bennett and Bejar (1998) argued that a computer-based test was a system consisting of a construct definition, test design, and task design; examinee interface; tutorial; test development tools; automated scoring; and reporting. Further, they noted that the interplay among system components needed to be accounted for in scoring-program design and validation because these components affect one another, sometimes in unanticipated ways. Well, it's still not only the scoring!

One of the key contributions of Evidence-Centered Design (ECD; chap. 2, this volume) is that it offers a strong conceptual framework for driving the development of complex assessment systems in a construct-centered way. The models emerging from an ECD approach to assessment design—student, evidence, and task—can drive the other components of the assessment also—the user interface, tutorial, test developer tools, reporting formats, tasks, and automated scoring—so that all the components of a computer-based test work synergistically.

In other words, the ECD approach suggests creating scoring as part of the design and validation of an *integrated* system. Such an approach is very different from the one that has often been taken, especially with automated essay scoring. Here, automated routines were typically created as general modules to be used with testing programs that already included essay components. In such a situation, the existing test provides the context into which the automated scoring system must fit. The construct definition (such as it may be), the examinee interface, the tasks, the rubric, and the human-generated operational scores become a target for the automated scoring system to hit *regardless* of how well-supported the underlying construct might be.

In honoring Harold Gulliksen, Messick (1989) noted that "if you do not know what predictor and criterion scores mean, you do not know much of anything in applied measurement (p. 13)." When we uncritically use human scores as the development model and validation criterion for automated programs, we find ourselves in almost that situation. If we successfully model the scores of a pair (if we're lucky) of human judges devoting (at most) a few minutes per essay, we also model any systematic biases humans bring to the scoring enterprise. This is an odd result, for automated scoring offers the opportunity to *remove* those biases. Why institutionalize them instead through our modeling methodology?

Further, if we do this modeling through step-wise regression—which some scoring mechanisms have routinely used—we cede control, at least to some degree, of the construct to whatever variables best model the particular raters that happened to score, and the particular examinees that happened to respond to, that prompt. We let a statistical, rather than a substantive, criterion decide which variables to choose and how to weight them in determining examinee performance.

A far more satisfying approach would be to go back to first principles, using ECD methods to define the characteristics of good performance in some relevant context (e.g., secondary school), and then design tasks, rubrics, and automated scoring mechanisms built around those characteristics.[2] In this approach, human scores are no longer the standard to be predicted. Rather, once ECD has been

---

[2] Iterative cycles would be anticipated, of course, in a continuing interplay among rational analysis, conjectures about construct-based elements of an assessment system, and empirical tests and model criticism (Mislevy, personal communication, September 10, 2003). This is the basis of any good validation program.

used to define the evidence needed to support claims for proficiency, human scoring is used only to check that the machine scoring is identifying and accumulating that evidence correctly.

I should be clear that the ECD approach does not forsake human judgment. It only uses it differently. That is, human judgment is employed to help define the characteristics of good domain performance (e.g., in writing, architectural design, medical problem solving), the behaviors that would be evidence of it, and the characteristics of tasks that would elicit those behaviors. With respect to scoring, human experts should do what they do best: choose the features of responses to include and their directional relationships to the underlying proficiency (Dawes, 1979). Experts may even be used to determine how to weight each feature because expert weighting may be more easily justified to disciplinary communities (e.g., writing instructors) than empirical weighting, and because experts generally produce weights that are nearly as good as empirically derived ones (Dawes, 1979).[3] Thus, in ECD, the emphasis on human judgment is *up front* in design, and not solely after-the-fact as an outcome to be predicted.

In defining the characteristics of good domain performance, we should be sure to take advantage of cognitive research on what makes for proficiency in that domain. The work on automated essay scoring, for example, has capitalized well on theory in computational linguistics (e.g., Burstein, Kukich, Wolff, Lu, & Chodorow, 1998) and on the psychology of knowledge representation (e.g., Landauer & Dumais, 1997). But there has been little, if any, cognitive *writing* theory incorporated in any of the automated essay scoring work to date even though these systems typically issue scores for writing proficiency.

AUTOMATED-SCORING RESEARCH NEEDS TO USE APPROPRIATE METHODS.

Although the work in some fields of automated scoring has incorporated measurement methods effectively, in other fields the research has not been as rigorously done. Rigor is particularly important for automated scoring because without scientific credibility, the chances for general use in operational testing programs are significantly diminished, especially with the recent emphasis on

---

[3] A second problem with weights derived through regression is that the best linear composite invariably puts greater weight on those features that work most effectively in prediction for the majority of candidates. It is possible that some well-written essays will emphasize features differently than a brute empirical weighting says they should and, thus, get lower machine scores than an astute human judge might give (Braun, personal communication, October 10, 2003).

scientifically based research as a prerequisite for the purchase and use of educational programs and products (Feuer, Towne, & Shavelson, 2002). Such rigor is essential whether the research is done in an experimental setting or is conducted in the context of an operational testing program. The methodological weaknesses include the most basic rudiments of scientific investigation. Some studies fail to describe the examinee population, the sampling method, the evaluation design, how the automated scoring program works, the data analysis methods, or even the results adequately enough to assess the credibility of the work. Other flaws are, perhaps, more subtle. These include reporting results from the sample used to train the scoring program rather than from a cross-validation; using only a single prompt, which offers little opportunity for generalization to *any* universe of tasks; failing to correct for chance agreement, which can be very high when scoring scales are short and the effective range used by human raters is shorter still; combining results across grade levels, producing spuriously high correlations; reporting findings only for a general population, without considering subpopulations; and reporting only exact-plus-adjacent agreement because this is the standard traditionally used for human rating.

Perhaps the most subtle but pernicious flaw is mistaking machine–human agreement for validation. Machine–human agreement is but a piece of evidence in the validity argument (Bennett & Bejar, 1998; Williamson, Bejar, & Hone, 1999). For automated scores, as for any other scores, the validity argument must rest on an integrated base of logic and data, where the data allows a comprehensive analysis of how effectively those scores represent the construct of interest and how resistant they are to sources of irrelevant variance (Messick, 1989). Exemplary in this regard, at least in automated essay scoring, is the work of Powers and colleagues, which represents the only comprehensive comparison of human vs. automated scoring vis-à-vis *multiple* external criteria (Powers, Burstein, Chodorow, Fowles, & Kukich, 2001), as well as the only analysis of the extent to which automated graders can be manipulated into giving scores that are either undeservedly high or low (Powers, Burstein, Chodorow, Fowles, & Kukich, 2000). Studies like these set a standard toward which automated scoring research should strive because they illustrate that it is *validity*—and not just rater agreement or reliability more generally—that should be the standard against which alternative scoring systems should be compared.

AUTOMATED-SCORING RESEARCH NEEDS TO BE PUBLISHED IN PEER-REVIEWED MEASUREMENT JOURNALS.

The results of automated scoring research in medical licensure, mathematics, computer science, and architectural design have been widely published in peer-reviewed measurement journals (e.g., Bejar, 1991; Bennett, Rock, Braun, Frye, Spohrer, & Soloway, 1990; Bennett & Sebrechts, 1996; Bennett, Sebrechts, & Rock, 1991; Clauser, Subhiyah, Nungenster, Ripkey, Clyman, & McKinley, 1995; Clauser, Margolis, Clyman, & Ross, 1997; Williamson, Bejar, & Hone, 1999). Perhaps because of commercial pressures or differences in the disciplinary communities responsible for development, the same cannot be said for automated essay scoring.[4] In this field, the research has appeared as conference papers, in conference proceedings, in linguistics journals, as book chapters, and as technical reports. These dissemination vehicles, while certainly respectable, don't typically get the same level of methodological scrutiny as the peer-reviewed measurement journals. That may be one reason why the automated essay scoring research, on average, hasn't been as rigorous from a measurement perspective as that in other fields. A fair amount of the automated essay scoring research is quite good and would only be improved through such publication.

FUTURE RESEARCH SHOULD STUDY THE USE OF MULTIPLE SCORING SYSTEMS.

The basic idea behind using multiple sources of evidence—be they items, raters, or occasions—is that systematic, valid sources of variance should cumulate and unsystematic, irrelevant ones should wash out (Messick, 1989). Thus, we often have multiple human raters grade the same student productions with the knowledge that, over the long run, the resulting scores will be more generalizable than if they had been rendered by a single judge. We can use the same principle with scoring programs in the hope that different approaches would complement one another by balancing weaknesses—that is, systematic but irrelevant and idiosyncratic sources of variance. We should not expect this approach to work if the automated graders are simply trivial variations of one another. In that case, they will share similar strengths and weaknesses. The greatest chance for success would seem to come from systems that are substantially different in their scoring approaches. In a successful multiple

---

[4] Ironically, work on automated essay scoring predates all other forms of automated scoring by several decades (e.g., Page, 1967).

system approach, the human grader might be able to play a quality-control role, checking only a sample of the machine-scored responses, as is done in the Architect Registration Examination, rather than rating all responses as a human still does for the essay section of the Graduate Management Admission Test.

AUTOMATED SCORING COULD HELP CHANGE THE FORMAT AND CONTENT OF ASSESSMENT

Large-scale assessment currently depends very heavily on one-time, multiple-choice tests. The reasons we use multiple-choice tests so widely are because they can be efficiently scored and because they produce a great deal of generalizable information in a short period. However, educators typically disdain them because they poorly reflect the format, and often the content, students must learn to succeed in a domain. That is, educators see multiple-choice questions as too distant in format and substance from the activities routinely undertaken in the study of school achievement domains. Because they are not closely tied to curriculum, such tests tend to offer little information of immediate use to students and teachers. As a result, we employ them largely for external accountability purposes and administer them as infrequently as possible to limit the disruption of classroom learning.

In conjunction with the Internet, automated scoring has the potential to lighten the influence of the one-time, multiple-choice testing event and better integrate assessment into the curriculum. The Internet provides the means to easily deliver standardized performance assessment tasks to the classroom (Bennett, 2001). Those tasks can be as simple as an essay prompt or they can be more complex, incorporating such dynamic stimuli as audio, video, and animation. Tasks can also be highly interactive, changing how they unfold depending upon the actions that the student takes – much as the simulation section of the United States Medical Licensing Examination does today (United States Medical Licensing Examination, 2003). They could also be designed so that they act—perhaps incidentally, perhaps explicitly—as learning experiences. Such tasks should be very attractive to educators and policy makers, as long as student performance can be automatically scored.

One could imagine such tasks being used in several ways. One way is simply as a means of allowing performance tasks to be used more often in one-time testing events. Performance tasks, like essays, are employed now to a limited degree at great expense and with substantial delay in reporting. Automated scoring has the potential to reduce the cost and delay, and thereby increase the attractiveness of using performance tasks as a component in one-time testing systems.

A second way is formatively; that is, as frequent practice, progress monitoring, or skill diagnosis measures, all in preparation for some culminating one-time assessment. A third possibility is to add a summative layer to this formative use by taking information from each periodic progress measure to supplement the data provided by the culminating assessment. A last possibility is to, at some point, do away with the culminating assessment entirely and let the periodic events bear the full formative and summative weight (Bennett, 1998).

Whether or not it is used in combination with a culminating assessment, any summative use of periodic performance assessment would require tasks built to measure critical domain proficiencies, enough tasks to provide generalizable results, and an evidence model capable of aggregating information across tasks in a meaningful way. Creating such assessments would not be cheaper than creating multiple-choice tests, although the intellectual discipline required for automated scoring should help make task creation more systematic and efficient (Mislevy, Steinberg, & Almond, 2002). In any event, the educational benefits might well outweigh the costs.

CONCLUSION

To sum up this commentary, we can move the field forward by remembering that it's *still* not only the scoring. The hard work in automated scoring is not in mimicking the scores of human raters; it's in devising a scoring approach—and more generally, an assessment—grounded in a credible theory of domain proficiency, be that domain writing, mathematics, medical problem solving, or architectural design. Second, we can move the field forward by conducting rigorous scientific research that helps build a strong argument for the validity of the scores our automated routines produce. Third, we can move the field forward by publishing the results of our research in peer-reviewed measurement journals where the quality of our work is critiqued from a measurement perspective and, hopefully, improved as a result. Regardless of the techniques we use—natural language processing, neural networks, statistical methods—automated scoring is first and last about providing valid and credible *measurement*. Without incorporating measurement principles, and submitting our methods and results to technical review, automated scoring is not likely to be either valid or credible. Fourth, we might move the field forward by attempting to use competing scoring approaches in combination, using multiple pieces of evidence to bolster the meaning of automated scores. Finally, we may be able to use automated scoring to create assessments that are more closely tied to the format and content of curriculum. Perhaps through this use of automated scoring, we can fundamentally alter the character of large-scale testing in ways that bring lasting educational impact.

ACKNOWLEDGMENTS

I thank Anat Ben-Simon, Isaac Bejar, Henry Braun, Dan Eignor, Bob Mislevy, and David Williamson for their comments on earlier drafts of this manuscript.

REFERENCES

Bejar, I. I. (1991). A methodology for scoring open-ended architectural design problems. *Journal of Applied Psychology, 76*(4), 522–532.

Bennett, R. E. (1998). *Reinventing assessment: Speculations on the future of large-scale educational testing.* Princeton, NJ: Policy Information Center, Educational Testing Service. Retrieved September 15, 2003, from ftp://ftp.ets.org/pub/res/reinvent.pdf

Bennett, R. E. (2001). How the Internet will help large-scale assessment reinvent itself. Education Policy Analysis Archives [On-line], *9*(5). Retrieved September 15, 2003, from http://epaa.asu.edu/epaa/v9n5.html

Bennett, R. E., & Bejar, I. I. (1998). Validity and automated scoring: It's not only the scoring. *Educational Measurement: Issues and Practice, 17*(4), 9–17.

Bennett, R. E., Rock, D. A., Braun, H. I., Frye, D., Spohrer, J. C., & Soloway, E. (1990). The relationship of expert-system scored constrained free-response items to multiple-choice and open-ended items. *Applied Psychological Measurement, 14*, 151–162.

Bennett, R. E., & Sebrechts, M. M. (1996). The accuracy of expert-system diagnoses of mathematical problem solutions. *Applied Measurement in Education, 9*, 133–150.

Bennett, R. E., Sebrechts, M. M., & Rock, D. A. (1991). Expert-system scores for complex constructed-response quantitative items: A study of convergent validity. *Applied Psychological Measurement, 15*, 227–239.

Burstein, J., Kukich, K., Wolff, S., Lu, C., & Chodorow, M. (August 1998). *Enriching automated essay scoring using discourse marking and discourse relations.* Paper presented at the 17th International Conference on Computational Linguistics, Montreal, Canada.

Clauser, B. E., Margolis, M. J., Clyman, S. G., & Ross, L. P. (1997). Development of automated scoring algorithms for complex performance assessments: A comparison of two approaches. *Journal of Educational Measurement, 34*, 141–161.

Clauser, B. E., Subhiyah, R. G., Nungenster, R. J., Ripkey, D. R., Clyman, S. G., & McKinley, D. (1995). Scoring a performance-based assessment by modeling the judgment process of experts. *Journal of Educational Measurement, 32*, 397–415.

Dawes, R. M. (1979). The robust beauty of improper linear models in decision making. *American Psychologist, 34*, 571–582.

Enbar, N. (1999). This Is E-Rater. It'll be scoring your essay today. *Business Week Online.* Retrieved September 15, 2003 from http://www.businessweek.com/bwdaily/dnflash/jan1999/nf90121d.htm

ePEN electronic performance evaluation network. (2003). Retrieved September 15, 2003 from http://www.pearsonedmeasurement.com/epen/index.htm

ETS online scoring network. (2003). Retrieved September 15, 2003, from http://www.ets.org/reader/osn/

Feuer, M. J., Towne, L., & Shavelson, R. J. (2002). Scientific culture and educational research. *Educational Researcher, 31*(8), 4–14.

Landauer, T. K., & Dumais, S. T. (1997). A solution to Plato's problem: The Latent Semantic Analysis theory of the acquisition, induction, and representation of knowledge. *Psychological Review, 104*, 211–240.

Messick, S. (1989). Validity. In R. L. Linn (Ed.), *Educational measurement* (3rd ed.; pp 13–103). New York: MacMillan.

Mislevy, R. J., Steinberg, L. S., Breyer, F .J., Almond, R. A., & Johnson,. L. (2002). Making sense of data from complex assessments. *Applied Measurement in Education, 15*, 363–378.

Page, E. B. (1967). The imminence of grading essays by computer. *Phi Delta Kappan, 48*, 238–243.

Powers, D. E., Burstein, J. C., Chodorow, M., Fowles, M. E., & Kukich, K. (2000). *Comparing the validity of automated and human essay scoring* (RR-00-10). Princeton, NJ: Educational Testing Service.

Powers, D. E., Burstein, J. C., Chodorow, M., Fowles, M. E., & Kukich, K. (2001). *Stumping e-rater™: Challenging the validity of automated essay scoring* (RR-01-03). Princeton, NJ: Educational Testing Service.

United States Medical Licensing Examination. (2003). *2004 USLME Bulletin: Preparing for the test.* Retrieved September 15, 2003, from http://www.usmle.org/bulletin/2004/preparingforthetest.htm#cbt

Williamson, D. M., Bejar, I. I., & Hone, A. S. (1999). 'Mental model' comparison of automated and human scoring. *Journal of Educational Measurement, 36*(2), 158–184.

Author Index

413

W

Y

Z

Subject Index

421

U

unidimensional, 4, 34, 194–195, 326
unidimensional model, 194
utility, 5, 75, 172, 192, 240, 323, 388

V

validity, 4–5, 8–9, 15–18, 20, 32, 50–51, 61,
69–73, 77, 83–85, 89, 95, 107, 110, 113–
116, 118–119, 125, 130, 138, 141–142,
153, 158–159, 162–164, 169, 172–173,
192, 222, 233, 250–252, 260, 270, 279,
283, 289, 291, 299–300, 305, 315, 324–
325, 334, 349, 375– 376, 379, 384–387,
394, 395, 398, 404–405, 407–408, 410
variance component, 61, 145–146, 153, 177
vector space methods, 317–318, 335, 337,
342, 385–387
vocabulary usage, 340–341

W

web-based online scoring, 403
weights of evidence, 31, 216, 287
work product, 2–3, 16, 22, 43–47, 49, 51–
52, 62–63, 65, 67, 76–77, 84–85, 88, 94–
97, 101, 107–110, 112, 114–115, 119,
170, 211–215, 225–226, 242, 244–246,
262, 265, 268, 272, 314, 317, 323, 376,
380–381, 383, 387, 389, 393